Venous Disorders

Ajay K. Khanna · Ravul Jindal
Editors

Venous Disorders

Current Concepts

Springer

Editors
Ajay K. Khanna
Department of General Surgery
Institute of Medical Sciences
Banaras Hindu University
Varanasi
India

Ravul Jindal
Vascular and Endovascular Surgery
Fortis Hospital
Mohali
India

ISBN 978-981-13-1107-9 ISBN 978-981-13-1108-6 (eBook)
https://doi.org/10.1007/978-981-13-1108-6

Library of Congress Control Number: 2018954830

This Springer imprint is published by the registered company Springer Nature Singapore Pte Ltd.
The registered company address is: 152 Beach Road, #21-01/04 Gateway East, Singapore 189721, Singapore

Preface

It has been estimated that more than 25 million people in the USA have superficial venous reflux in their legs, and perhaps 7 million exhibit serious complications such as chronic edema, skin changes, and ulceration. Perhaps in excess of 500,000 Americans suffer from debilitating chronic venous ulcers. Though exact figures for Indian scenario is not available but as of the large population in India, the number of cases are exorbitant. Such ulcers are notoriously difficult to heal using usual wound management measures. Over the past several years, much has been learned about the pathophysiology of venous insufficiency, and in the last few years new and exciting treatment modalities have been developed. These new methods of resolving venous hypertension in the superficial veins of the lower extremities are safe and offer better patient outcomes with significantly less patient inconvenience than prior surgical remedies. Today varicose veins can be treated with new and promising treatment modalities which include venous ablation procedures using radiofrequency, laser, and foam and glue sclerotherapy. While these procedures have been available only in the last few years, a growing body of data supports their effectiveness. Most patients require a combination of treatment methods depending on the point of highest venous reflux, the presence of bulging varicosities, the presence of incompetent perforator veins, and the depth of subcutaneous tissue overlying the muscle fascia. Radiofrequency or laser ablation in combination with microphlebectomy and foam sclerotherapy and the recent ones such as mechanochemical treatment and glue treatment has been shown to achieve excellent clinical and cosmetic outcomes.

Venous ulcers are debilitating and notoriously difficult to heal by usual wound management measures. Over the past several years, much has been learned about the pathophysiology of venous insufficiency, and in the last few years new and exciting treatment modalities have been developed. Though compression remains the sheet anchor of the treatment of venous ulcer, many new and different modalities are available for this difficult problem. These new methods of resolving venous hypertension are safe and offer better patient outcomes with significantly less patient inconvenience.

For DVT, traditional treatment regimens including anticoagulation, venous compression stockings, and leg elevation often are insufficient for patients with significant pain and swelling from extensive venous thrombosis. Recent breakthroughs in minimally invasive interventional radiology techniques, however, are improving the prognosis of DVT. Catheter-directed thrombolysis is an emerging treatment alternative for selected patients with extensive, symptomatic DVT. Primary and recurrent venous thromboembolic disease (VTE, deep venous thrombosis, and pulmonary embolism) remains a significant source of morbidity and mortality in the hospitalized patient. Nonspecific subjective complaints and lack of specific objective findings related to acute deep venous thrombosis (DVT) and pulmonary embolism (PE) complicate the diagnosis. There remains no single serum marker available to exclusively confirm the diagnosis of VTE. While D-dimer is highly sensitive and useful for diagnostic exclusion, it lacks the specificity necessary for diagnostic confirmation resulting in the need for a variety of additional studies (i.e., duplex ultrasound, venography, V/Q scanning, helical thoracic and pelvic CT scans, and pulmonary angiography). There is evolving research supporting the utility of various plasma markers as novel "biomarkers" for VTE including selectins, microparticles, interleukin-10, and other cytokines.

This book discusses various aspects of superficial veins and deep veins and has chapters on hemodynamics of venous circulation in lower limb, deep venous reflux novel biomarkers in deep vein thrombosis, infra-popliteal DVT, relevance of wave length in laser treatment in varicose veins, pelvic congestion syndrome, May-Thurner syndrome, nutcracker syndrome, endothermal heat-induced thrombosis, recurrent varicose veins, venous trauma, one stop vein clinic, alternatives for venous ulcer treatment, venous anatomy, therapeutic options in lymphedema, nerve damage during endovenous thermal ablation, newer oral anticoagulants, compression therapy for venous ulcer, sclerotherapy for varicose veins , thrombolysis for DVT, post-thrombotic syndrome, etc. All chapters have been written by experts in this field who have extensive knowledge in this subject. It is not possible to cover everything related to venous problem in the book but whatever the best available are incorporated in this book.

This book will be a rewarding experience for postgraduates and practicing vein physicians and surgeons and is written by experts in various fields. This book contains many figures and the readers will really enjoy reading the various chapters. Both the editors (AK, RJ) have been engaged in vascular practice for a long period and have treated many patients with venous disorders with the newly available Gazettes in the armamentarium of treatment of venous disorders.

I acknowledge the help of Dr. Naren Agarwal of Springer, India, for accepting my proposal readily and in bringing this book to fruition. It is a pleasure working with Dr. Naren Agarwal and this is my second exposition with him. First was when we brought out a book on *Ulcers of the Lower Extremity* by Springer in 2016, which came out beautifully and was taken as one of the important additions to the literature in this field.

I am indebted to my family Dr. Anuradha, Dr. Divya, and Dr. Soumya who provided me all the moral support and will forgive me for any negligence which was unavoidable. I am really thankful to my Coeditor Dr. Ravul Jindal who is now the president of the Venous Association of India and remained as a source of inspiration in bringing out this book.

We dedicate this book to our patients who really has taught us the practical principles of management of their disease.

This book will be really useful to all clinicians dealing with venous disorders and also to postgraduate residents being trained in surgical residency. This book will provide a fertile seed for ongoing basic and clinical research.

Varanasi, India Ajay K. Khanna
Mohali, India Ravul Jindal

Contents

1 **Anatomy of the Venous System of the Lower Limbs** 1
Jean-François Uhl and Claude Gillot

2 **Hemodynamic Aspects of Chronic Venous Disease** 21
Seshadri Raju

3 **Deep Venous Reflux** 29
Arjun Jayaraj

4 **Recurrent Varicose Veins** 39
Mark S. Whiteley

5 **Relevance of Wavelength in Laser Treatment of Varicose Veins** 51
Harinder Singh Bedi and Yudhishtar Singh Bedi

6 **Sclerotherapy for Varicose Veins** 63
Tarun Grover

7 **Nerve Injury due to Endovenous Thermal Ablation for Varicose Veins** 71
Shoaib F. Padaria

8 **Endothermal Heat-Induced Thrombosis** 83
Vijay Thakore, Hiral Varnami, and Karan Thakore

9 **Deep Vein Thrombosis: The Disease** 89
Devendra Dekiwadia

10 **Post-Thrombotic Syndrome** 105
Devendra Dekiwadia, Birju Patel, and Dilip Vaghasia

11 **Isolated Infrapopliteal Deep Venous Thrombosis** 117
Madhuri Gore

12 **Novel Biomarkers in Deep Vein Thrombosis** 129
Ajay K. Khanna, Manbendra Vaidya, and Soumya Khanna

13 **Newer Oral Anticoagulants** 137
Ravul Jindal and Piyush Chaudhary

14 **Therapeutic Alternatives for Venous Ulcer** **147**
Fernando Vega Rasgado

15 **Compression Therapy for Venous Ulcer** **159**
Giovanni Mosti

16 **Pelvic Congestion Syndrome** **171**
Devendra Dekiwadia, Birju Patel, and Dilip Vaghasia

17 **May-Thurner Syndrome** **183**
Soumya Khanna and Ajay K. Khanna

18 **Nutcracker Syndrome** **191**
Ajay Savlania and Shivanesan Pitchai

19 **Venous Trauma** **201**
Arvind Kohli and Gurjit Singh

20 **Therapeutic Options in Lymphedema** **205**
Waldemer Lech Olszewski and Marzanna Teresa Zaleska

21 **One-Stop Vein Clinic: The Ideal Option** **225**
R. Bootun, T. R. A. Lane, and A. H. Davies

About the Editors

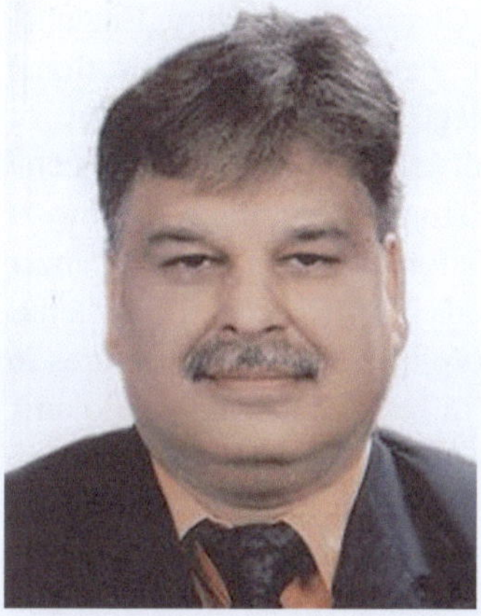

Ajay K. Khanna MS, FAMS, FACS, FICS, FACRSI, MNAMS, MBA, DSc, FRSTMH, FAIS, FUICC, FUWAI, FFIM, FMAS PDCR is professor of surgery and former Head of the Department of General Surgery at the Institute of Medical Sciences, Banaras Hindu University, Varanasi. The author has a teaching experience of more than 35 years and has been awarded Young Outstanding Teacher and Eminent Surgical Teacher awards. He served as president of Varanasi Surgical Society, president of Uttar Pradesh chapter of the Association of Surgeons of India (ASI), Governing Council member of ASI, vice president of ACRSI, and executive member of ASI, AMASI, VAI, ATVSI, IASO. He has delivered more than 15 orations: Dr. S.P. Srivastava Memorial Oncology Oration, UP Chapter of ASI; Dr. S.N. Mathur Oration of UP Chapter of ASI; Roshan Lal Subharti Oration of UP ASI; S.C. Misra Memorial Oration of UP Chapter ASI; Dr. A.K. Mehrotra Oration of UP ASI; T P Banerjee Symposium Orator of UP ASI; Prof. P. N. Chuttani Oration of National Academy of Medical Sciences; Dr. R. Prasad Oration of Jharkhand ASI; Dr. S.P. Srivastava Oration of UP IMA; S P S Memorial Oration of NIMA; R M Tewari Oration of Jharkhand ASI; P K Sen Memorial Oration of ASI; Karnik Memorial Lecture of ICS; Khubchandani Oration of ASI (ACRSI); N L Bordia Oration of ATCVSI; P C Dubey Oration of Lucknow Surgeons Club. He received various fellowship awards, viz. Clinical Research Fellowship and Registrar at the Department of Surgery, University of Wales College of Medicine, Cardiff, Wales, UK; Metrogyl Travelling Fellowship by Gastrointestinal Research Society; Commonwealth Scholarship; Indo-Czechoslovakian Cultural Exchange Program; Best Poster award at the World Congress of Collegium Internationale Chirurgiae Digestivae; Fellowship of Matsumae International Foundation, Japan; Fellow UICC International Cancer Technology Transfer Fellowship, USA; Best Paper award at U.P. Chapter of the Indian Society Of Gastroenterology; R M Kasliwal award of National Academy of Medical Sciences; Indo-Italian Cultural Exchange Fellowship; International Collaboration/Exchange Programme of INSA, Young Outstanding Surgical teacher, UP chapter of ASI; Eminent Surgical Teacher Award, UP ASI; and Best Poster prize at 10th VAICON. His name appears in *Asia's Who's Who reference book*, Marquis Who's Who in the World, *Five Hundred Leaders of Influence*, International Directory of Distinguished Leadership, Man of the Year, American Biographical Institute, International Cultural Diploma of Honor by American Biographical Institute 2000, millennium Medal of Honor by American Biographical Institute, Member of ABIs' Research Board of Advisors, Twentieth Century Admirable Achievers (Distinguished Who' Who), Member of the American Association for the Advancement of Science 2002, Marquis Who's Who in Medicine and Healthcare 2002, Indo-Asian Who's Who, Asian/American Who's Who, and International Professional of the Year—2005 by International Biographical Centre, Cambridge, England. He is Fellow of United Writers Association, Fellow of Indian National Science Academy, Fellow of American College of Surgeons, Fellow of International College of Surgeons, Fellow of Association of Colorectal Society of India, Fellow of Royal Society of Tropical Medicine, Fellow of Association of Surgeons of India, Fellow of Union for International Cancer Control, and Fellow of Minimal Access Surgeons of India. Prof. Khanna has delivered more than 100 CME lectures and more than 100 Guest lectures in various national and international conferences in India, USA, Japan, Poland, Egypt, etc. He has more than 350 publications in various national and international journals and 50 chapters in various books to his credit. He is the editor of three books: *Current Seminars in Surgery*, *Manual of Vascular Surgery*, and *Ulcers of the Lower Extremity*. He has attended more than 200 national and international conferences and presented more than 250 presentations. He has guided more than 50 theses for MS course. He is an examiner for MBBS, MS, BDS, DNB, and FNB in minimal access surgery. He is a fellow/member of 33 societies. He is a widely traveled person and has worked in various well-reputed institutes in almost all the major countries of the world. He is a devoted teacher and very active academician and is well praised by all his students. He started the vascular surgery in the department of Surgery at BHU. He is the joint editor of the *Indian Journal of Surgery*. He has organized more than 25 conferences and workshops. He was the chief inspector for Quality Assurance Review of the Department of Clinical Surgical Sciences, the University of the West Indies, St. Augustine Campus, Trinidad and Tobago, and is in the Expert Selection Committee of UPSC, Uttar Pradesh; BPKIMS, Dharan, Nepal; Aligarh Muslim University, Aligarh; KGMU, Lucknow; Public Service Commission, J & K; MCI Inspector; DNB Inspector; IGIMS, Patna; PGI, Chandigarh; and Indian Institute of Information Technology, Allahabad.

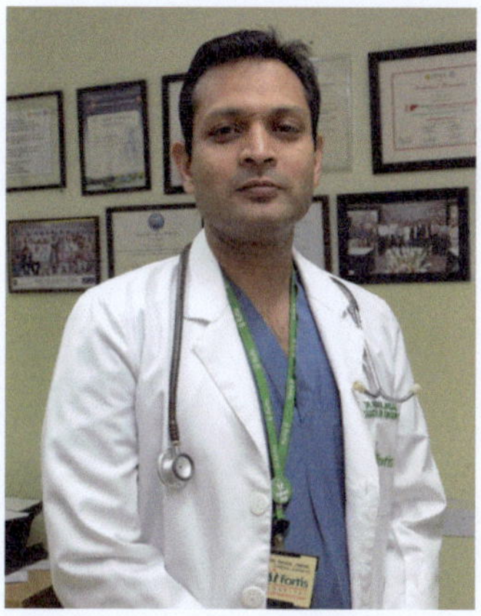

Ravul Jindal MS, DNB, FRCS, FAMS, FIVS is presently director of vascular and endovascular surgery, Fortis Hospital, Mohali. He is working in the field of surgery for the past 21 years and is with Fortis for 12 years. His areas of expertise include peripheral arterial and venous interventions. Dr. Ravul Jindal completed his MBBS from Mahatma Gandhi Institute of Medical Sciences, Sewagram, and MS in General Surgery from PGIMER, Chandigarh. He was awarded a Diplomate of the National Board in General Surgery, New Delhi. After completing his senior residency at PGIMER, Chandigarh, he went on to do his Fellowship in Vascular Surgery at St Mary's Hospital, London, UK. He also completed his FRCS from the Royal College of Surgeons of Edinburgh. St Mary's hospital is world renowned for vascular surgery and is affiliated to Imperial College. Penicillin was discovered by Alexander Fleming in this hospital. Dr. Jindal is actively involved in the national vascular bodies and is a life member of the Vascular Society of India and *President of the Venous Association of India* (www.venous.in). He is also an executive member of the International Compression Club (ICC) and council member of L'Union Internationale de Phlebologie (UIP). He has vast experience in open and endovascular surgeries, with expertise in endovascular management of aortic aneurysms, revascularization in diabetic foot, and varicose veins. His special interests are the laser treatment of varicose veins where patients are treated as day care without any surgical incisions. He popularized the treatment of diabetic foot, endovascular treatment of aortic aneurysms, and laser ablation of varicose veins in this part of the world. He also introduced the MOCA Technique (mechanico-chemical ablation of varicose veins) and Glue Closure Technique to treat varicose vein for the first time in the country, which are nonthermal ways of managing varicose veins. Dr. Jindal is involved in research, presentation of papers at national and international meetings, and has a number of publications to his credit. He has written more than 10 book chapters as the first author in international books in the field of vascular surgery and is credited with more than 30 publications in various international journals.

Contributors

Harinder Singh Bedi Cardiovascular Sciences of Ludhiana Mediways Hospital, Ludhiana, Punjab, India

Yudhishtar Singh Bedi USC, Los Angeles, CA, USA

R. Bootun Section of Vascular Surgery, Charing Cross Hospital, Imperial College London, London, UK

Piyush Chaudhary Vascular and Endovascular Surgery, Fortis Hospital, Mohali, India

A. H. Davies Section of Vascular Surgery, Charing Cross Hospital, Imperial College London, London, UK

Devendra Dekiwadia Dekiwadia Hospital, Rajkot, Gujarat, India

Claude Gillot URDIA Anatomy Research Unit EA 4465, Paris Descartes University, Paris, France

Madhuri Gore Consultant Surgeon, Former Professor and Chief of Surgery, LTMG Hospital, Mumbai, India

Tarun Grover Division of Vascular and Endovascular Surgery, Medanta Medicity Hospital, Gurugram, Haryana, India

Arjun Jayaraj RANE Center for Venous and Lymphatic Diseases at St. Dominic Hospital, Jackson, MS, USA

Ravul Jindal Vascular and Endovascular Surgery, Fortis Hospital, Mohali, India

Ajay K. Khanna Department of General Surgery, Institute of Medical Sciences, Banaras Hindu University, Varanasi, India

Soumya Khanna Institute of Medical Sciences, Banaras Hindu University, Varanasi, India

Arvind Kohli Department of CTVS, GMC, Jammu, India

T. R. A. Lane Section of Vascular Surgery, Charing Cross Hospital, Imperial College London, London, UK

Giovanni Mosti Angiology Department, MD Barbantini Clinic, Lucca, Italy

Waldemer Lech Olszewski Central Clinical Hospital, Ministry of Internal Affairs, Warsaw, Poland

Shoaib F. Padaria Department of Vascular Sciences, Jaslok Hospital and Research Centre, Mumbai, India

Birju Patel Dekiwadia Hospital, Rajkot, Gujarat, India

Shivanesan Pitchai Sree Chitra Tirunal Institute for Medical Sciences and Technology, Trivandrum, India

Seshadri Raju The Rane Center, Jackson, MS, USA

Ajay Savlania Postgraduate Institute of Medical Education and Research, Trivandrum, India

Gurjit Singh Division of CTVS, JK Medicity Hospital, Jammu, India

Karan Thakore Department of Surgery, Karamsad Medical College, Baroda, Gujarat, India

Vijay Thakore Angiocare VINS Hospital, Baroda, Gujarat, India

Jean-François Uhl URDIA Anatomy Research Unit EA 4465, Paris Descartes University, Paris, France

Dilip Vaghasia Dekiwadia Hospital, Rajkot, Gujarat, India

Manbendra Vaidya Institute of Medical Sciences, Banaras Hindu University, Varanasi, India

Hiral Varnami Angiocare VINS Hospital, Baroda, Gujarat, India

Fernando Vega Rasgado Instituto Mexicano de Flebología, Academia Mexicana de Flebología y Linfología, Clínica de Várices y Ulceras de México, Mexico City, Mexico

Mark S. Whiteley The Whiteley Clinic, London, UK

The Whiteley Clinic, Guildford, UK

The Whiteley Clinic, Bristol, UK

Marzanna Teresa Zaleska Department of Applied Physiology, Mossakowski Medical Research Center, Polish Academy of Sciences, Warsaw, Poland

Anatomy of the Venous System of the Lower Limbs

1

Jean-François Uhl and Claude Gillot

Abbreviations

AAGSV	Anterior accessory of the GSV
CVD	Chronic venous disease
GSV	Great saphenous vein
LNVN	Lymph node venous networks of the groin
SSV	Small saphenous vein

1.1 Introduction

The embryogenesis of the venous network of the lower limbs explains the main variations of the venous network superficial veins, perforating veins, and deep venous system. It is likely that the number of the so-called primitive chronic venous disease could be explained by unknown underlying anatomical abnormalities [1].

The muscular veins play an important role, due to the effect of the muscular pumps by their activation of the deep venous return and the aspiration of the superficial system via the perforator veins. They always act at the same level. This explains the anatomical fixity of most of the perforators and the interest of their knowledge [2].

The color duplex is essential in any patient with chronic venous disease (CVD) to provide anatomical and hemodynamical data. Direct CT venography is a useful complement to get more detailed morphological information and a 3D map of the whole venous network [3].

These new imaging techniques are a useful complement to the classical descriptive anatomy. They improve our anatomical knowledge of the veins, which is useful for radiologists, angiologists, as well as vascular surgeons and students. The final aim is to better perform venous mapping which is the keystone for any treatment.

1.2 The New Terminology of the Veins

A new terminology of the venous system was defined by a consensus conference of experts during the UIP Congress of Rome [4] in order to provide a common language between anatomists, radiologists, angiologists, and surgeons. The international nomenclature is summarized on the Fig. 1.1 (veins) and Fig. 1.2 (perforator veins).

J.-F. Uhl (✉) · C. Gillot
URDIA Anatomy Research Unit EA 4465, Paris Descartes University, Paris, France

A. K. Khanna, R. Jindal (eds.), *Venous Disorders*, https://doi.org/10.1007/978-981-13-1108-6_1

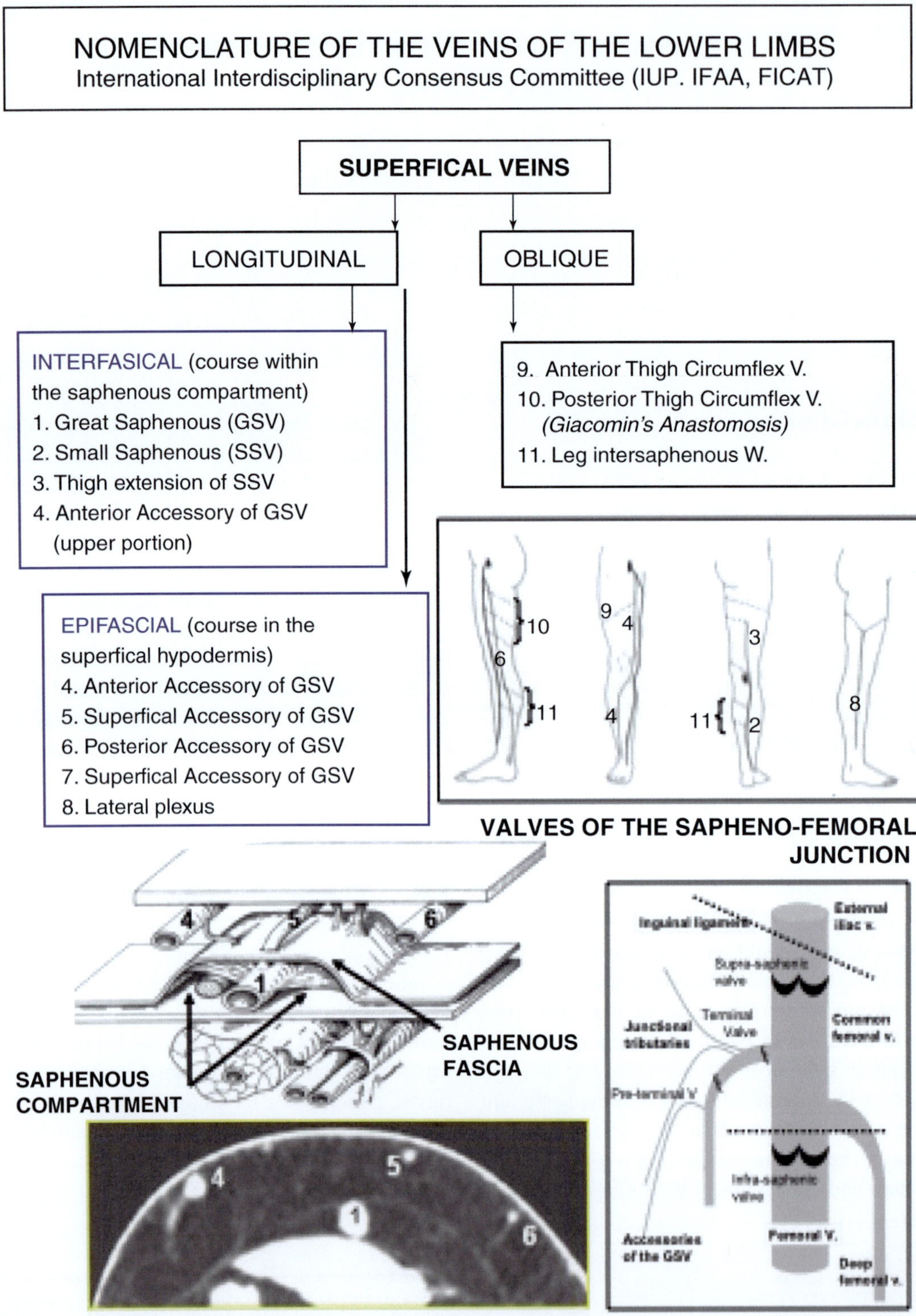

Fig. 1.1 International nomenclature of the veins of the lower limb (from A. Caggiati)

NOMENCLATURE of PERFORATING VEINS (PV) (main eponyms in brackets)

1. DORSAL FOOT PV
2. MEDIAL FOOT PV
3. LATERAL FOOT PV
4. PLANTAR FOOT PV
5. MEDIAL ANKLE PV
6. ANTERIOR ANKLE PV
7. LATERAL ANKLE PV
8. PARATIBLAL PV *(SHERMAN, BOYD)*
9. POSTERIOR TIBIAL PV *(COCKETT)*
10. ANTERIOR LEG PV
11. LATERAL LEG PV
12. MEDIAL GASTROCNEMIUS PV *(GILLOT)*
13. LATERAL GASTROCNEMIUS PV
14. INTERGEMELLAR PV *(MAY)*
15. PARA-ACHILLEAN PV *(BASSI)*
16. MEDIAL KNEE PV
17. SUPRAPATELLAR PV
18. LATERAL KNEE PV
19. INFRAPATELLAR PV
20. POPLITEAL FOSSA PV *(DOOD, THIERI)*
21. PV OF THE FEMORAL CANAL *(DOOD)*
22. INGUINAL PV
23. ANTERIOR THIGH PV
24. LATERAL THIGH PV
25. POSTERO-MEDIAL THIGH PV
26. SCIATIC PV
27. POSTERO-LATERAL PV *(HACH)*
28. PUDENDAL PV
29. SUPERIOR GLUTEAL PV
30. MID GLUTEAL PV
31. LOWER GLUTEAL PV

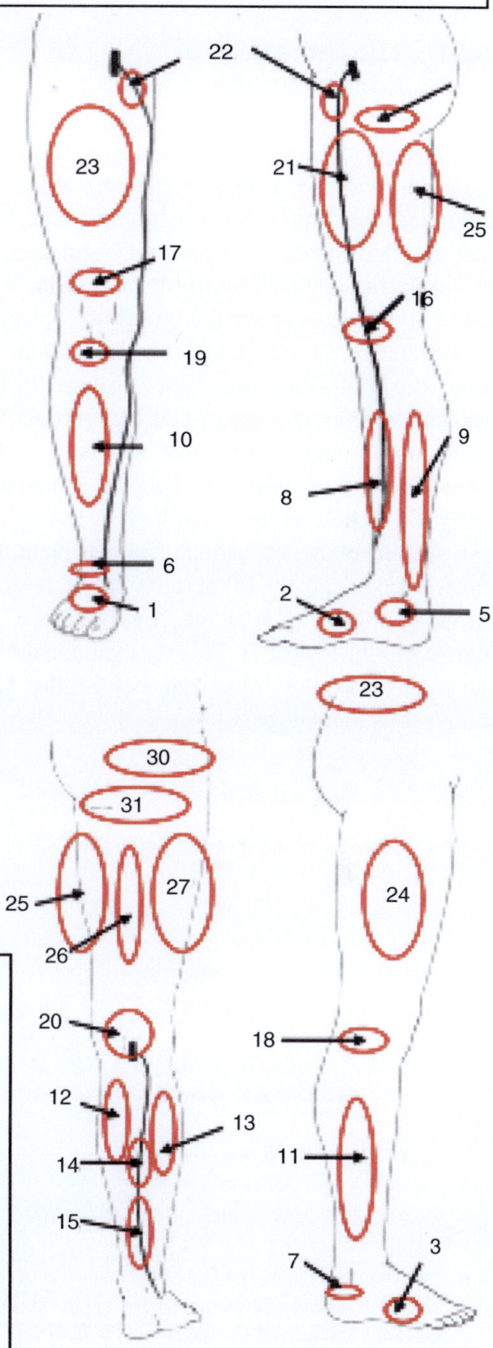

Main references:

Caggiati A, Bergan JJ, Gloviczki P, Jantet G, Wendell-Smith CP, Partsch. Nomenclature of the veins of the lower limbs: an international interdisciplinary consensus statement. J Vasc Surg. 2002;36(2):416–22.

Caggiati A, Bergan JJ, Gloviczki P, Eklof B, Allegra C, Partsch H. Nomenclature of the veins of the lower limb: extensions, refinements, and clinical application. J Vasc Surg. 2005;41(4):719–24.

Cavezzi A, Labropoulos N, Partsch H, Ricci S, Caggiati A, Myers K, Nicolaides A, Smith PC. Duplex ultrasound investigation of the veins in chronic venous disease of the lower limbs–UIPconsensus document. Part II. Anatomy. Eur J Vasc Endovasc Surg. 2006;31(3):288–99.

Fig. 1.2 Nomenclature of the perforator veins (from A. Caggiati)

1.3 The Superficial Venous System

1.3.1 The Three Venous Compartments (Fig. 1.3)

The subcutaneous tissues of the lower limbs are organized with two connective fasciae along the thigh and leg: superficially below the skin, formerly called "fascia superficialis," and deeper, the deep fascia layer or muscular fascia, also called aponeurosis above the muscles.

These two fascia layers are continuous all along the limb. They are closely related to the saphenous veins: the superficial layer covers the saphenous trunks, while the tributaries, also called epifascial veins, are located subcutaneously. By definition between the two fascia layers, we have the saphenous compartment [5] easily recognized by echography in transversal slices, giving the sign of the "Egyptian eye" as shown in Fig. 1.4 [6, 7]. This was validated by a consensus meeting organized before the UIP congress of San Diego [8].

1.3.2 The Short Saphenous Vein (SSV)

Origin: The SSV is formed by two roots: the lateral perforators and the lateral malleolar plexus; the origin of the vein is often a plexus; there is commonly no lateral marginal vein (Fig. 1.5). The sural nerve is stuck to the SSV from the ankle to mid-calf.

The termination types of the SSV: The SSV termination or arch ends into the popliteal vein. The saphenous popliteal junction is frequently located close to the lateral aspect of the tibial nerve.

There are five possible termination types for the SSV [9] according to the presence (A and B) or the absence (C, D, and E) of SPJ (Fig. 1.6).

Important point: *The SSV is located close to the nerves* at different levels which are high-risk zones for the treatment of SSV, particularly by thermal ablation. In clinical practice, the clinician needs to be aware of danger zones in treatment of venous disease with SSV surgical approach and endovenous procedures. This is

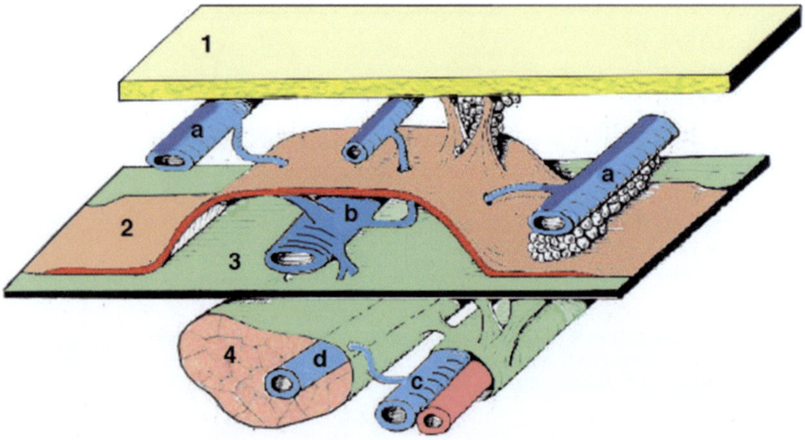

Fig. 1.3 The three compartments of the venous system of the lower limb, separated by three layers: (1) the skin, (2) the saphenous fascia, and (3) the muscular fascia. In the deep plan, under the muscular fascia, is located the deep venous system: deep trunks (**c**) and muscular veins (**d**) inside the muscles (4). In the saphenous compartment (saphenous eye), between the two fascia layers are located the saphenous trunks (**b**). Under the skin is located the tributaries (**a**) of the saphenous trunks

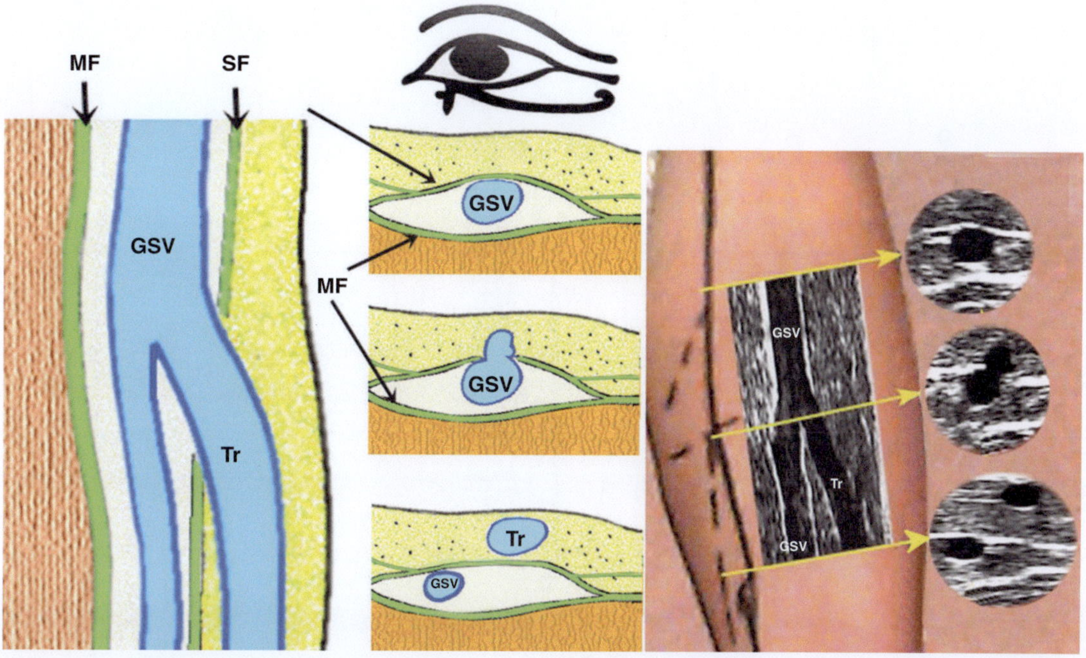

Fig. 1.4 The "Egyptian eye," echographic view of the saphenous compartment. *MF* muscular fascia, *SF* saphenous fascia, *GVS* great saphenous vein, *Tr* tributary of GVS

Fig. 1.5 The lateral perforators of the foot and origin of the small saphenous vein (SS). Dorsal superficial arch (DA), malleolar plexus (MP), fifth metatarsal bone (M5), common trunk of the lateral foot perforator veins (C), retrotendinous perforator vein (R or cunean Cu), intertendinous perforator vein (I), inframalleolar perforator vein (S), fibular perforator (P)

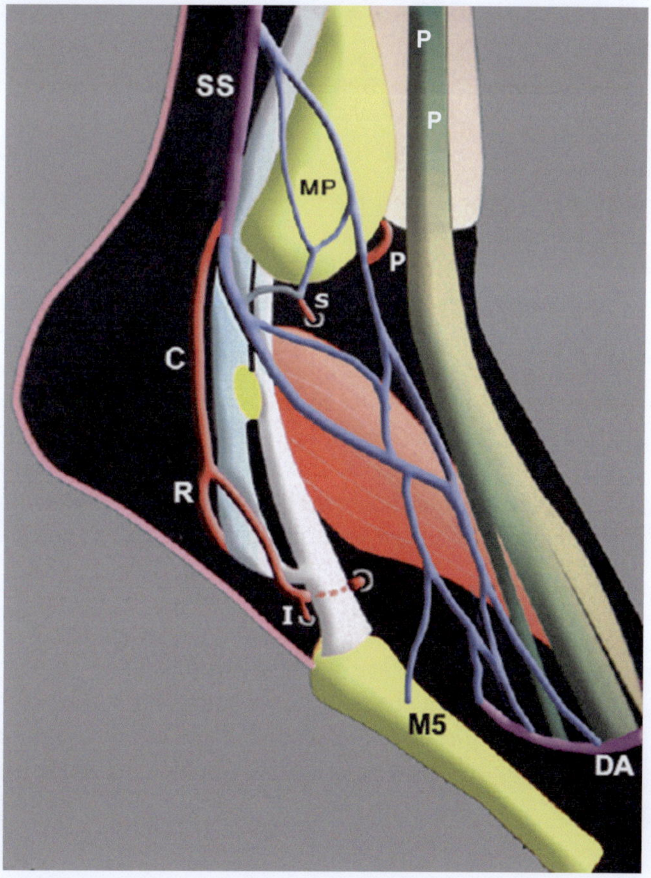

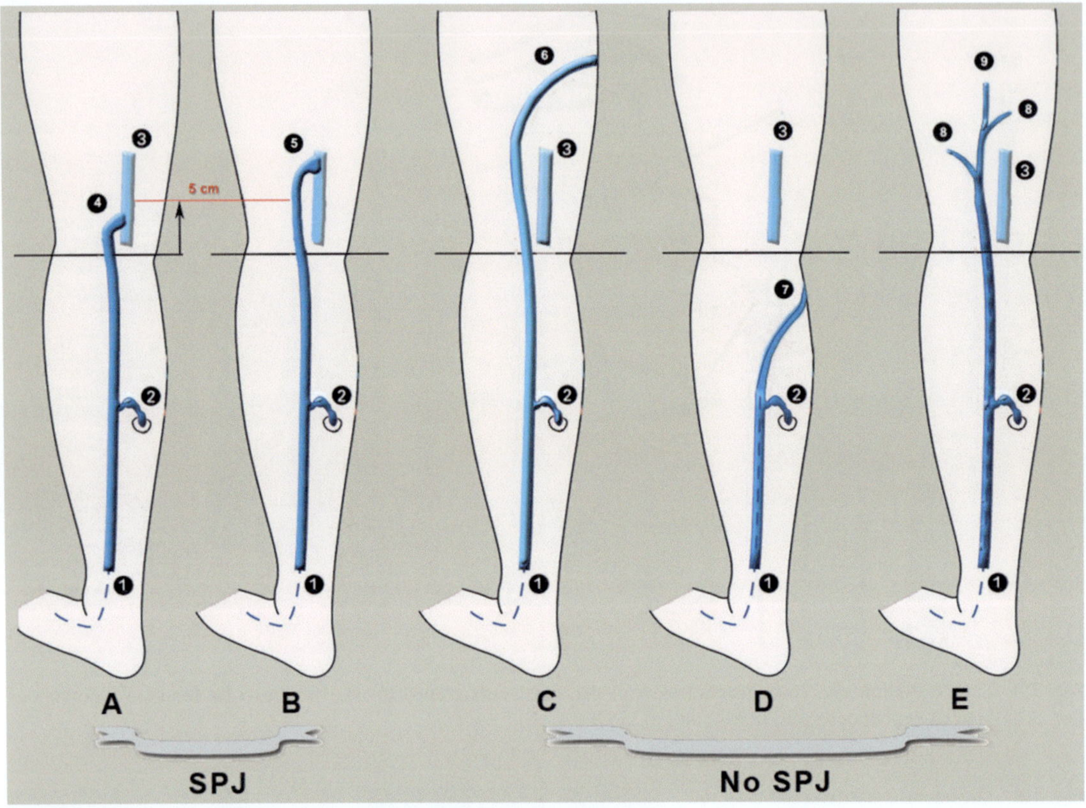

Fig. 1.6 The five different types of termination of the short saphenous vein (SSV). With a saphenous popliteal junction (SPJ): A (modal arch) and B (high SPJ more than 5 cm above the crease). Without SPJ: C (Giacomini continuation), D (short type), E (plexiform termination)

particularly true: [10] At the lower third of the calf, the sural nerve is stuck to the SSV trunk.

- At the apex of the calf (formation of the sural nerve by its two tibial and fibular branches)
- In the popliteal fossa crossing the tibial nerve and commonly the nerve of the medial gastrocnemius muscle (Fig. 1.5)

The surgeons should be aware of these risky zones to avoid nerve trauma during the treatment of SSV.

The anatomical knowledge of the sural nerve pedicle (Fig. 1.7) is also useful to avoid the risk of injection of the SSV artery. These anatomical features explain the usefulness of ultrasonographic mapping prior to any treatment and as a control during any invasive procedure of SSV.

The thigh or deep extension of the SSV: Also named postaxial or thigh or dorsal or cranial extension of the SSV (companion vein of the postaxial nerve of the embryo), it is located below the muscular fascia, close to the femoral posterior cutaneous nerve (Fig. 1.8).

It is connected to the deep muscular veins of the thigh (semimembranosus and biceps).

It commonly extends with the Giacomini vein (inter saphenous anastomosis) to join the GSV below the groin.

1.3.3 The Great Saphenous Vein (GSV) [11]

Identification: The identification of the GSV is made by color duplex: it is easily located inside

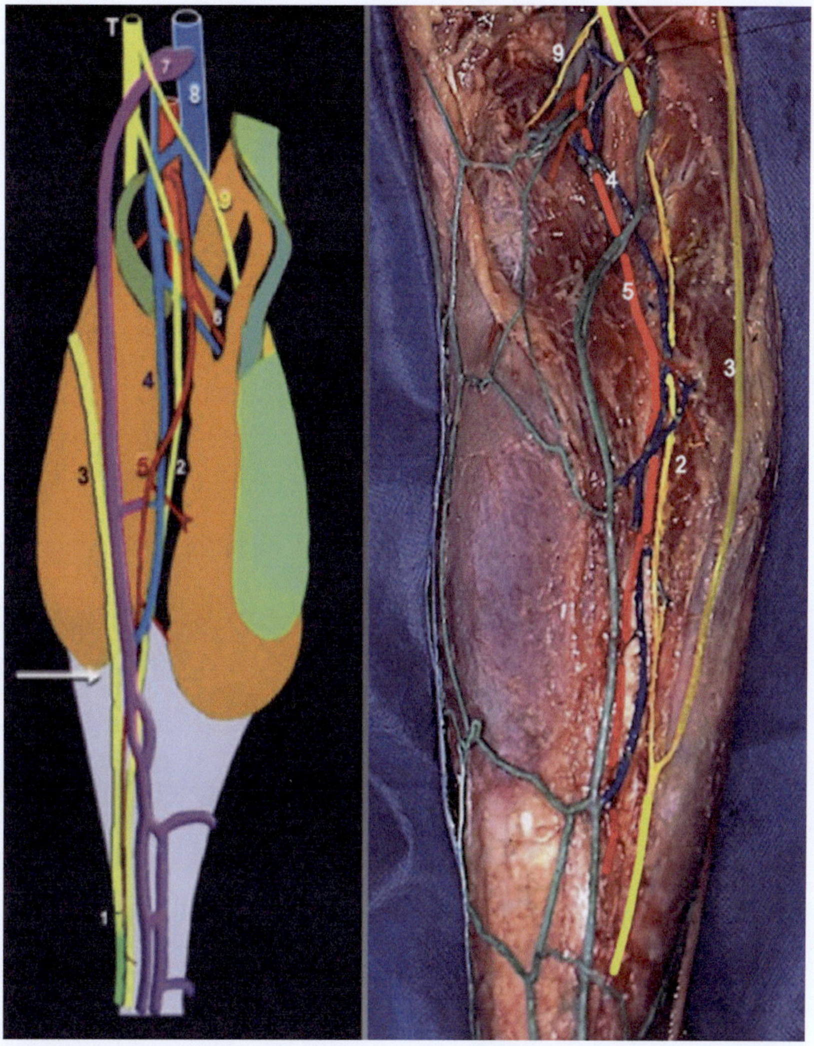

Fig. 1.7 The sural nerve pedicle. Left: drawing of the sural nerve pedicle. The "common" sural nerve (1) is formed at the apex of the calf (wire arrow) by the medial branch (2) coming from the tibial nerve (T) and the lateral one (3) coming from the common fibular nerve. The inter-gastrocnemial vein or vein of the sural nerve (4) is located just below the deep fascia of the SSV (7) next to the small saphenous artery (5). Please notice the vicinity of the tibial (T) and medial gastrocnemial nerve (9) close to the arch of the SSV (7). 8 = popliteal vein 6 = medial gastrocnemial pedicle. Right: Anatomical dissection of the calf showing the same

the saphenous compartment or echographic "eye," as in Fig. 1.2.

Origin: Begins by three roots below the anterior part of the tibial malleolar area with (Figs. 1.9 and 1.14):

- The medial marginal vein of the foot
- The inframalleolar perforator
- The dorsal communicating vein of the foot joining the anterior tibial veins

The termination of the GSV (arch or French "crosse") is always located in the inguinal crease.

Complex connections exist at the root of the thigh; each of them could be the leak point of a truncal reflux of the GSV at the thigh level (Fig. 1.10): medially, with the pudendal and perineal network [1–3], upward with the tributaries of the abdominal wall (b) or iliac area (a), and downward with the Giacomini vein (f) and the posterior accessory saphenous vein (g).

A number of variations of these tributaries have been described, but the important point is the presence of a constant segment delimited by the two last valves of the GSV termination: the terminal valve (close to the saphenous

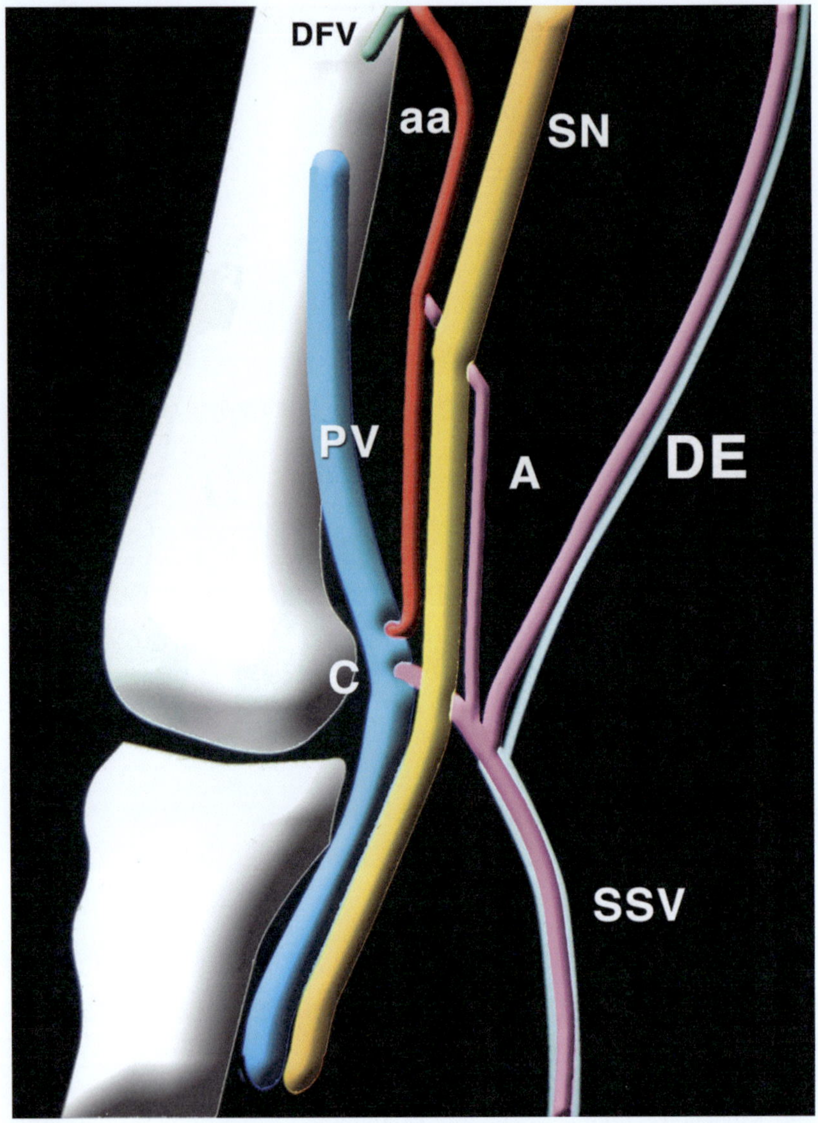

Fig. 1.8 The deep or thigh extension of the SSV (DE) also has accompanying nerve: the femoral posterior cutaneous nerve. It should be distinguished from the deep venous arcades (A and aa) located along the great sciatic nerve, connected to the deep femoral vein (DFV) upward

femoral junction or ostium) and the preterminal valve, located 15–25 mm below. All tributaries of the GSV end into this intervalvular segment.

Anatomy and hemodynamics of this intervalvular segment are mostly important to be checked. This could be assessed by duplex between the terminal reflux (Fig. 1.11) and the preterminal one (Fig. 1.12) [12, 13].

1.3.4 The Anterior Accessory Great Saphenous Vein (AAGSV)

Its origin is usually made by lateral branches of the knee or of the lateral leg. The AAGSV then crosses the anterior aspect of the thigh to join the inguinal area. Located subcutaneously, it goes through the fascia 10–12 cm below the inguinal fold, located here inside its own

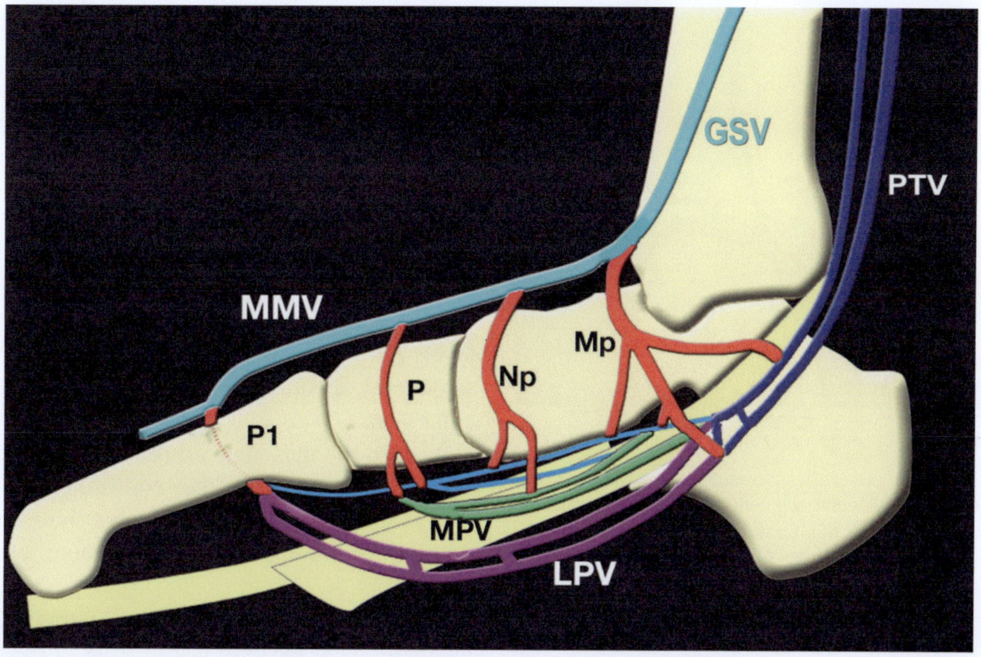

Fig. 1.9 Origin of the GSV at the ankle and medial perforators of the foot. Great saphenous vein (GSV), posterior tibial veins (PTV), lateral plantar veins (LPV), medial plantar veins (MPV), perforator of the first metatarsal (P1), malleolar perforator (Mp), navicular perforator (Np), medial marginal vein of the foot (MMV), anterior perforator of the foot (P). Please notice that the direction of the blood in the medial perforators is paradoxal: from the deep system toward the superficial system (medial marginal vein)

Fig. 1.10 Crossroad connections of the GSV termination at the root of the thigh: Perineal (2, 3) and pudendal (1) anastomoses. Superficial circumflex iliac vein (Ci), abdominal subcutaneous (Epi), external pudendal (Pu), anterior accessory saphenous vein (AAS), great saphenous vein (GSV), Giacomini vein (G), posterior accessory saphenous vein (PAS), terminal valve (TV), and preterminal valve (PTV)

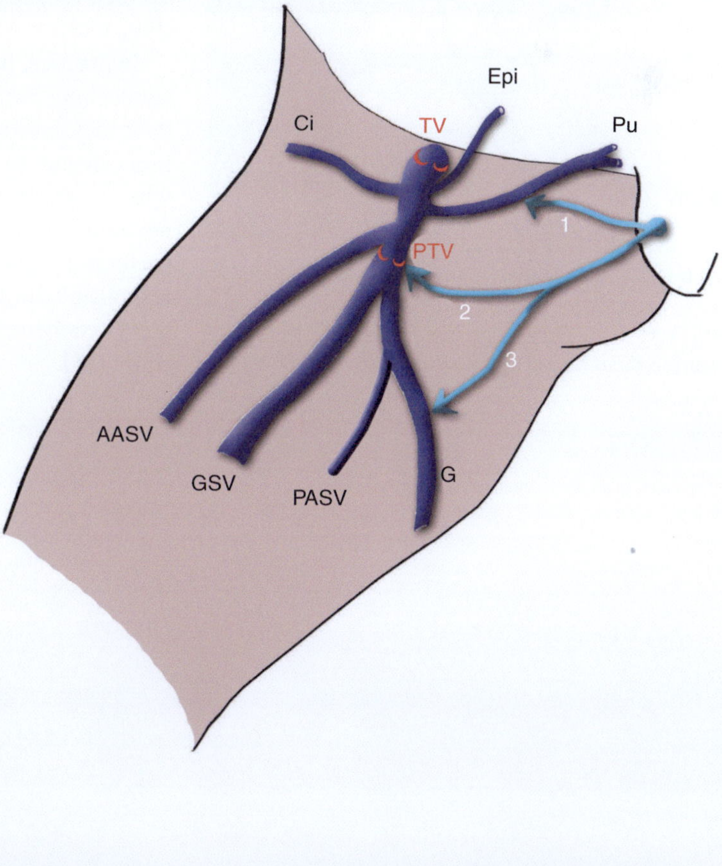

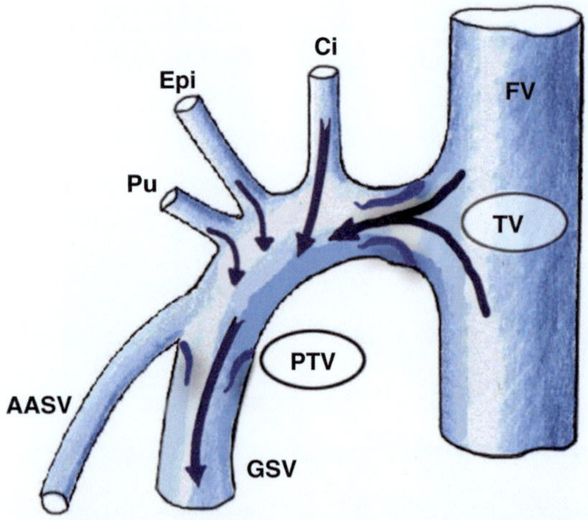

Fig. 1.11 Intervalvular segment of the GSV termination with tributaries: case of a terminal reflux down to the GSV trunk. Superficial circumflex iliac vein (Ci), abdominal subcutaneous (Epi), external pudendal (Pu), anterior accessory saphenous vein (AAS), great saphenous vein (GSV), terminal valve (TV), preterminal valve (PTV), femoral vein (FV)

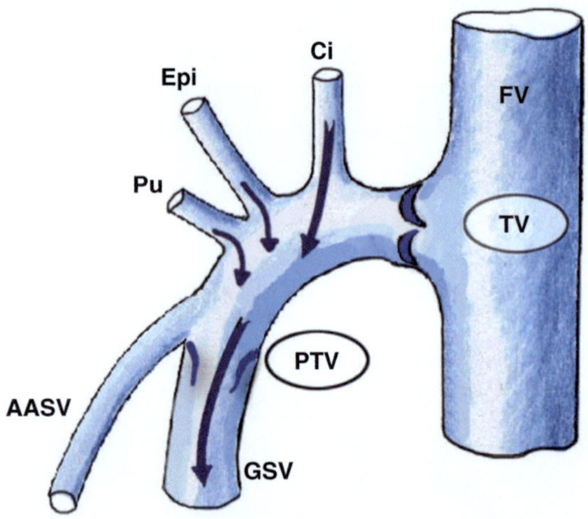

Fig. 1.12 Intervalvular segment of the GSV termination with tributaries: case of a preterminal reflux of the GSV trunk

saphenous compartment. It is differentiated from the GSV by the alignment sign: the vein is located in the same sagittal axis of the femoral vein.

1.4 The Perforators Veins

The perforator veins join the superficial to the deep system. The theory of the hemodynamical levels [14] explains their location always at the same level, according to the anatomy of the muscular veins.

In fact, the muscular veins are mostly important for hemodynamics: they constitute the active part of the deep system because of their aspiration power on the superficial system via the perforators.

For efficacy reasons, the perforators have a relatively fixed location just in front of the muscular veins in order to optimize the venous drainage. This explains the constancy of their anatomical pattern. These anatomical considerations are useful for the investigators in daily practice. The Atlas book of Gillot [2] shows their average location according to the tibia's length (Fig. 1.13).

In practice, the PVs are not single and straight connections from the deep to the superficial system: they are frequently plexus shaped dividing into several tortuous branches and connected with the muscular veins (Fig. 1.13). These connections also make truly subfascial interperforator anastomoses which are probably responsible for the high recurrence rate after surgical treatment, as reported in a 3 years follow-up study [15].

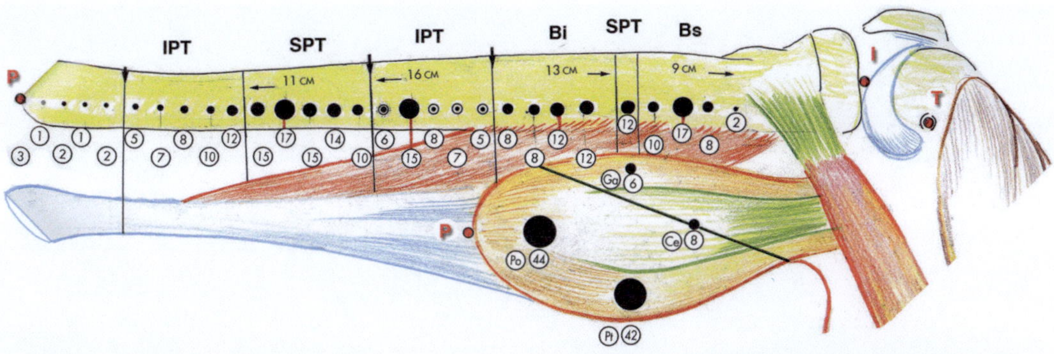

Fig. 1.13 The levels of the leg and calf perforators (from the Atlas book of Gillot). Ankle (A) less than 5 cm, inferior posterior tibial (IPT) 5–9 cm, inferior posterior tibial (IPT) 10–15 cm, inferior paratibial (IPT), superior paratibial (SPT). The groups of the calf PV: polar (Po) posterior (Pt), central (Ce), and anterior (Ga)

It is important to highlight the role of the *lymph node perforators of the groin.*

The lymph node venous networks of the groin (LNVN) are characterized by three features:

- Their trans-nodal route
- Their network shape connections with the GSV and mostly the AAGSV
- The existence of direct perforators that join the common femoral vein by [16]

They should be checked during any assessment of CVD patients. They can be found, thin and competent, in any healthy individual. They could be seen in primary CVD, but are more commonly found in REVAS following groin surgery, and are associated with multiple sinuous neovascular channels. Their presence is an absolute contraindication for any surgical approach of the groin:

Echo-guided sclerotherapy is recommended.

1.5 The Deep Venous System

Is located by definition below the muscular fascia, including two parts:

1.5.1 The Deep Venous Trunks

Begin at the foot with the *foot pump* located in the plantar veins [17].

The lateral plantar veins are bigger and join the plexus-shaped medial plantar at the calcaneus plexus. This originates the two *posterior tibial veins* (Fig. 1.9). These veins are commonly making a network at the lower part of the leg (Figs. 1.14 and 1.15), which is a mechanism against reflux.

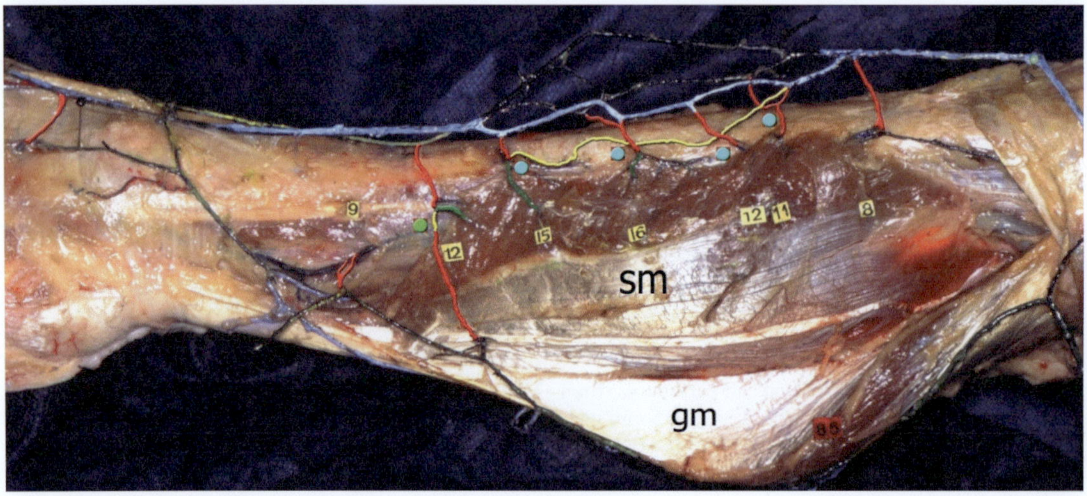

Fig. 1.14 Anatomical dissection (medial view of a right leg). The medial perforators of the leg are colored in red (see blue circles). They are connected to the branches of the great saphenous vein (light blue) and connected between them by an inter-perforator anastomosis (in yellow)

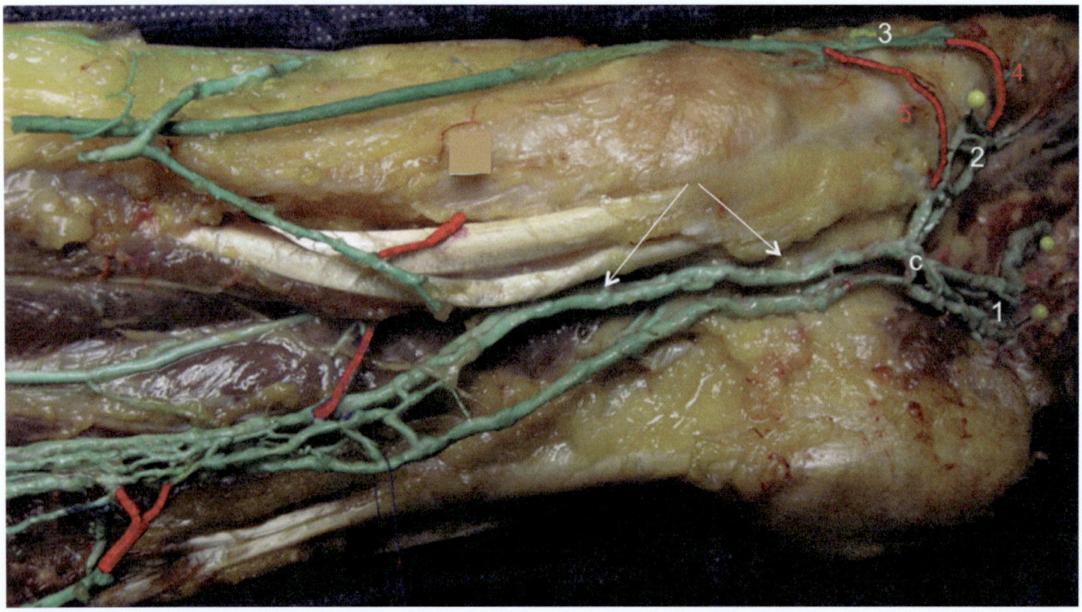

Fig. 1.15 Anatomical dissection with latex injection and colored segmentation: The plexus of the posterior tibial veins. The medial plantar veins (1) join the lateral ones (2) at the level of the calcaneus plexus (c). They drain the blood into the medial marginal vein (3) by the medial perforators. They are not arranged in a plexus in the lower part, showing two veins (arrows)

Dorsally, the anterior tibial veins come from an anastomosis with the submalleolar perforator.

Laterally, the two *fibular veins* are small veins running upward inside the fibrous fibula's canal at the lower part of the leg. They become bigger veins above the arcade of the hallux flexor longus after receiving the huge lateral veins of the soleus muscle (Fig. 1.16).

The *popliteal vein* is formed by two roots [14, 18]: lateral one coming from the fibular and medial from the posterior tibial. They could join at different levels and so receive the anterior tibial veins in different ways as shown on the Fig. 1.17. Up to the adductor arcade, the popliteal vein becomes *the femoral vein*, usually coming with a small collateral canal.

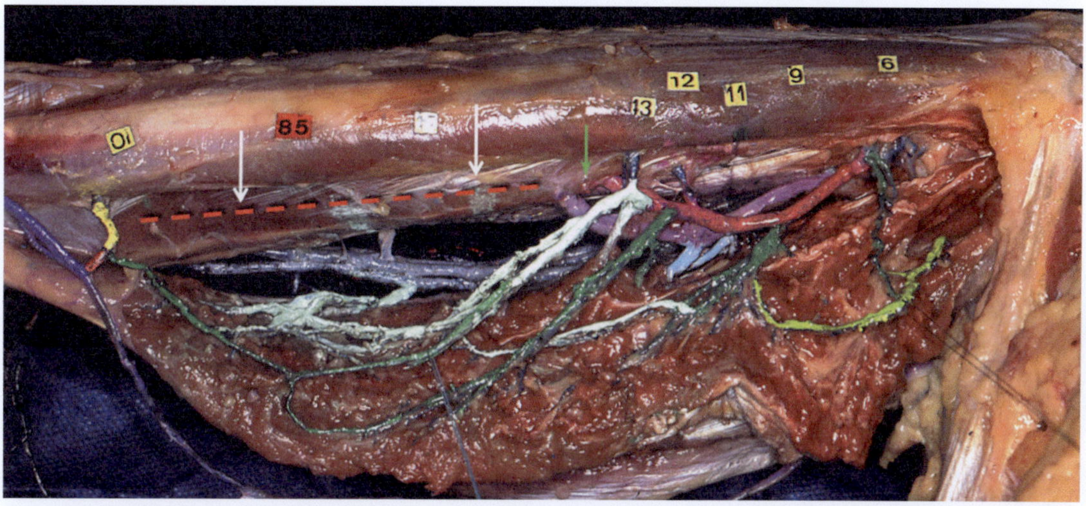

Fig. 1.16 The two fibular veins go up into the fibular canal (dotted line): the upper limit of this fibrous and bony canal is marked by the arcade of the hallux flexor longus (green arrow). The fibular veins (in red) receive at this level the huge lateral veins of the soleus muscle

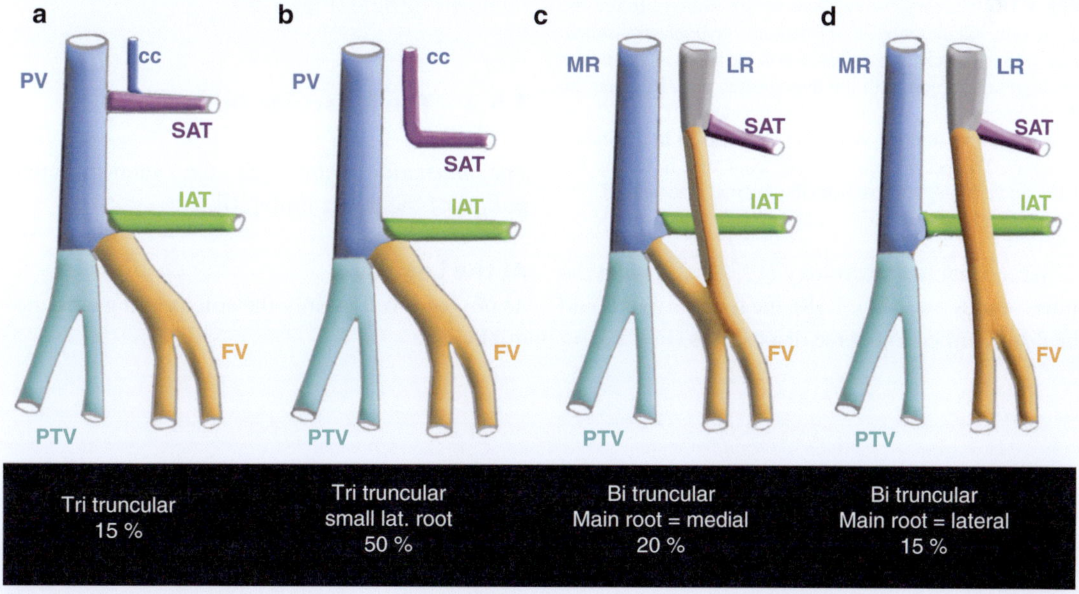

Fig. 1.17 The four different arrangements of the roots of the popliteal vein (Gillot). (**a**) Tritruncular dispositive, (**b**) idem with small lateral root, (**c**) bitruncular with main medial, (**d**) bitruncular with main lateral root. *PV* popliteal vein, *MR* medial root, *LR* lateral root, *SIAT* superior anterior tibial vein, *IAT* inferior anterior tibial vein, *PTV* posterior tibial vein, *FV* fibular vein, *cc* collateral canal

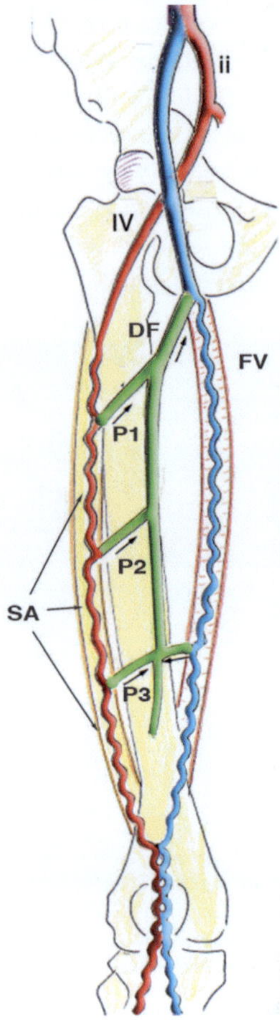

Fig. 1.18 The three venous axis in the embryo. In red the axial vein. Commonly, it will become hypoplastic, sciatic arcade (SA) which is a small arcade in the adult. Please notice the high connection with the hypogastric vein. In green the deep femoral (DF), with its three perforators (P1, P2, P3). In blue the modal femoral vein (FV) is dominant in the modal anatomy. The persistence of a big axial vein is fed by the ischiatic vein (IV) coming from the internal iliac vein (II)

According to embryology [19, 20, 21], with the three venous axes (Fig. 1.18), the femoral axis could be distinguished into three dispositives (Fig. 1.19).

The three main variations of the femoral vein are [22]:

- Modal type of a big femoral vein along the artery and nerve inside the femoral canal.
- Unitruncular dispositive made of a big axial vein draining into the deep femoral vein and a hypoplastic femoral vein. (This axio-femoral trunk is characterized by its particular location, running vertically along the sciatic nerve.)
- Bitruncular dispositive with both veins of similar diameter.

The adductor canal (or Hunter's canal) is a narrowed area with rigid walls located at the femoropopliteal junction. Its role in the venous outlet syndrome is probably underestimated [23]. In clinical vascular practice, investigators should keep in mind that a duplex ultrasound at the precise level of the outlet (11–13 cm from the condyle) should be routine, checking for:

1. A possible extrinsic compression of the venous axis inside the canal
2. A dilatation of the derivative routes, particularly the venous arcades of the semimembranosus muscle (Fig. 1.24).

1.5.2 The Muscular Veins

The muscular veins and the veno-muscular pumps of the lower limb [20].

At the Leg Level

At the leg level: mainly the soleus and gastrocnemial veins

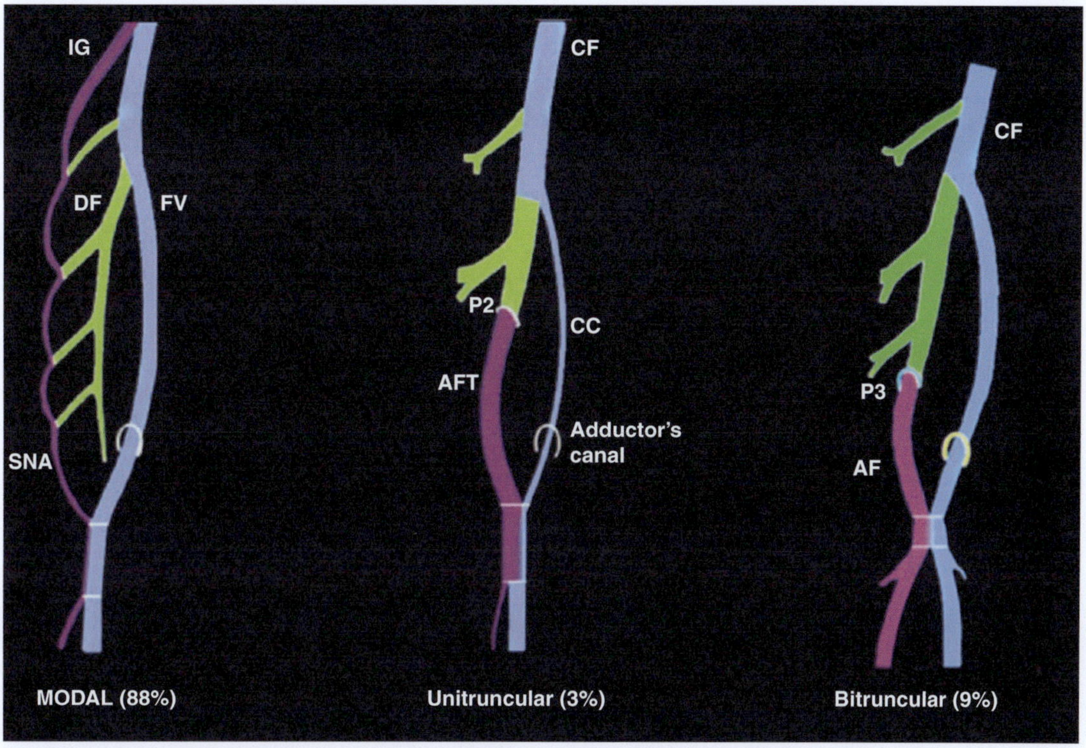

Fig. 1.19 Anatomical variations of the femoral vein. Modal anatomy is the most common (88%); the axial vein is reduced to a small sciatic nerve arcade (SNA) along the ischiatic nerve, connected to the pelvis by the inferior gluteal vein IG. In the case of the nonregression of the axial vein, it could give either an axio-femoral trunk in 3% (with a hypotrophic femoral vein reduced to a small collateral canal, cc) or a bitruncular dispositive (9%) with both axes of similar diameter. *DF* deep femoral vein, *CF* common femoral vein, *IG* inferior gluteal vein, *P2*, *P3* deep femoral vein perforators

The *veins of the soleus* are divided into two parts. The lateral is the bigger; its huge veins are draining vertically into the fibular veins above the arcade of the hallux flexor longus. The medial part is smaller, draining horizontally into the tibial posterior veins (Figs. 1.20, 1.21, and 1.22).

The *gastrocnemial veins* include the medial veins (bigger, in light blue) and the lateral ones.

For both muscles, the vascular pedicle is emerging from the hilum and ends in the lateral aspects of the popliteal vein (Fig. 1.23). A common trunk of the medial veins with the SSV is found in 30% of the cases.

Important point, the origin of the gastrocnemial veins takes place at the lower part of the muscles from perforator veins by a termino-terminal connection.

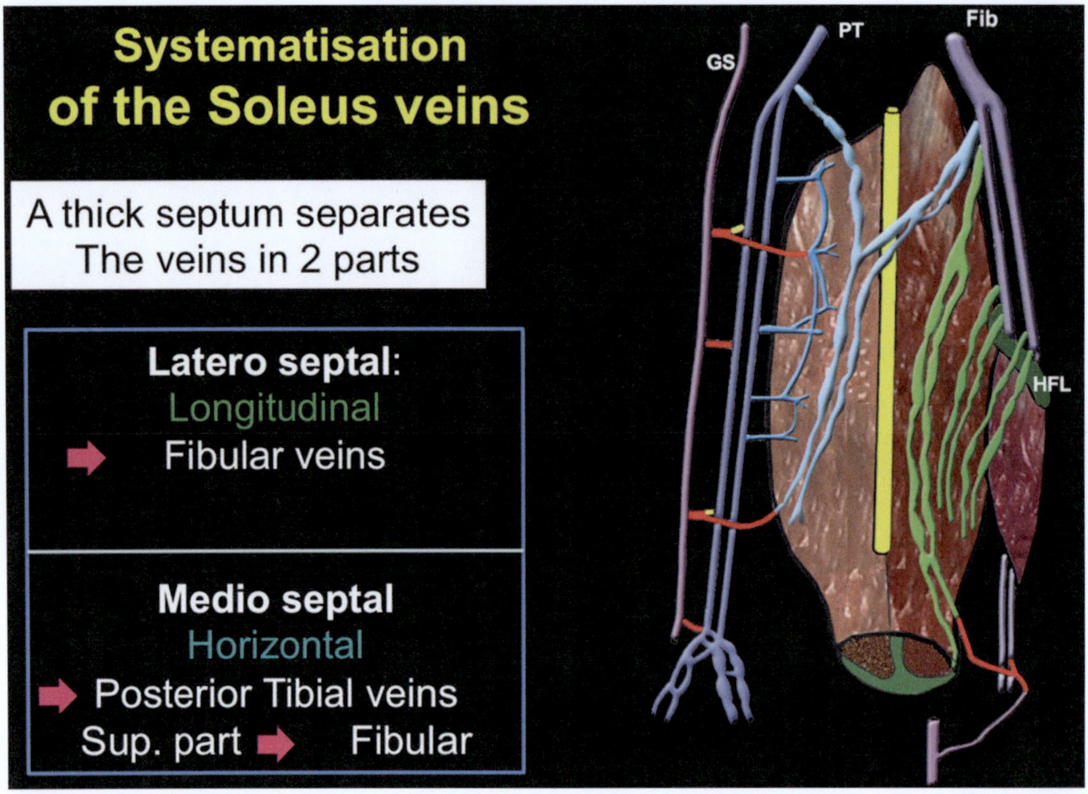

Fig. 1.20 Systematization of the veins of the soleus muscle. Laterally (bigger) draining vertically in the fibular veins above the arcade of the hallux flexor longus (HFL). Medially draining horizontally in the posterior tibial veins (PT). Please notice the medial leg perforators. Of the great saphenous vein (GS) territory

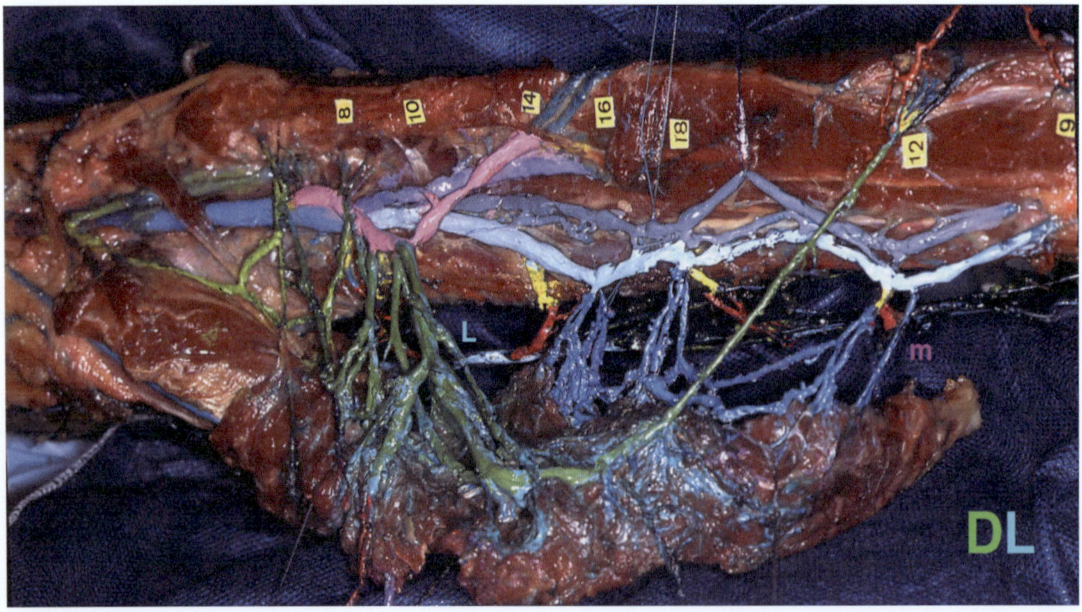

Fig. 1.21 Anatomical dissection after latex injection and colored segmentation (lateral view of a right leg): the veins of the soleus muscle. The lateral veins (in blue) are bigger, ending in the fibular veins (in pink). The medial veins of the soleus (in green) end in the posterior tibial (in light blue). Please notice the hemodynamical levels shown on the yellow labels on the top

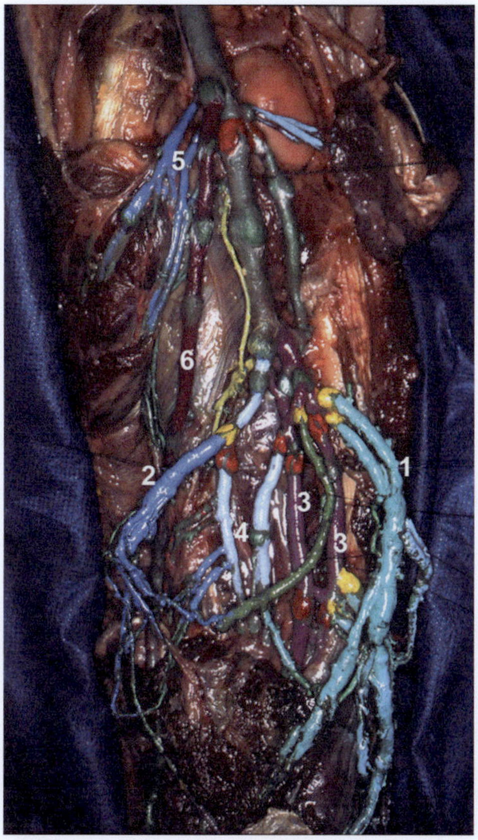

Fig. 1.22 Veins of the soleus: Anatomical dissection after latex injection and colored segmentation (posterior view of a right calf). The lateral veins of the soleus (1) are colored in light blue, the lateral ones in dark blue (2). The valves are colored in yellow. 3 = fibular veins, 4 = posterior tibial veins, 5 = medial gastrocnemial veins, 6 = SSV

Medially, the polar perforator is joining the SSV. This explains the common path of reflux observed for the GSV trunk, a communicating vein of the calf providing a powerful aspiration effect toward the gastrocnemial pump.

At the Thigh Level

The veins of two muscles play a role semimembranosus and biceps posteriorly and the quadriceps at the anterior aspect of the thigh.

The *veins of the semimembranosus* muscle are made of huge arcades providing a pump which connects the popliteal vein to the deep femoral vein (Fig. 1.24). So, in case of an obstacle on the femoropopliteal axis, these arcades act like a safety valve.

The *veins of the biceps* located laterally are making smaller arcades.

These both venous networks (biceps and semimembranosus) frequently are connections with the upper part of the thigh extension of the SSV.

The *veins of the quadriceps* muscle are draining at the root of the thigh in the circumflex tributaries of the deep femoral vein.

Physiological Point of View

On the *physiological point of view*, these muscular veins are the veno-muscular pumps of the lower limb, the true peripheral heart for the venous return. The first pump is the foot pump located in the plantar veins, explaining the role of the foot static disorders in worsening the chronic venous disorders [24]. But the main one and most powerful are the *calf pump*, including the soleus pump at the leg level, and the gastrocnemius pump at the popliteal level.

The activation of these pumps is a chain of events from the foot, leg, popliteal, and thigh successive muscular activations.

The anatomy of these pumps also explains the hemodynamical levels of the perforator veins, located at those particular levels for efficacy reasons.

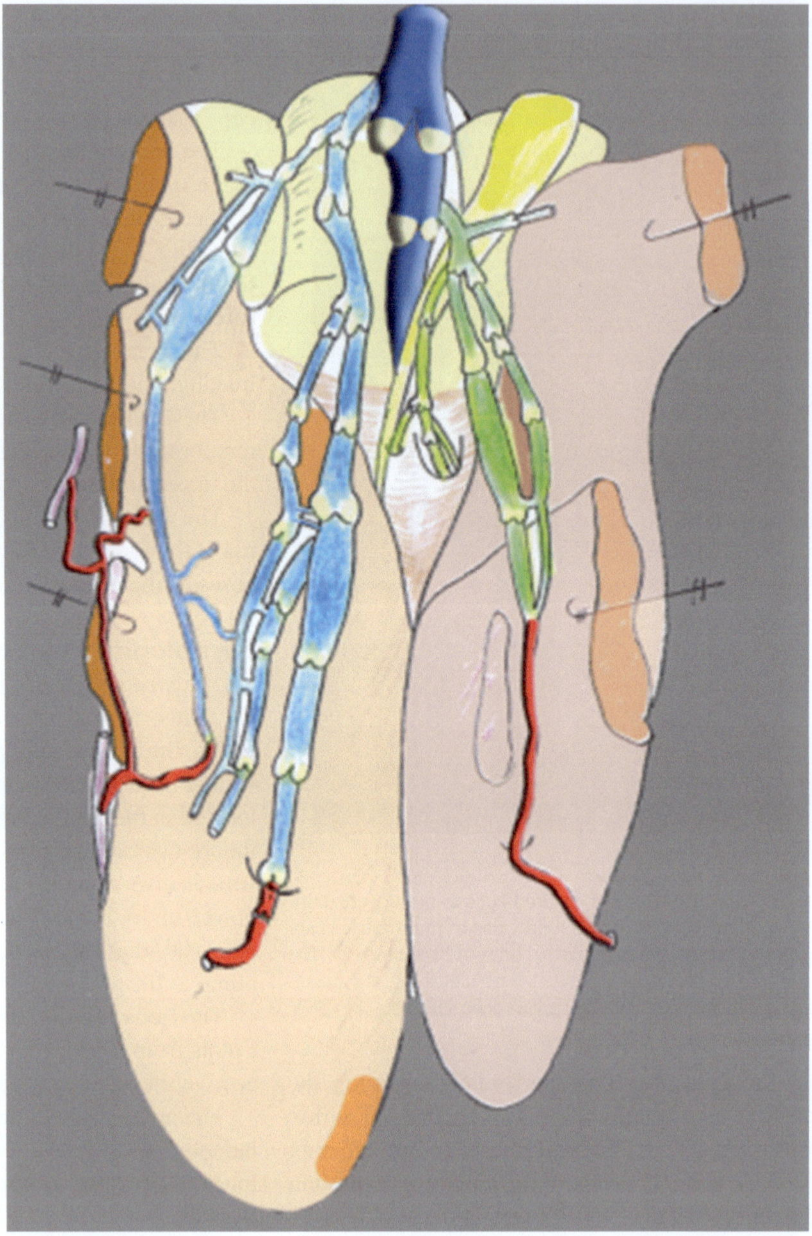

Fig. 1.23 The gastrocnemial veins. The medial veins (bigger) are colored in light blue: two main trunks joining in a unique collector ending in the popliteal vein (dark blue). The lateral veins are smaller, colored in green. Please notice that these veins originate from the lower part of the muscle by a termino-terminal anastomosis with perforators (in red)

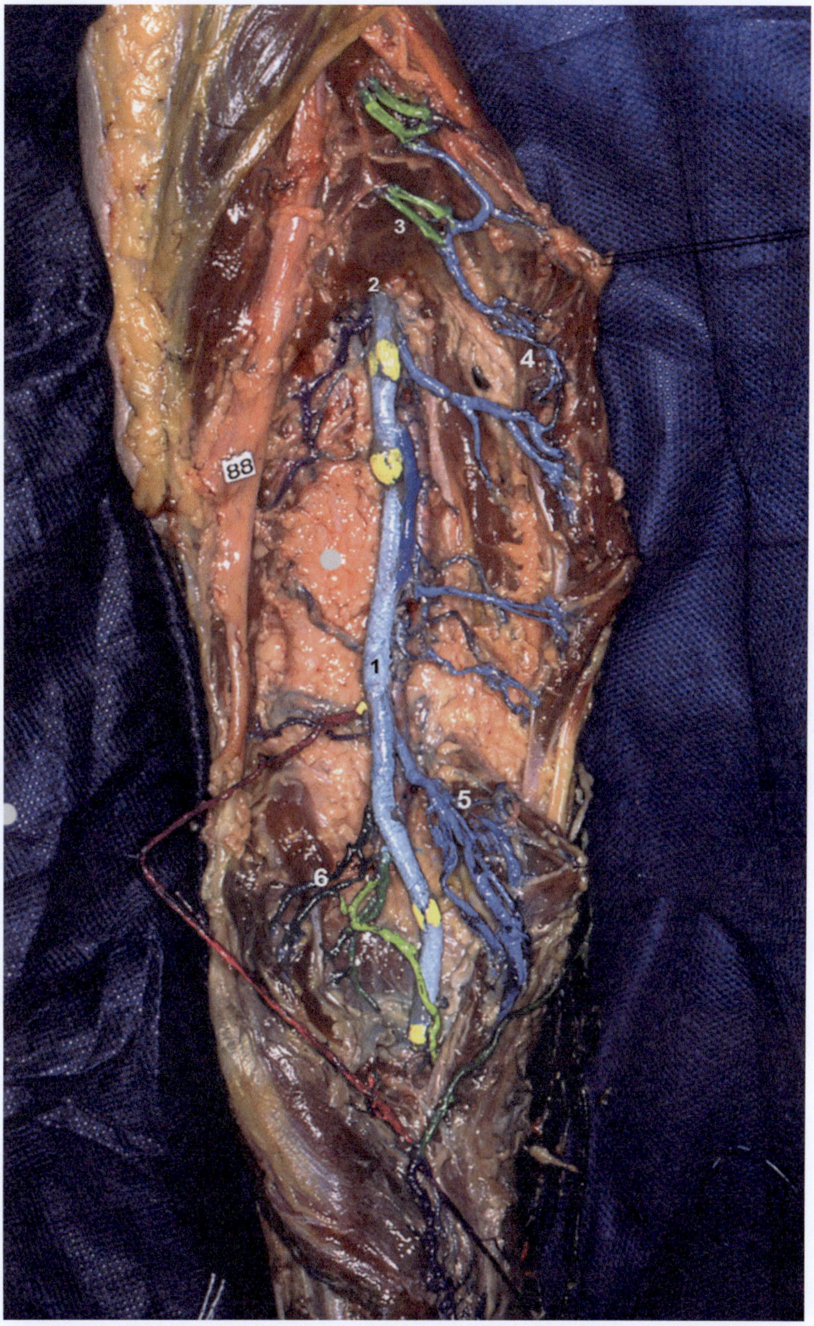

Fig. 1.24 The venous arcades of the semimembranosus muscle (anatomical dissection after latex injection and colored segmentation). This dissection clearly shows that the arcades (in blue) connect the popliteal vein (1) to the deep femoral vein (3, in green) and so bypass Hunter's canal hiatus (2). 1 = popliteal vein, 2 = femoropopliteal junction at Hunter's hiatus, 3 = deep femoral vein, 4 = arcades of the semimembranosus muscle, 5 = medial gastrocnemial veins, 6 = lateral gastrocnemial veins

References

1. Gaweesh AS, Kayed MH, Gaweesh TY, Shalhoub J, Davies AH, Khamis HM. Underlying deep venous abnormalities in Patients with unilateral chronic venous disease – a pilot study using direct injection CT venography. Phlebology. 2013;28:426–31.
2. Gillot C. Multimedia Atlas of the superficial venous networks of the lower limb Editions Phlébologiques Françaises-Corlet Editeur, Cabourg France, 1994 out of print (a CD-Rom version is available from Ganzoni company). 1994.
3. Uhl JF, Chahim M, Verdeille S, Martin-bouyer Y. The 3D modeling of the venous system by MSCT venography technique, indications and results. Phlebology. 2013;27:270–88.
4. Caggiati A, Bergan JJ, Gloviczki P, Jantet G, Wendell-Smith CP, Partsch H, International Interdisciplinary Consensus Committee on Venous Anatomical Terminology. Nomenclature of the veins of the lower limbs: an international interdisciplinary consensus statement. J Vasc Surg. 2002;36:416–22.
5. Caggiati A, Ricci S. The long saphenous vein compartment. Phlebology. 1997;12:107–11.
6. Bailly M. Cartographie CHIVA. In Editions Techniques Encyclopédie Médico-chirurgicale. Paris; 43-161-B; 2005. p. 1–4.
7. Lemasle P, Uhl JF, Lefebvre-Vilardebo M, Baud JM. Proposal of an echographic definition of the great saphenous vein and of the accessory saphenous veins at the thigh level. Phlebologie. 1996;49(3):279–85.
8. Coleridge-Smith P, Labropoulos N, et al. Venous disease of the lower limbs—UIP Consensus Document. Part I. Basic principles. Eur J Vasc Endovasc Surg. 2006;31:83–92.
9. Lemasle P, Uhl JF, Lefebvre-Vilardebo M, Tamisier D, Baud JM, Cornu-Thénard A. Confrontation écho-chirurgicale de la terminaison de la saphène externe dans le cadre de la chirurgie d'exérèse: résultats préliminaires. Phlebologie. 1996;49(3):279–86.
10. Uhl JF, Gillot C. Anatomy and embryology of the small saphenous vein: nerve relationships and implications for treatment. Phlebology. 2013;28(1):4–15.
11. Gillot C. The arch of the great saphenous vein. Anatomical basis and technique of high ligation. Phlebologie. 1994;47(2):117–33.
12. Pieri A, Vannuzzi A, Duranti A, et al. Rôle central de la valvule pré-ostiale de la veine saphène interne dans la genèse des varices tronculaires des membres inférieurs. Phlebologie. 1995;48:227–9.
13. Cappelli M, Molino Lova R, Ermini S, Zamboni P. Hemodynamics of the sapheno-femoral junction. Patterns of reflux and their clinical implications. Int Angiol. 2004;23(1):25–8.
14. Gillot C. Biradicular origin of the popliteal vein. Phlebologie. 1987;40(4):1001–18.
15. Van Rij A, Hill G, Gray C, Christie R, et al. A prospective study of the fate of venous leg perforators after varicose vein surgery. J Vasc Surg. 2005;42:1156–62.
16. Uhl JF, Lo Vuolo M, Labropoulos N. Anatomy of the lymph node venous networks of the groin and their investigation by ultrasonography. Phlebology. 2016;31(5):334–43.
17. Uhl JF, Gillot C. Anatomy of the foot venous pump: physiology and influence on chronic venous disease. Phlebology. 2012;27:219–30.
18. Gillot C. Popliteal venous arrangements: hypotheses and certainties. Phlebologie. 1998;51(1):65–74.
19. Uhl JF, Gillot C. Embryology and three-dimensional anatomy of the superficial venous system of the lower limbs. Phlebology. 1995;22(5):194–206.
20. Uhl JF, Gillot C. Anatomy of the veno-muscular pumps of the lower limb. Phlebology. 2015;30(3):180–93.
21. Uhl JF. Focus on embryogenesis of the venous system of the lower limbs. Phlebolymphology. 2015;22(2):55–62.
22. Uhl JF, Gillot C, Chahim M. The anatomical variations of the femoral vein. J Vasc Surg. 2010;52:714–9.
23. Uhl JF, Gillot C. Anatomy of the hunter's canal and its role in the venous outlet syndrome of the lower limb. Phlebology. 2015;30(9):604–11.
24. Uhl JF, Gillot C, Chahim M. Foot static disorders: a major risk factor of CVD? Phlebology. 2012;27:13–8.

Hemodynamic Aspects of Chronic Venous Disease

2

Seshadri Raju

2.1 Introduction

The hemodynamics of chronic venous disease differs significantly from arterial insufficiency. Often, arterial concepts are inappropriately applied to venous pathology. In some instances, such as, for example, saphenous reflux, applicable hemodynamics is unique and has no parallel in arterial practice. In this chapter, we focus on four areas of chronic venous disease: (1) quantifying saphenous reflux, (2) defining critical venous stenosis, (3) grading severity of iliac vein stenosis ("area method"), and (4) hemodynamics of venous collaterals and venous bypass.

2.2 Quantifying Saphenous Reflux

At the present time, saphenous reflux is defined by the duration of reflux; reflux duration >500 ms is considered significant reflux [1]. This is obviously a qualitative parameter as the quantity of reflux of similar duration will vary in quantity if the velocity and reflux and the size of the vein are different. The hemodynamics of saphenous reflux is to hasten calf refill after exercise, shortening the venous filling time (VFT). This can be measured by the ambulatory venous pressure measurement test traditionally performed with ten tiptoe stands to exercise the calf pump. A VFT of 20 s is considered normal; mild abnormality, 16–20 s; moderate, 10–15 s; and severe, <10 s, respectively. Dysfunction of the calf pump often coexists with saphenous reflux and in some cases precedes it in silent fashion [2]. Excluding cosmetic cases where saphenous ablation is performed for other reasons such as to prevent recurrence of branch varicosities, the purpose of ablation in symptomatic patients (CEAP class 3–6) is to unload the calf pump from reflux. Such an indication would obviously require some way to quantify reflux, not merely define it qualitatively for proper selection of patients. The refluxing volume is derived by the formula: Reflux duration in seconds X Reflux velocity in cm/sec. X lumen area (sq cm) of the saphenous vein at the measuring point (traditionally 2 cm below the saphenofemoral junction). The area is derived from the duplex diameter, and a circular vein lumen is assumed. Errors inherent in the duplex methodology and assumptions are minor and can be neglected without major impact on the reported observations.

The normal calf pump volume is about 100 cm^3, and half or more will be ejected with a single toe-stand maneuver. This ejected volume (EV) and ejection fraction (EF) as percentage of resting calf volume can be measured using a commercially available air plethysmographic instrument (APG; ACI medical, Los Angeles, CA). It is reasonable to assume that a quantitative reflux volume of about 30 cm^3 or about 50% EV is necessary to adversely affect calf pump function. It is then possible to

S. Raju
The RANE Center, Jackson, MS, USA

A. K. Khanna, R. Jindal (eds.), *Venous Disorders*, https://doi.org/10.1007/978-981-13-1108-6_2

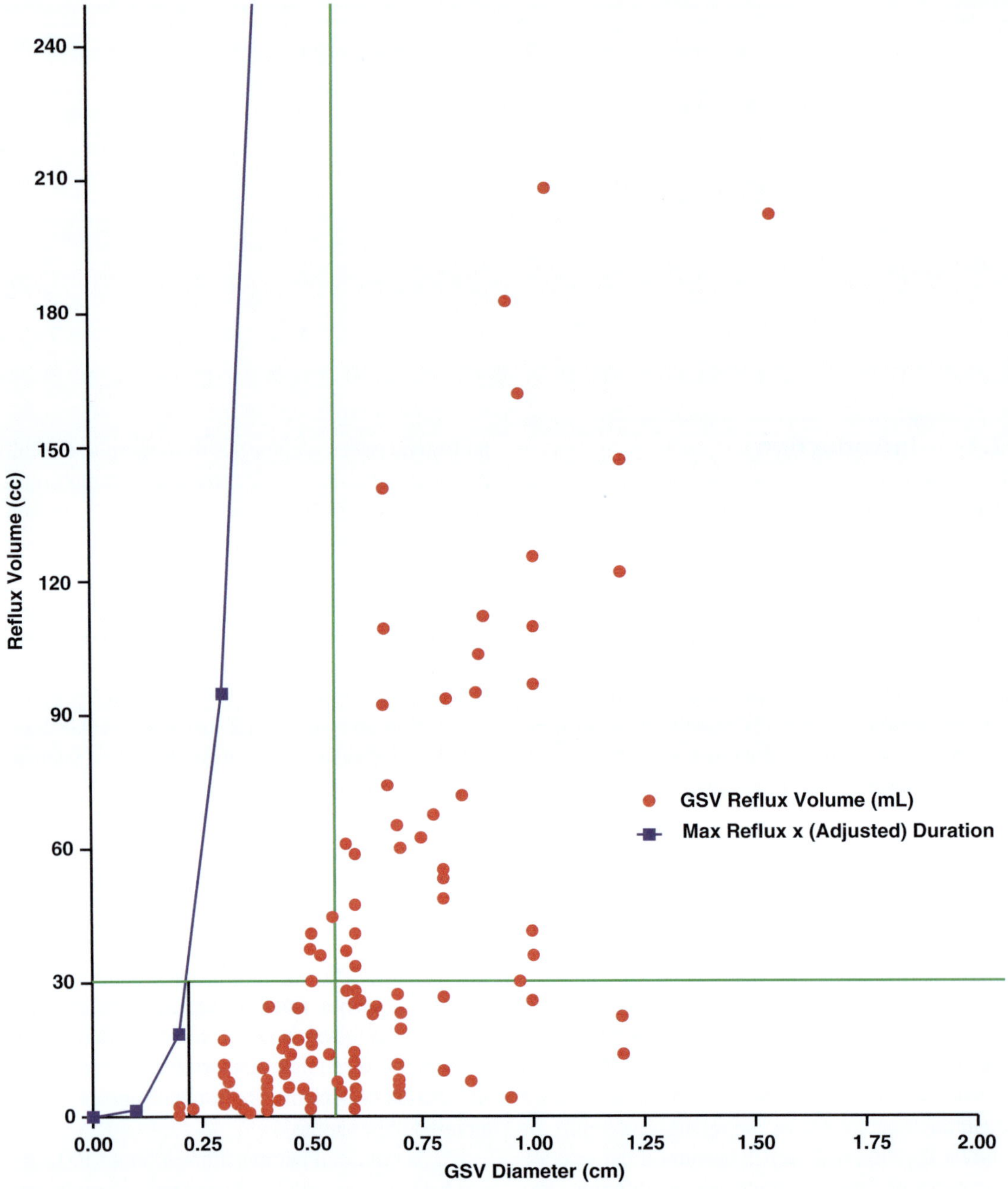

Fig. 2.1 Relationship of measured reflux volume and saphenous size. All except three limbs (0.5 cm, 0.5 cm, and 0.52 cm, respectively) with a saphenous diameter <0.55 cm had reflux volumes of ≥30 cm³. However, the reverse was not true; roughly half the limbs with saphenous diameter ≥5.5 mm had measured reflux volumes <30 cm³ and the other half >30 cm³. Maximum reflux potential of various saphenous sizes is shown as a line (blue). Actual measured reflux volume was much less than the maximum potential. See text for explanation

explore the physical attributes of the refluxing saphenous vein (mainly size) that will allow this quantity of reflux to unbalance the calf pump. We can also correlate the effect of quantitative reflux on ambulatory venous pressure and VFT.

In an analysis of 119 limbs with isolated saphenous reflux, saphenous size was shown to be a critical factor controlling quantity of reflux (Fig. 2.1) [2]. *A quantitative reflux of >30 cm³ was possible only if the size of the saphenous vein exceeded 5.5 mm. This means that ablation of a saphenous vein less than this threshold size may not lead to durable functional results.* Navarro and colleagues also identified 5.5 mm as the threshold saphenous size to be associated with hemodynamic calf impairment [3].

A careful examination of Fig. 2.1 shows that a saphenous size >5.5 mm does not automatically mean that a large quantitative reflux is present; some of the large saphenous veins indeed carry trivial reflux. Typically, either the reflux velocity or its duration is small in these large veins. The paradox of a large saphenous vein with a small reflux can be explained by the small size and number of reentry perforators that feed the saphenous reflux into the calf pump. They offer high resistance to reflux flow even though the saphenous vein can carry a larger reflux volume if adequate runoff was available to drain the reflux into the calf. Quantifying reflux is superior to mere qualitative detection of reflux for proper clinical assessment.

Ambulatory venous pressure measurement can further illuminate the hemodynamic impact of saphenous reflux. The correlation between VFT and measured quantity of reflux in a cohort of 66 limbs with isolated saphenous reflux is shown in Fig. 2.2. As expected, most limbs with a reflux quantity of <30 cm^3 have normal VFT, and those with reflux >30 cm^3 have shortened VFT. Some exceptions should be noted.

VFT was normal in eight limbs despite quantitative reflux >30 cm^3, apparently due to adequate compensation by the calf pump. Contrawise, a shortened VFT was present in 17 limbs even though reflux was <30 cm^3. It can be inferred that calf pump disease was likely the reason for the abnormal VFT in these limbs separate from the trivial reflux present.

It is clear that the interaction between saphenous reflux and the calf pump is the critical pathophysiologic mechanism, not the presence of reflux per se. Ambulatory pressure measurement and air plethysmography are crucial tools for understanding the complexities of the interaction between reflux and the calf pump. Unfortunately, evaluation of saphenous reflux in clinical practice has devolved into using only the duplex examination.

2.3 Definition of Critical Venous Stenosis

The critical element in arterial stenosis is perfusion, the adequacy of which is gauged by downstream perfusion pressure; a "critical" stenosis of 70% or greater is required to impact perfusion. Flow is generally unaffected in venous stenosis except in extreme cases when nearly all of the outflow is thrombosed (phlegmasia cerulea dolens).The critical element in venous stenosis is back (peripheral) pressure—the trigger for microvascular injury and CVD manifestations [4, 5]. There is not a direct relationship between percentage stenosis and back pressure (see later) because of the intercession of the pressure-volume relationship of the peripheral venous bed in pressure determination. For this reason, there is not a set percentage stenosis that is "critical" as in the arterial system. In addition to the aforementioned pressure-volume relationship, there are also several central mechanisms that influence peripheral venous pressure [5].

Central mechanisms that impact peripheral venous pressure include (1) arterial inflow into the limb, (2) right atrial pressure, (3) intra-abdominal pressure, and (4) stenosis of the iliac-caval outflow tract draining the limb. Clinical examples for these, respectively, are (1) A-V fistula, (2) congestive heart failure, (3) morbid obesity, and (4) May-Thurner syndrome or post-thrombotic iliac vein stenosis. Peripheral venous pressure is elevated in these situations, often accompanied by edema or skin manifestations.

2.4 Grading Severity of Iliac Vein Stenosis ("Area Method")

The arterial flow into the lower limb is a constant fraction of cardiac output which itself is uniform among individuals with only minor variation related to body mass and surface area [6, 7]. It is also remarkable that the venous effluent at the venous end of the capillary emerges with a uniform postcapillary pressure of ≈17 mmHg. Since the volume and pressure of the limb venous flow are fixed, coalescing into a single outflow trunk (common iliac vein, CIV), it follows that CIV will

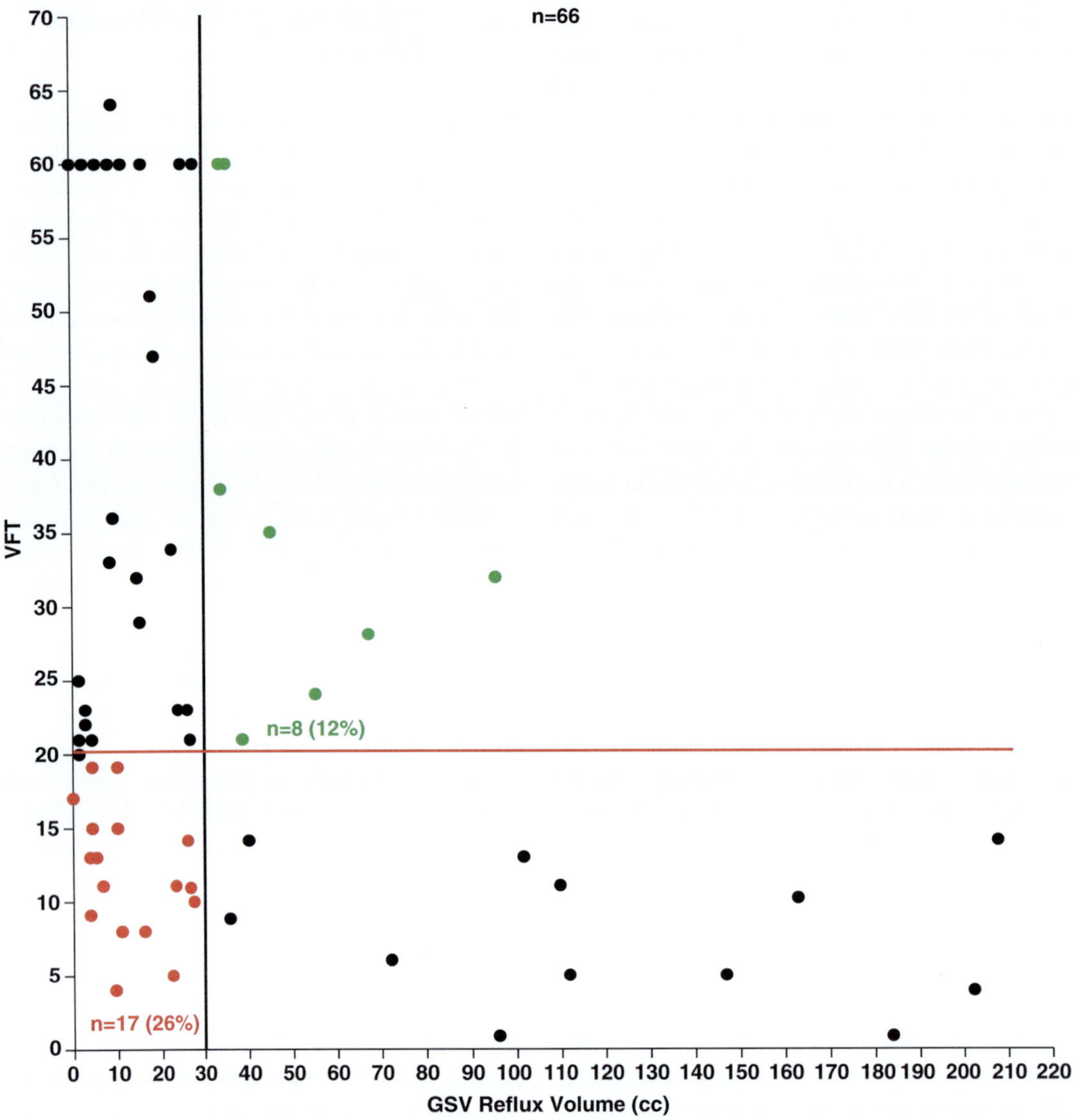

Fig. 2.2 Relationship between measured reflux volume and venous filling time (VFT) of ambulatory venous pressure. The data set is divided into four rectangles based on intersecting lines marking the 30 cm^3 reflux volume and 20 s VFT, which is considered "normal." Limbs (62%) in the outer rectangles along the *x* and *y* axis have concordant VFT, i.e., normal VFT if the reflux volume is <30 cm^3 and abnormal VFT when reflux volume exceeds this threshold. Twelve percent of limbs above the red VFT line have normal VFT despite reflux volume exceeding the 30 cm^3 threshold. Twenty-six percent of limbs (innermost rectangle on X-Y intersection) have abnormally shortened VFT despite a relatively small volume of reflux <30 cm^3. The discordant VFT in the last two groups is due to identifiable reflux buffering mechanisms and intrinsic calf pump abnormalities, respectively, in many of the limbs (see text)

have an optimal luminal area to keep the peripheral venous pressure in the normal range (<11 mmHg). One can derive this optimal or "ideal" diameter by a variety of methods, including, for example, the Poiseuille equation which relates pressure and flow to the radius (πr^4). There is reliable data on the size of the common femoral vein from large population surveys where duplex examination was used [8]. One can project the expected size of the common iliac vein from this data using the scaling law of Murray [9]. We can assume from telelogic reasons that such an "ideal" diameter of iliac venous outflow will coincide with iliac vein caliber found in normal individuals. Morphometric data from CT images or IVUS planimetry in normal individuals can also be used provided there is no May-Thurner type of stenosis which occurs in as many as 2/3 of the population in silent form [10, 11]. Average estimates of optimal lumen size (+20% to account for body mass variation) for the various iliac vein segments derived from these methods are shown in Table 2.1. These are minimal values. Outflow stenosis can be considered to be present if the iliac vein size observed by IVUS or duplex is less than the thresholds shown in Table 2.1. Obviously, this method of grading stenosis severity is different from common practice in the arterial system. A "critical" threshold of percentage stenosis is not used since the venous back pressure will vary in individuals with the same percentage stenosis depending upon the individual pressure-volume relationship (Fig. 2.3). Another departure from common arterial practice is that percentage stenosis is not calculated based on the adjacent "normal" segment as comparator. This is because long diffuse stenosis (Rokitansky stenosis) without focal cues is frequently present in post-thrombotic iliac vein stenosis [12]. In that event, the segment is not truly "normal" but stenotic; if used as a comparator, an underestimation of the stenosis will occur. All of this means that a decision to correct an iliac vein stenosis should not be based on a set threshold value but on IVUS findings and clinical presentation. Correction of <50% IVS area stenosis has yielded symptom relief [13]. The use of peripheral venous pressure to guide decision-making seems logical, but current data to support this is lacking.

Table 2.1 Recommended range (n + 20%) of target diameter and area values for the iliac-femoral segments

Vessels	Diameter (mm)	Area[a] (mm)
IVC	17–24	N/A[b]
CIV	16–20	200–240
EIV	14–17	150–180
CFV	12–14	110–135

[a]Suggested area ranges are +20% over base value and do not mathematically correspond to suggested diameter ranges.
[b]Only transverse diameter is used as IVC and is usually partially collapsed into an oval rather than a circle.

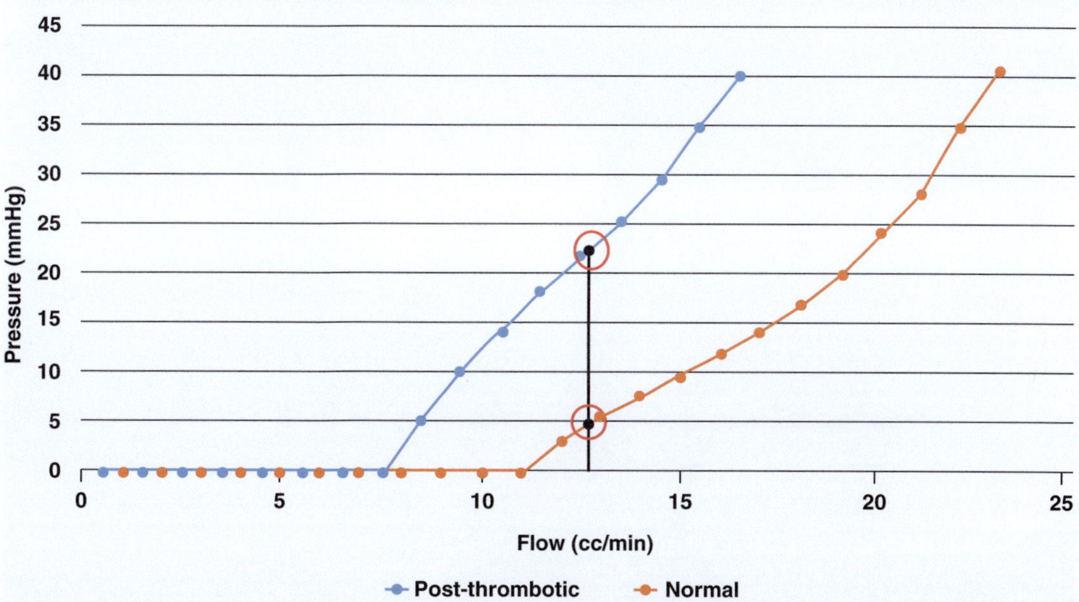

Fig. 2.3 Hypothetical pressure-volume curves in two individuals that vary because of post-thrombotic changes. Given the same flow volume (13 cm³/min; X axis), the pressures are different: 24 mmHg in post-thrombotic and 5 mmHg in the normal vein. The intercession of the pressure-volume curve in the determination of the pressure means that a fixed percentage value of stenosis to define criticality is not possible in venous flow

2.5 Hemodynamics of Venous Collaterals and Venous Bypass

It is a common observation that even extensive collaterals "disappear" in completion venograms immediately after iliac vein stenting (Fig. 2.4). We have also observed that many patients with seemingly extensive collateralization continue to be symptomatic but obtain relief after iliac vein stenting [14]. This is strong evidence that even extensive collateralization does not provide adequate outflow to decompress the peripheral venous tree and lower the pressure. An explanation for this paradox can be found in the Poiseuille equation: $F = \Delta P^* \pi r^4/8l\eta$. The radius of the vessel enters the equation in the 4th power. The surprising influence of vessel radius by several orders of magnitude in peripheral resistance is well-known but has received scant attention in venous flow. A cartoon representation of the number of collaterals of a given size required to replace a normal sized common iliac vein is shown in Fig. 2.5.

The enormous power of the geometric factor underlying conductance should give pause to the notion underlying the Palma veno-venous bypass. The attractiveness of this bypass as a concept, since its description by Eduardo Palma, was largely based on its venographic appearance. A well-constructed Palma bypass can be visually seen on venography to "bypass" the obstructed iliac vein. The perception is clearly one based on perfusion, not reduction of peripheral venous (back) pressure. Most of the literature related to the Palma procedure report outcomes in terms of patency, not reduction of pressure in the limb. The literature predates description of venous clinical severity scores. Clinical outcome is reported in generic terms (e.g., "good" or "satisfactory"), but not in objective terms. Based on Poiseuille equation, one can hazard a guess that most patients are likely to have residual symptoms following a Palma bypass utilizing a saphenous vein of 4–6 mm in size. Without question, these bypasses can enlarge over time (a temporary A-V fistula may help) and

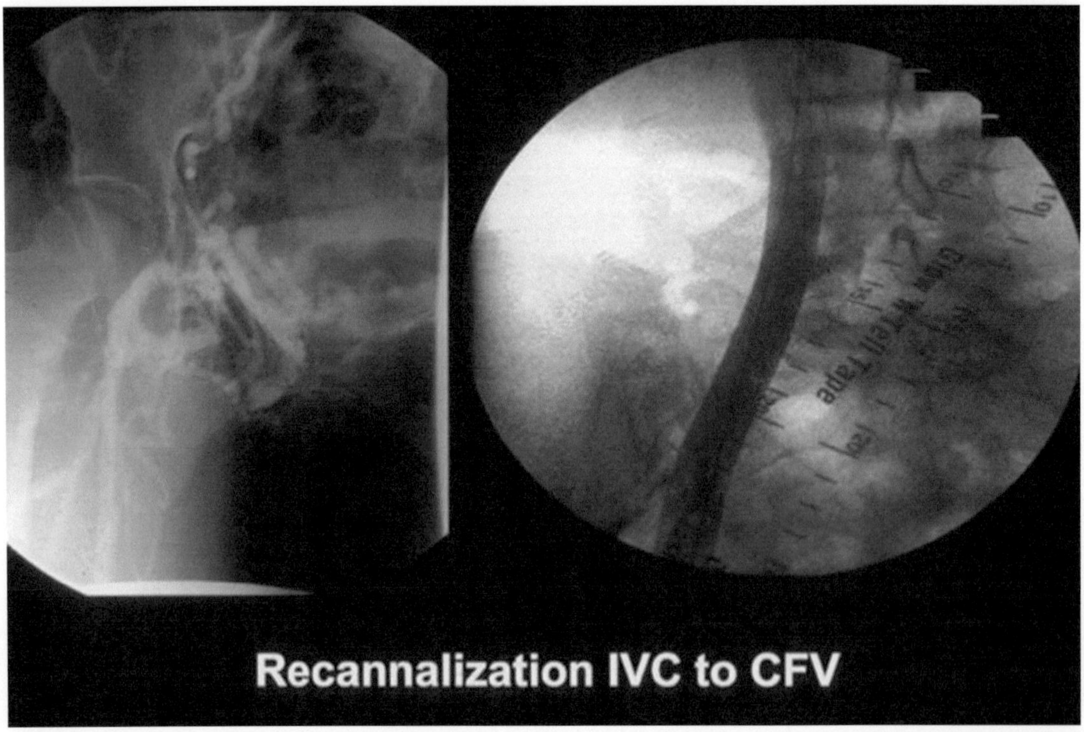

Fig. 2.4 Disappearance of collaterals following iliac vein stenting

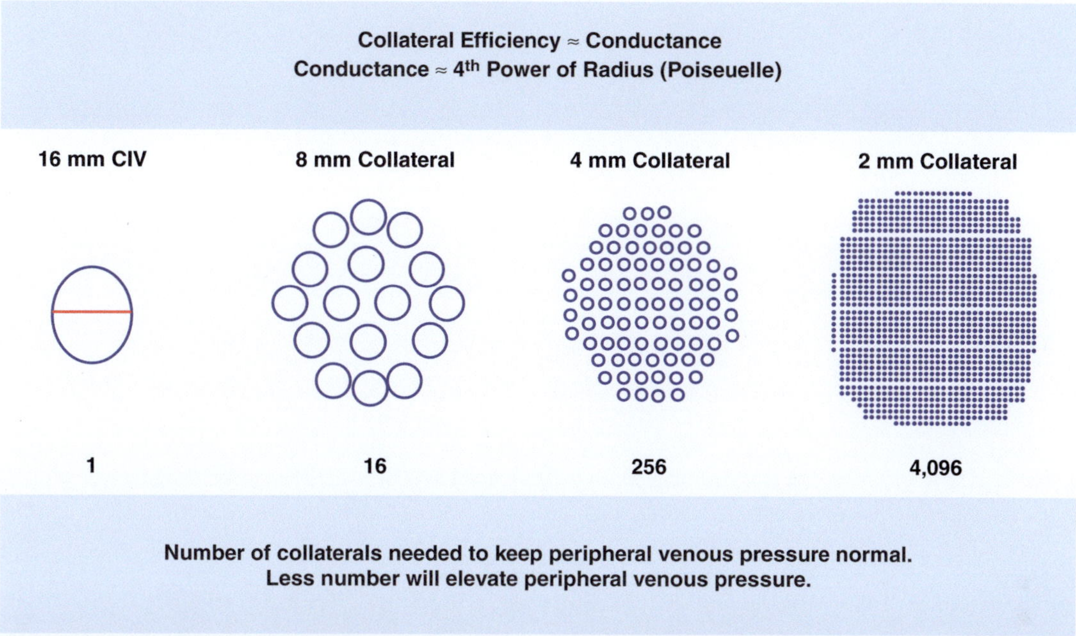

Fig. 2.5 A cartoon depicting the power of the geometric factor in the Poiseuille equation. Number of collaterals 1–8 mm in calib required to equal the conductance of a 16 mm CIV to maintain peripheral venous pressure in the dame normal range. Peripheral venous pressure is unlikely to be normalized even with extensive collateralization. Certainly, a 4–6 mm size Palma bypass has little chance of normalizing peripheral venous pressure in the presence of an occluded common iliac vein

approach the caliber of CIV. It is, however, more common to see kinks and persistent collaterals after performance of the Palma bypass.

References

1. Gloviczki P, Gloviczki ML. Guidelines for the management of varicose veins. Phlebology. 2012;27(Suppl 1):2–9.
2. Raju SWJM, Jones T. Quantifying saphenous reflux. J Vasc Surg. 2015;3:8–17.
3. Navarro TP, Delis KT, Ribeiro AP. Clinical and hemodynamic significance of the greater saphenous vein diameter in chronic venous insufficiency. Arch Surg. 2002;137(11):1233–7.
4. Pascarella L, Schonbein GW, Bergan JJ. Microcirculation and venous ulcers: a review. Ann Vasc Surg. 2005;19(6):921–7.
5. Raju S, Kirk O, Davis M, Olivier J. Hemodynamics of 'critical' venous stenosis and stent treatment. J Vasc Surg. 2013;1:1–8.
6. Hall JE. Guyton and hall textbook of medical physiology. 13th ed. Philadelphia: Elsevier; 2016. p. 1145.
7. Nichols W, O'Rourke M, Vlachopoulos C. McDonald's blood flow in arteries: theoretical, experimental and clinical principles. 6th ed. Boca Raton: CRC Press; 2011.
8. Fronek A, Criqui MH, Denenberg J, Langer RD. Common femoral vein dimensions and hemodynamics including Valsalva response as a function of sex, age, and ethnicity in a population study. J Vasc Surg. 2001;33(5):1050–6.
9. Sherman TF. On connecting large vessels to small. The meaning of Murray's law. J Gen Physiol. 1981;78(4):431–53.
10. Fukaoka M, Okada M, Sugimoto T. Assessment of lower extremity venous function using foot venous pressure measurement. Br J Surg. 1999;86:1149–54.
11. Kibbe MR, Ujiki M, Goodwin AL, Eskandari M, Yao J, Matsumura J. Iliac vein compression in an asymptomatic patient population. J Vasc Surg. 2004;39(5):937–43.
12. Raju S, Davis M. Anomalous features of iliac vein stenosis that affect diagnosis and treatment. J Vasc Surg Venous Lymphat Disord. 2014;2(3):260–7.
13. Raju S, Oglesbee M, Neglen P. Iliac vein stenting in postmenopausal leg swelling. J Vasc Surg. 2011;53(1):123–30.
14. Neglen P, Raju S. Intravascular ultrasound scan evaluation of the obstructed vein. J Vasc Surg. 2002;35(4):694–700.

Deep Venous Reflux

3

Arjun Jayaraj

Chronic venous insufficiency (CVI) encompasses an extensive range of clinical manifestations from limb swelling to non-healing ulcers. Etiologies for CVI in the deep venous system include reflux, venous obstruction, or a combination of the two. Of these, reflux alone or in combination with obstruction is the contributing factor in the overwhelming majority (70–90%) of instances [1–7]. Such reflux involving the deep vein (DVR) can result from primary or secondary etiologies. The occurrence of DVR varies in different populations. While the precise number is hard to determine due to difference in metrics used, an excess of 30–60% of DVR is believed to be primary in origin [8–12]. Secondary DVR arises as a result of deep vein thrombosis (DVT) involving the extremity. Often the two can coexist in the same patient [13]. Primary DVR arises due to stretching/elongation of the valve cusps or dilation of the affected venous segment. A developmental etiology has also been recognized due to symptoms predating the age of actual presentation, often as early as teenage years [14]. Trauma has also been presented as a cause. Degeneration of the fibroelastic tissue of the valve that gradually develops over time is deemed the most plausible cause in a majority of patients [14]. This chapter explores the pathophysiology and management of DVR.

3.1 Pathophysiology

Symptomatic DVR is likely to involve multiple mechanisms being overwhelmed. The latter include compensatory collateral pathways, involving superficial veins/perforator veins in addition to calf pump function. When reflux overwhelms such mechanisms, symptoms manifest. Coexistence of deep venous obstruction with DVR reinforces the pathology with earlier occurrence of symptoms than would be the case if obstruction did not exist. With regard to progression of DVR, it has been postulated that an initial incompetent valve high in the femoral vein creates an excess stress on the valve below and leads to it becoming incompetent. For clinical manifestations, the reflux must involve multiple venous segments in the thigh and calf (axial reflux) as opposed to segmental reflux. A functioning, competent popliteal valve is considered a barrier to the development of severe symptoms, even in the presence of reflux involving the entire femoral vein since it protects the calf pump from the deleterious effect of reflux. This is particularly true for patients with venous ulcer (C6 disease) in whom Danielsson et al. noted axial distribution of reflux in a majority of patients (79%). In their series, no patient had isolated DVR below the knee with primary etiology as the predominant

A. Jayaraj
RANE Center for Venous and Lymphatic Diseases at St. Dominic Hospital, Jackson, MS, USA

A. K. Khanna, R. Jindal (eds.), *Venous Disorders*, https://doi.org/10.1007/978-981-13-1108-6_3

cause [4]. Shami and colleagues have also explored the role of DVR in patients with venous ulcers and noted that DVR was present in as many as 47% of such limbs [15]. Secondary DVR resulting from DVT often involves not only the thrombosed segment but also the adjacent segment(s). As Caps et al. have pointed out, permanent valvular damage can occur even in the absence of thrombosis of the deep venous segment. The precise mechanism has not been identified, but the release of inflammatory mediators and localized vein dilation has been proposed as potential contributing factors [16]. The most frequent pathophysiology in secondary DVR is direct damage to the vein valve cusps by the thrombus.

The role of the competent popliteal valve is still debated. Historically, the "gatekeeper" role of this valve has been elucidated by several authors [17, 18]. However, more recent work by Neglen et al. has shown the popliteal valve not to be a less important determinant of venous hemodynamics or clinical severity. The authors note that reflux in additional segments must also be considered [19].

The differences in morphology of the vein wall and valve structure in patients with primary and secondary reflux have been reported by Kistner et al. [13]. Raju and colleagues have reported their findings on valve station changes in 149 patients undergoing valve reconstruction surgery using grades 0–5 to denote the same (Fig. 3.1). Grade

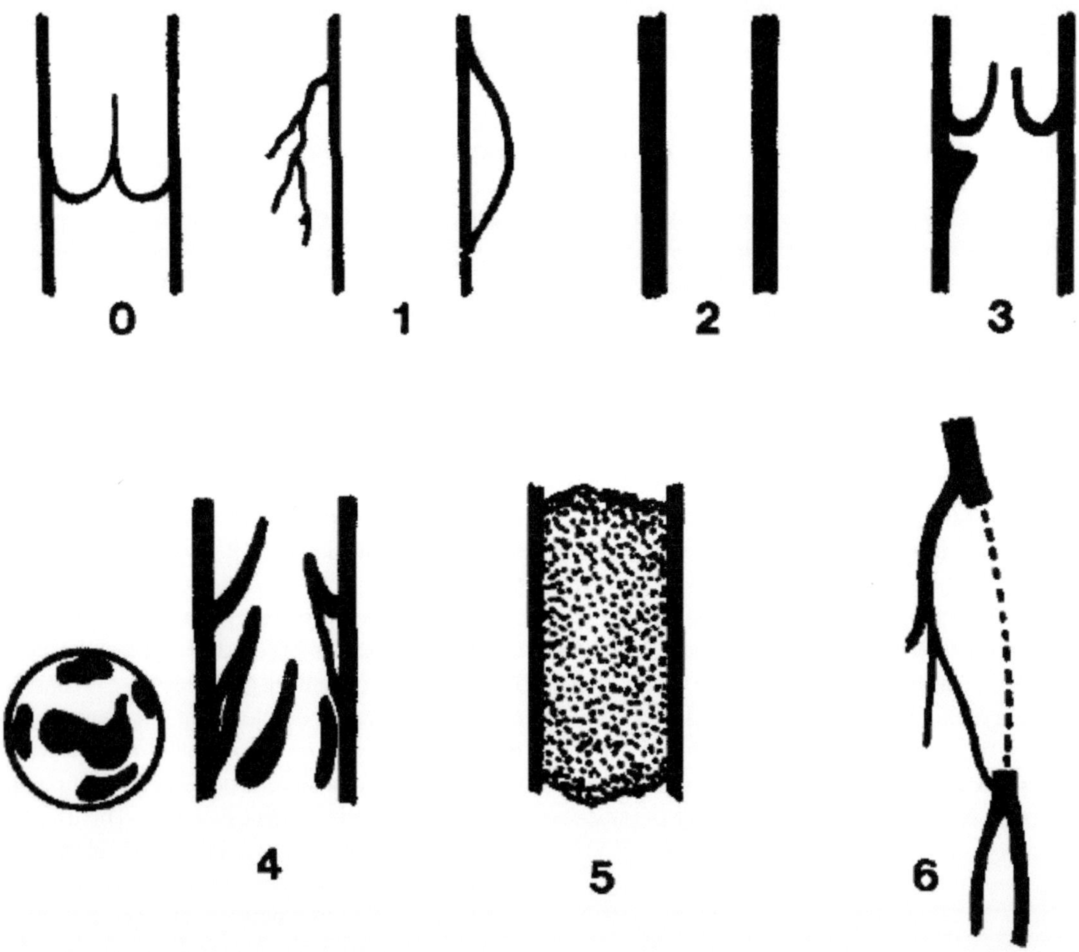

Fig. 3.1 Valve station grading system. Grade 0—normal-appearing valve station. Grade 1—increased collaterals/tributaries. Grade 2—venous valve thickening/fibrosis at valve station. Grade 3—thickening of valve cusps and/or intima. Grade 4—intraluminal trabeculae. Grade 5—thrombosis/occlusion. Grade 6—postthrombotic dissolution/disappearance (From Raju S, Fredericks RK, Hudson CA, Fountain T, Neglén PN, Devidas M. Venous valve station changes in "primary" and postthrombotic reflux: an analysis of 149 cases. Annals of Vascular Surgery. 2000;14(3):193. With permission from Annals of Vascular Surgery)

0/1 is mainly seen in primary DVR, while grade 4/5 is usually present in secondary DVR. Grade 2/3 can be seen in primary or secondary DVR [20]. However, it must be borne in mind that while valve station changes do affect reconstruction technique, they do not affect clinical outcomes. Dr. O'Donnell's group has reported on the significant role that DVR plays in the progression of CVI. Clinical severity increases with an increase in DVR (higher CEAP clinical class correlates with worsening axial reflux) [21]. This has been supported by other studies [22, 23]. Additional pathophysiological factors contributing to DVR have also been explored. Sarin et al. elucidated the role of flow in medial calf vein perforators with distal compression during the relaxation phase as a contributor to the severity of venous disease [24].

3.2 Diagnosis

Lurie and colleagues have described four stages of the venous valve cycle—opening, equilibrium, closing, and closed phases. The equilibrium phase results in flow separation and creation of a vortex along the valve cusp that prevents stasis inside the valve packet. These investigators concluded that the main axial jet stream facilitates outflow according to the authors [25]. The ability of the valve to maintain the closed phase determines occurrence of reflux. Metrics such as valve closure time/reflux time (VCT/RT) have been postulated and used to grade reflux. But VCT/RT is more qualitative than quantitative indices. The severity of reflux cannot be gauged by such metrics, especially because they do not correlate with hemodynamic and clinical parameters. However, other metrics such as peak reflux velocity (PRV) and time-averaged flow (TAF) have demonstrated good correlation with both hemodynamic parameters and clinical severity in multiple studies [19, 26]. Thus, while a wide range of metrics exist for DVR, the most relevant ones appear to be PRV and TAF, assessed using venous duplex. Reflux in the deep veins of the lower extremity is typically evaluated in the standing position [27] using the cuff deflation technique put forth by van Bemmelen et al. [28]. Based on studies by Masuda et al. and Araki et al., the standing cuff deflation technique appears to be a superior method when compared to other techniques, including Valsalva maneuver [29, 30]. The most common criteria used for defining reflux are derived from data published by multiple groups [28, 31, 32] including Labropoulous et al. and have since been incorporated into the clinical practice guidelines of the Society for Vascular Surgery and the American Venous Forum [33, 34]. Per the guidelines, DVR is defined as reflux lasting for 500 ms or more in the deep veins below the knee and the deep femoral vein and lasting for 1000 ms or more in the femoral and popliteal veins. The current role of descending phlebography in assessing reflux is deemed only of historical importance now with duplex technology having supplanted it [35, 36].

In addition to venous duplex, other methods that help shed light on DVR include air plethysmography (APG) and ambulatory venous pressure (AVP). APG helps determine a variety of parameters that quantify calf pump function in addition to determining the venous filling index, a highly sensitive indicator of severe venous disease and reflux in general [22]. AVP was once the traditional gold standard for assessing DVR. However, AVP is impacted by other factors including calf pump function [37] and is therefore more of a global index of calf function than a specific measure of DVR. It cannot be used to evaluate success of treatment thereof, as normalization occurs in only a fraction of treated limbs despite good clinical outcome [14]. The presence of medial calf perforator vein flow with distal compression during relaxation phase is also an indicator of more severe venous disease including DVR, as noted previously [24]. Diagnosis of concomitant deep venous obstruction should focus on determining etiology of obstruction, in addition to determining flow patterns in and out of the affected segment. Such testing includes multiple studies including noninvasive testing (venous duplex ultrasound (DUS), air plethysmography (APG), and computerized tomographic venogram [CTV]/magnetic resonance venogram [MRV] and invasive testing (ascending venogram and intravascular ultrasound). DUS serves as a screening tool and helps determine the extent of stenosis or occlu-

Table 3.1 Normal luminal area and corresponding diameter cut offs for the common femoral, external iliac and common iliac veins respectively

Vein	Luminal area (mm^2)	Diameter (mm)
CFV	125	12
EIV	150	14
CIV	200	16

CFV common femoral vein, *EIV* external iliac vein, *CIV* common iliac vein

sion based on luminal diameters, besides providing reflux data. Normal luminal diameter cutoffs used for the common femoral vein (CFV), the external iliac vein (EIV), and the common iliac vein (CIV) are 12 mm, 14 mm, and 16 mm, respectively (Table 3.1). The corresponding areas used for the three segments are 125 mm^2, 150 mm^2, and 200 mm^2, respectively. Air plethysmography provides information on calf pump function, the competence of which serves as one of the factors determining development of chronic venous insufficiency. CTV/MRV helps illuminate venous anatomy and provides information on compression/occlusion and collateral circulation. Ascending venography provides data on flow patterns and may be helpful, especially in patients with prior deep vein thrombosis.

3.3 Treatment

DVR, as noted previously, can exist in isolation or coexist with superficial venous reflux (SVR) and/or deep venous obstruction (DVO). Treatment should be tailored accordingly.

3.3.1 Isolated Deep Venous Reflux

Symptomatic patients (lifestyle limiting severe pain, swelling, skin changes, and/or ulceration) with DVR that is not responsive to conservative treatment should be considered for surgical intervention. The latter categories include valvuloplasty, valve transplant, transposition of incompetent venous segment, and valve substitution. The femoral vein is usually the site for such interventions, although the popliteal vein can also be used.

Valvuloplasty

Valvuloplasty techniques include internal valvuloplasty, external valvuloplasty, and external banding (Figs. 3.2, 3.3, 3.4, and 3.5). Internal valvuloplasty involves the use of a venotomy at the level of commissure [*longitudinal transcommisural*] [38], above commissure [*supracommissural*] [39] or a venotomy that starts above and extends to the level of commissure (*supra-T commissural*) [40] to suture approximate the cusps and thereby restore valvular competence. External valvuloplasty involves suture of valve attachment lines from the outside to facilitate competence of the valve cusps without the use of a venotomy. This can be accomplished using an external commissural suture, an external/internal suture, or an angioscopically directed external suture [41–45]. The advantage of external valvuloplasty is that it enables repair of multiple valves at the same operation. External banding involves the use of a PTFE, Dacron, or fascia-based sleeve to create a band around the incompetent valve that is tightened until competence is attained.

While long-term data for external valvuloplasty are not available, multiple series have noted good results for internal valvuloplasty in as many as 75% patients at 5 years [9, 11, 12, 46–48]. The results were superior when performed for primary DVR as compared to secondary DVR. Overall internal valvuloplasty repair has remained competent for 8–15 years in 60–73% of cases with continued good clinical results reflected in such patients [47, 48]. Regarding external banding valvuloplasty (EBV), a recent study by Ma and colleagues noted an improved clinical picture (VCSS score improvement), hemodynamic status (reflux time/reflux volume), and venous ulcer healing (average 18 days) with low complication and symptom recurrence rate in 1252 limbs that underwent popliteal vein external banding for severe CVI over a 15-year period [49]. Another study by Camilli et al. reported on 54 patients with primary DVR who underwent femoral vein EBV with a mean follow-up of 38 months. Complete resolution of deep reflux was noted in 41 patients (76%), significant improvement in 8 (14.8%), and no change in 5 (9.2%) [50].

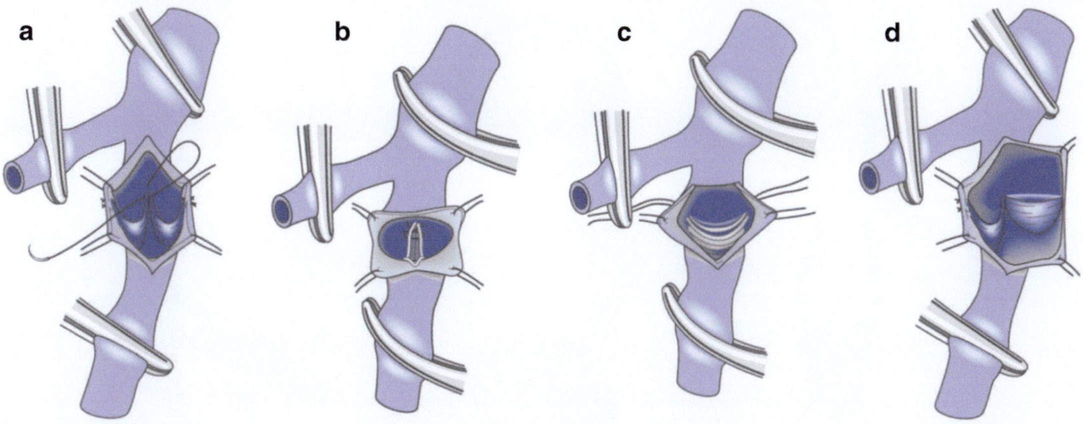

Fig. 3.2 Internal valvuloplasty (**a**) Kistner technique—transcommisural. (**b**) Raju technique—supravalvular transverse venotomy. (**c**) Sottiurai technique—supra T-commissural incision. (**d**) Tripathi technique—trapdoor incision to improve valve cusp visualization during repair (Reprinted with permission from Dalsing MC. Deep Venous Valve Reconstruction in Chronic Venous Insufficiency. Rutherford's Vascular Surgery 7th Edition)

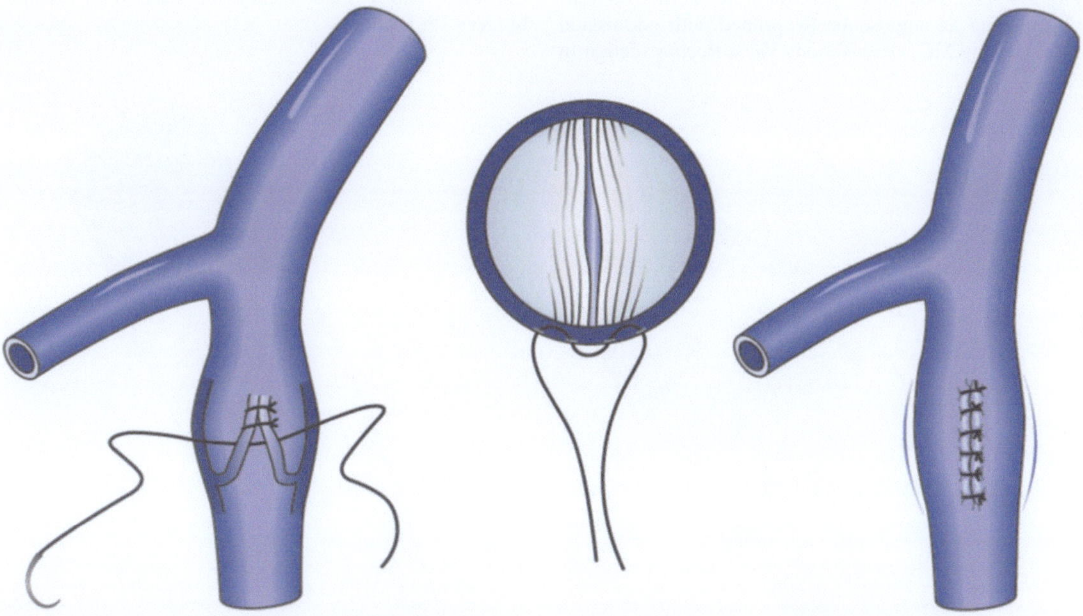

Fig. 3.3 External valvuloplasty—suture of valve attachment lines from the outside to enable competence of the valve cusps without the use of a venotomy (Reprinted with permission from Dalsing MC. Deep Venous Valve Reconstruction in Chronic Venous Insufficiency. Rutherford's Vascular Surgery 7th Edition)

Valve Transplant

Valve transplantation involves harvesting a 2–3 cm segment of axillary/brachial vein with a competent valve and transplanting it to the femoral vein (after resection of appropriate segment of femoral vein) just below its confluence with the profunda vein. This transplant can also be performed at the level of the popliteal vein.

Reported outcomes vary between groups and over time. Clinical success has ranged from 40% at 12 months to 92% at 64 months of follow-up [9–11, 48, 51–54]. There are data to suggest that clinical success deteriorates over the long term as noted by

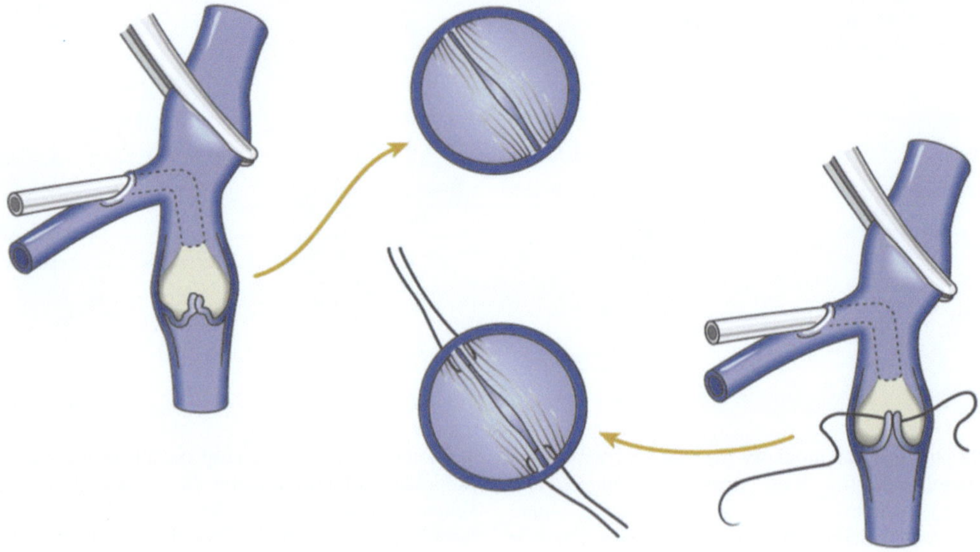

Fig. 3.4 Precision suture placement in external valvuloplasty using an angioscope (Reprinted with permission from Dalsing MC. Deep Venous Valve Reconstruction in Chronic Venous Insufficiency. Rutherford's Vascular Surgery 7th Edition)

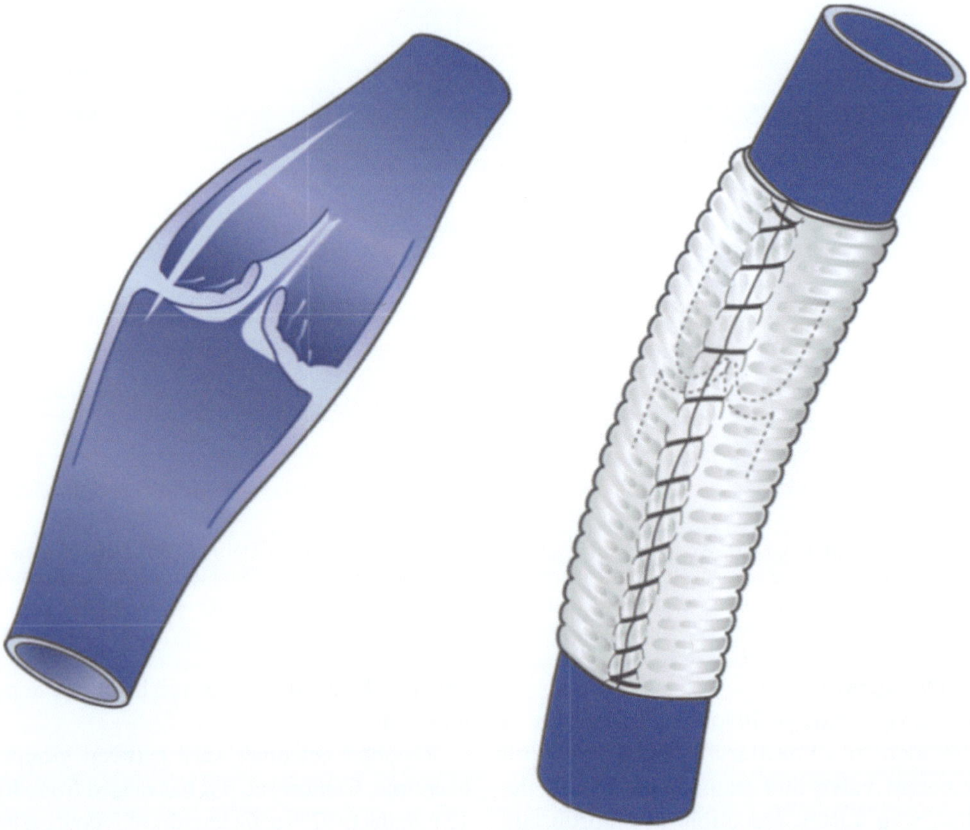

Fig. 3.5 External banding with consequent conversion of an incompetent valve (left) to a competent valve post banding (right) (Reprinted with permission from Dalsing MC. Deep Venous Valve Reconstruction in Chronic Venous Insufficiency. Rutherford's Vascular Surgery 7th Edition)

Taheri et al. whose clinical success fell from 75% at 5 years to 55% at 10 years [53]. Eklof et al. have suggested that the popliteal vein recipient site is perhaps the better option, given the better size match of the axillary vein to the popliteal vein than to the femoral vein. The authors also feel that a competent valve at the popliteal level safeguards against both femoral and profunda femoral vein reflux into the calf [55]. Bry et al. reported on results in 15 patients undergoing axillary-to-popliteal vein valve transplantation and observed a 93% symptom improvement and a 62% cumulative ulcer-free survival on late follow-up [mean 5.3 years] [56].

Transposition of Incompetent Venous Segment

Transposition is performed by placing the incompetent venous system distal to the competent valve. Since the femoral system is most commonly the incompetent system and the profunda femoris valve remains competent, the incompetent femoral vein can be transected and reimplanted distal to the competent profunda femoris valve. The great saphenous vein can also be used as a site for such outflow.

Outcomes reported following transposition surgery have also been varied, with good results reported in 25% at 18-month follow-up to 40% at 120-month follow-up [9, 11, 12, 57]. As Eklof et al. point out, such outcomes are similar to results after valve transplantation but poorer to outcomes after valvuloplasty, given that transposition and transplantation are primarily used in patients with secondary DVR who generally have a worse prognosis than that following valvuloplasty, which is mainly used in patients with primary DVR [55].

Valve Substitution

Novel techniques of valve substitution include methods to create a new in situ valve, use of artificial valve, and cryopreserved vein valves. Additionally, mechanical and bioprosthetic venous valves that can be implanted by using a transcatheter technique have been used on an experimental basis. These valves consist of single, double, or triple cusp leaflets made of synthetic or biological materials attached to a carrier or frame [58]. Bioengineered, autologous cell-based, endothelialized valve constructs are currently being researched and may open up a new therapeutic paradigm for management of patients with severe DVR [59]. The challenge will be to prevent thromboembolic complications. Improving outcomes in patients with secondary DVR also remains a continuing challenge. While individual experience and patient factors may determine the precise technique used for valve intervention for primary DVR, data from Masuda et al. and Raju et al. suggest that from a durability standpoint, internal valvuloplasty should be considered first, followed by external banding, then external valvuloplasty, and finally valve transplant [12, 13, 47]. The options for secondary DVR are more limited as previously noted.

3.3.2 Deep Venous Reflux in the Setting of Deep Venous Obstruction (DVO)

Treatment of the deep venous stenosis alone is often sufficient for symptomatic patients with combined DVR and DVO [6, 60]. Such treatment is accomplished by an endovascular route with open surgery reserved for patients who are not candidates for a percutaneous approach or those who have failed the same. Endovascular intervention involves angioplasty and stenting of the entire disease segment and is performed under general anesthesia. The latter is required secondary to the severe pain/discomfort that patients may experience with angioplasty. With the patient in the supine position and under ultrasound guidance, access to the mid-thigh femoral vein is obtained and a 11 Fr. Access sheath placed (10 cm). A venogram is then performed if not contraindicated by the patient's renal function. Intravascular ultrasound (IVUS) interrogation is then performed using 8.3 Fr IVUS probe (Phillips Volcano, San Diego, CA). The entire femoroiliocaval segment is then interrogated to identify the presence and extent of lesion(s). Any reduction in the luminal area below that noted in Table 3.1 requires treatment in the symptomatic patient. Angioplasty is carried out using an 18 mm angioplasty balloon in a sequential fashion of the common femoral, external iliac, common iliac, and distal IVC segments. Stenting is then performed using 18–20 mm

Wallstents (Boston Scientific, Marlborough, MA) of the diseased segments. Careful attention must be paid during IVUS interrogation since at times larger caliber stents may have to be used. To provide additional radial strength across the iliocaval confluence which is a choke point, a 25 mm Gianturco Z stent (Cook Medical, Bloomington, IN) is deployed using a 14 mm Cook Shuttle sheath (Cook Medical, Bloomington, IN). The majority of this stent is within the Wallstent with just a few mm extending beyond the edge of the Wallstent. Post dilation of the entire stent stack is then carried out using the previously used angioplasty balloon. Completion IVUS interrogation is then carried out to ensure that all areas of disease have been successfully treated and that there is good stent apposition. A completion venogram is then performed to ensure adequacy of flow through the reconstructed segments.

Seager et al. in their systematic review of endovenous stenting in chronic venous disease secondary to iliac vein obstruction supported consideration of stenting given safety profile and encouraging results [61]. In a series of 982 patients undergoing femoroiliocaval stenting, Neglen et al. reported primary, primary assisted, and secondary patencies of 79%, 100%, and 100% for non-thrombotic lesions and 57%, 80%, and 86% for postthrombotic syndrome, respectively [62]. The Mayo Clinic group described their stent experience in 91 patients with postthrombotic disease and noted primary, primary assisted, and secondary patencies at 36 months of 71%, 90%, and 95%, respectively [63]. De Graaf and colleagues recounted their experience of stenting across the iliocaval confluence and observed primary, primary assisted, and secondary patencies at 3 years of 70%, 73%, and 78% for self-expanding stents [64].

3.3.3 Deep Venous Reflux in the Setting of Superficial Venous Reflux (SVR)

Treatment of the superficial venous reflux alone is often helpful in providing patients with DVR and SVR symptomatic relief. This is contemporarily accomplished by endovenous techniques. The latter include thermal techniques such as radiofrequency ablation and laser ablation in addition to nonthermal non-tumescent techniques, e.g., mechanochemical ablation (MOCA). These topics are covered in Chaps. 5, 6, and 7. Abolition of SVR should be considered as the initial line of treatment in patients who do not have concomitant DVO. While abolition of SVR may have a greater impact on segmental DVR as opposed to axial DVR, clinical improvement may be adequate to preclude further treatment. Marston et al. have suggested using DVR reflux velocity to select patients for superficial ablation in cases of combined superficial/deep reflux. In 75 limbs, significant clinical and hemodynamic (air plethysmography) improvement was noticed when DVR had a maximum reflux velocity of 10 cm/s or less. The authors suggest that superficial ablation may be worthwhile when deep reflux is below this threshold, especially when associated segmental deep reflux is confined to the root segment at the origin of superficial reflux [i.e., femoral or popliteal in cases of great or small saphenous veins, respectively] [26]. Such findings echo prior observations that saphenous ablation abolishes associated deep venous reflux in some patients, presumably by eliminating saphenous reflux load into the deep system. These investigators conclude that such treatment may work by causing less dilatation of the deep veins and consequent restoration of valvular competence [65–67].

Conclusion

Deep venous reflux is relatively common in patients with chronic venous insufficiency and often coexists with other superficial venous, perforator, and/or deep venous pathology. Attention must be paid to this at the time of diagnosis to provide appropriate treatment to the symptomatic patient in the process ensuring the best possible outcome.

References

1. Moore DJ, Himmel PD, Sumner DS. Distribution of venous valvular incompetence in patients with the postphlebitic syndrome. J Vasc Surg. 1986;3(1):49–57.
2. Shull KC, Nicolaides AN, Fernandes é Fernandes J, Miles C, Horner J, Needham T, et al. Significance of

popliteal reflux in relation to ambulatory venous pressure and ulceration. Arch Surg. 1979;114(11):1304–6.
3. Hanrahan LM, Araki CT, Rodriguez AA, Kechejian GJ, LaMorte WW, Menzoian JO. Distribution of valvular incompetence in patients with venous stasis ulceration. J Vasc Surg. 1991;13(6):805–11. discussion 11–2
4. Danielsson G, Arfvidsson B, Eklof B, Kistner RL, Masuda EM, Satoc DT. Reflux from thigh to calf, the major pathology in chronic venous ulcer disease: surgery indicated in the majority of patients. Vasc Endovasc Surg. 2004;38(3):209–19.
5. Johnson BF, Manzo RA, Bergelin RO, Strandness DE Jr. Relationship between changes in the deep venous system and the development of the postthrombotic syndrome after an acute episode of lower limb deep vein thrombosis: a one- to six-year follow-up. J Vasc Surg. 1995;21(2):307–12. discussion 13
6. Neglen P, Thrasher TL, Raju S. Venous outflow obstruction: an underestimated contributor to chronic venous disease. J Vasc Surg. 2003;38(5):879–85.
7. Raju S, Darcy MD, Neglen P. Unexpected major role for venous stenting in deep reflux disease. J Vasc Surg. 2009;51(2):401–8.
8. Eriksson I, Almgren B. Influence of the profunda femoris vein on venous hemodynamics of the limb. Experience from thirty-one deep vein valve reconstructions. J Vasc Surg. 1986;4(4):390–5.
9. Cheatle TR, Perrin M. Venous valve repair: early results in fifty-two cases. J Vasc Surg. 1994;19(3):404–13.
10. Raju S, Fredericks R. Valve reconstruction procedures for nonobstructive venous insufficiency: rationale, techniques, and results in 107 procedures with two- to eight-year follow-up. J Vasc Surg. 1988;7(2):301–10.
11. Sottiurai VS. Comparison of surgical modalities in the treatment of recurrent venous ulcer. Int Angiol. 1990;9(4):231–5.
12. Masuda EM, Kistner RL. Long-term results of venous valve reconstruction: a four- to twenty-one-year follow-up. J Vasc Surg. 1994;19(3):391–403.
13. Kistner RL, Eklof B, Masuda EM. Deep venous valve reconstruction. Cardiovasc Surg. 1995;3(2):129–40.
14. Kistner RL. Primary venous valve incompetence of the leg. Am J Surg. 1980;140(2):218–24.
15. Shami SK, Sarin S, Cheatle TR, Scurr JH, Smith PD. Venous ulcers and the superficial venous system. J Vasc Surg. 1993;17(3):487–90.
16. Caps MT, Manzo RA, Bergelin RO, Meissner MH, Strandness DE. Venous valvular reflux in veins not involved at the time of acute deep vein thrombosis. J Vasc Surg. 1995;22(5):524–31.
17. Brittenden J, Bradbury AW, Allan PL, Prescott RJ, Harper DR, Ruckley CV. Popliteal vein reflux reduces the healing of chronic venous ulcer. Br J Surg. 1998;85(1):60–2.
18. Rosfors S, Lamke LO, Nordström E, Bygdeman S. Severity and location of venous valvular insufficiency: the importance of distal valve function. Acta Chir Scand. 1990;156(10):689–94.
19. Neglen P, Egger JF, Olivier J, Raju S. Hemodynamic and clinical impact of ultrasound-derived venous reflux parameters. J Vasc Surg. 2004;40(2):303–10.
20. Raju S, Fredericks RK, Hudson CA, Fountain T, Neglén PN, Devidas M. Venous valve station changes in "primary" and postthrombotic reflux: an analysis of 149 cases. Ann Vasc Surg. 2000;14(3):193–9.
21. Welch HJ, Young CM, Semegran AB, Iafrati MD, Mackey WC, O'Donnell TF. Duplex assessment of venous reflux and chronic venous insufficiency: the significance of deep venous reflux. J Vasc Surg. 1996;24(5):755–62.
22. Neglen P, Raju S. A rational approach to detection of significant reflux with duplex Doppler scanning and air plethysmography. J Vasc Surg. 1993;17(3):590–5.
23. Labropoulos N, Delis K, Nicolaides AN, Leon M, Ramaswami G. The role of the distribution and anatomic extent of reflux in the development of signs and symptoms in chronic venous insufficiency. J Vasc Surg. 1996;23(3):504–10.
24. Sarin S, Scurr JH, Smith PD. Medial calf perforators in venous disease: the significance of outward flow. J Vasc Surg. 1992;16(1):40–6.
25. Lurie F, Kistner RL, Eklof B, Kessler D. Mechanism of venous valve closure and role of the valve in circulation: a new concept. J Vasc Surg. 2003;38(5):955–61.
26. Marston WA, Brabham VW, Mendes R, Berndt D, Weiner M, Keagy B. The importance of deep venous reflux velocity as a determinant of outcome in patients with combined superficial and deep venous reflux treated with endovenous saphenous ablation. J Vasc Surg. 2008;48(2):400–5. discussion 5–6
27. Szendro G, Nicolaides AN, Zukowski AJ, Christopoulos D, Malouf GM, Christodoulou C, et al. Duplex scanning in the assessment of deep venous incompetence. J Vasc Surg. 1986;4(3):237–42.
28. van Bemmelen PS, Bedford G, Beach K, Strandness DE. Quantitative segmental evaluation of venous valvular reflux with duplex ultrasound scanning. J Vasc Surg. 1989;10(4):425–31.
29. Masuda EM, Kistner RL, Eklof B. Prospective study of duplex scanning for venous reflux: comparison of Valsalva and pneumatic cuff techniques in the reverse Trendelenburg and standing positions. J Vasc Surg. 1994;20(5):711–20.
30. Araki CT, Back TL, Padberg FT, Thompson PN, Duran WN, Hobson RW. Refinements in the ultrasonic detection of popliteal vein reflux. J Vasc Surg. 1993;18(5):742–8.
31. Sarin S, Sommerville K, Farrah J, Scurr JH, Coleridge Smith PD. Duplex ultrasonography for assessment of venous valvular function of the lower limb. Br J Surg. 1994;81(11):1591–5.
32. Masuda EM, Kistner RL. Prospective comparison of duplex scanning and descending venography in the assessment of venous insufficiency. Am J Surg. 1992;164(3):254–9.
33. Labropoulos N, Giannoukas AD, Delis K, Mansour MA, Kang SS, Nicolaides AN, et al. Where does venous reflux start? J Vasc Surg. 1997;26(5):736–42.

34. Gloviczki P, Comerota AJ, Dalsing MC, Eklof BG, Gillespie DL, Gloviczki ML, et al. The care of patients with varicose veins and associated chronic venous diseases: clinical practice guidelines of the Society for Vascular Surgery and the American Venous Forum. J Vasc Surg. 2011;53(5 Suppl):2S–48S.
35. Neglen P, Raju S. A comparison between descending phlebography and duplex Doppler investigation in the evaluation of reflux in chronic venous insufficiency: a challenge to phlebography as the "gold standard". J Vasc Surg. 1992;16(5):687–93.
36. Baker SR, Burnand KG, Sommerville KM, Thomas ML, Wilson NM, Browse NL. Comparison of venous reflux assessed by duplex scanning and descending phlebography in chronic venous disease. Lancet. 1993;341(8842):400–3.
37. Raju S, Fredericks R, Lishman P, Neglen P, Morano J. Observations on the calf venous pump mechanism: determinants of postexercise pressure. J Vasc Surg. 1993;17(3):459–69.
38. Kistner R. Surgical repair of a venous valve. Straub Clin Proc. 1968;34:41–3.
39. Raju S, Berry MA, Neglen P. Transcommissural valvuloplasty: technique and results. J Vasc Surg. 2000;32(5):969–76.
40. Sottiurai VS. Technique in direct venous valvuloplasty. J Vasc Surg. 1988;8(5):646–8.
41. Gloviczki P, Merrell SW, Bower TC. Femoral vein valve repair under direct vision without venotomy: a modified technique with use of angioscopy. J Vasc Surg. 1991;14(5):645–8.
42. Kistner R. Surgical technique of external venous valve repair. Straub Clin Proc. 1990;55:15–6.
43. Hoshino S, Satakawa H, Iwaya F, Igari T, Ono T, Takase S. External valvuloplasty under preoperative angioscopic control. Phlebologie. 1993;46(3):521–9.
44. O'Donnell TF Jr. The role of angioscopic valve repair for primary valve incompetence (PVI). Hawaii Med J. 2000;59(6):266–8.
45. Welch HJ, McLaughlin RL, O'Donnell TF Jr. Femoral vein valvuloplasty: intraoperative angioscopic evaluation and hemodynamic improvement. J Vasc Surg. 1992;16(5):694–700.
46. Raju S, Hardy JD. Technical options in venous valve reconstruction. Am J Surg. 1997;173(4):301–7.
47. Raju S, Fredericks RK, Neglen PN, Bass JD. Durability of venous valve reconstruction techniques for "primary" and postthrombotic reflux. J Vasc Surg. 1996;23(2):357–66. discussion 66–7
48. Eriksson I. Reconstructive surgery for deep vein valve incompetence in the lower limb. Eur J Vasc Surg. 1990;4(3):211–8.
49. Ma T, Fu W, Ma J. Popliteal vein external banding at the valve-free segment to treat severe chronic venous insufficiency. J Vasc Surg. 2016;64(2):438.e1–45.e1.
50. Camilli S, Guarnera G. External banding valvuloplasty of the superficial femoral vein in the treatment of primary deep valvular incompetence. Int Angiol. 1994;13(3):218–22.
51. Nash T. Long term results of vein valve transplants placed in the popliteal vein for intractable postphlebitic venous ulcers and pre-ulcer skin changes. J Cardiovasc Surg. 1988;29(6):712–6.
52. Iafrati M, O'Donnell TF. Surgical reconstruction for deep venous insufficiency. J Mal Vasc. 1997;22(3):193–7.
53. Taheri SA, Lazar L, Elias S, Marchand P, Heffner R. Surgical treatment of postphlebitic syndrome with vein valve transplant. Am J Surg. 1982;144(2):221–4.
54. Raju S, Neglen P, Doolittle J, Meydrech EF. Axillary vein transfer in trabeculated postthrombotic veins. J Vasc Surg. 1999;29(6):1050–62. discussion 62–4
55. Eklof BG, Kistner RL, Masuda EM. Venous bypass and valve reconstruction: long-term efficacy. Vasc Med. 1998;3(2):157–64.
56. Bry JD, Muto PA, O'Donnell TF, Isaacson LA. The clinical and hemodynamic results after axillary-to-popliteal vein valve transplantation. J Vasc Surg. 1995;21(1):110–9.
57. Johnson ND, Queral LA, Flinn WR, Yao JS, Bergan JJ. Late objective assessment of venous value surgery. Arch Surg. 1981;116(11):1461–6.
58. Pavcnik D, Uchida B, Kaufman J, Hinds M, Keller FS, Rösch J. Percutaneous management of chronic deep venous reflux: review of experimental work and early clinical experience with bioprosthetic valve. Vasc Med. 2008;13(1):75–84.
59. Weber B, Hafner J, Willenberg T, Hoerstrup SP. Bioengineered valves for the venous circulation. Expert Rev Med Devices. 2016;13(11):1005–11.
60. Raju S, Darcey R, Neglen P. Unexpected major role for venous stenting in deep reflux disease. J Vasc Surg. 2010;51(2):401–8. discussion 8
61. Seager MJ, Busuttil A, Dharmarajah B, Davies AH. A systematic review of endovenous stenting in chronic venous disease secondary to iliac vein obstruction. Eur J Vasc Endovasc Surg. 2016;51(1):100–20.
62. Neglen P, Hollis KC, Olivier J, Raju S. Stenting of the venous outflow in chronic venous disease: long-term stent-related outcome, clinical, and hemodynamic result. J Vasc Surg. 2007;46(5):979–90.
63. Kurklinsky AK, Bjarnason H, Friese JL, Wysokinski WE, McBane RD, Misselt A, et al. Outcomes of venoplasty with stent placement for chronic thrombosis of the iliac and femoral veins: single-center experience. J Vasc Interv Radiol. 2012;23(8):1009–15.
64. de Graaf R, de Wolf M, Sailer AM, van Laanen J, Wittens C, Jalaie H. Iliocaval confluence stenting for chronic venous obstructions. Cardiovasc Intervent Radiol. 2015;38(5):1198–204.
65. Padberg FT Jr, Pappas PJ, Araki CT, Back TL, Hobson RW. Hemodynamic and clinical improvement after superficial vein ablation in primary combined venous insufficiency with ulceration. J Vasc Surg. 1996;24(5):711–8.
66. Sales CM, Bilof ML, Petrillo KA, Luka NL. Correction of lower extremity deep venous incompetence by ablation of superficial venous reflux. Ann Vasc Surg. 1996;10(2):186–9.
67. Walsh JC, Bergan JJ, Beeman S, Comer TP. Femoral venous reflux abolished by greater saphenous vein stripping. Ann Vasc Surg. 1994;8(6):566–70.

Recurrent Varicose Veins

4

Mark S. Whiteley

Visible varicose veins affect approximately 10–15% of the adult population, with a similar percentage of people suffering from superficial venous incompetence (also known as chronic venous incompetence or superficial venous reflux) which is essentially the same disease but without visible varicosities [1–3].

Traditionally, medicine has regarded varicose veins as "only cosmetic". It has become clear over the last couple of decades that leaving varicose veins untreated results in deterioration in about 4.7% of patients per year resulting in potential complications including bleeding, superficial venous thrombosis (commonly called superficial thrombophlebitis) and of course inflammatory skin damage around the lower leg [4]. This inflammatory skin damage is variably diagnosed clinically as venous eczema, lipodermatosclerosis, haemosiderin deposition and, if the epidermis breaks down, venous leg ulcer.

Varicose veins are treated in many different ways. However, there are currently two main schools of thought as to how to treat them. The first, and probably most widespread, is to remove or ablate the underlying refluxing veins and then remove the varicosities to improve the cosmetic result and to prevent thrombosis in the redundant varices. The second, emanating from France and Italy, is termed "haemodynamic surgery" where refluxing vessels are strategically ligated, allowing the venous reflux to continue but to drain into the deep system via perforating veins. The most well-known version of this is Claude Franceschi's CHIVA [5].

During my time treating patients with venous diseases, I have found it less useful getting caught up in the nuances of different ideologies and much more sensible to approach things from first principles. This has been a particularly useful approach with the advent of venous duplex ultrasonography and endovenous surgery. A great many theories as to why varicose veins occur and why they might recur after treatment have faded as it has become clear that they are not correct in view of the measurements we can now take and the techniques we can now perform.

So let us think about the principles.

Varicose veins are almost always a product of venous reflux. Of course, there are varicosities associated with deep vein obstruction when the superficial vein is being used as a bypass. Stasis in veins can also cause inflammation resulting in the appearance of chronic venous incompetence, but once again, this is a separate problem.

Therefore, we will concentrate on the major cause of varicose veins, which is a result of venous reflux disease.

The principles of treatment are to ensure accurate imaging to identify all of the points of

M. S. Whiteley
The Whiteley Clinic, London, UK

The Whiteley Clinic, Guildford, UK

The Whiteley Clinic, Bristol, UK
e-mail: mark@thewhiteleyclinic.co.uk

A. K. Khanna, R. Jindal (eds.), *Venous Disorders*, https://doi.org/10.1007/978-981-13-1108-6_4

significant venous reflux, to then remove the venous reflux and finally to remove the varicosities themselves, in order to prevent thrombosis and painful thrombophlebitis in the redundant venous dilations (varices).

Recurrent varicose veins occur when this process has been performed successfully (at least clinically), and yet in the future, varicose veins reappear in the same limb.

So why would varicose veins recur after successful treatment?

There are three reasons why varicose veins may recur after treatment:

1. Failure to treat the correct vein or veins—the initial treatment did not treat the underlying venous reflux, allowing varicosities to recur.
2. The correct veins were treated, but using techniques that allowed recurrent reflux to appear in the same vein in the future and hence allow varicosities to recur.
3. The underlying reflux was successfully and permanently treated, but new reflux develops in previously normal veins in the same limb—i.e. disease progression.

We can now look at each of these three causes of recurrent varicose veins in turn.

4.1 Failure to Treat the Correct Vein or Veins

It seems incredible that in today's world, we would treat patients with inadequate imaging or information. However, this is a daily occurrence in every country in the world.

There are several reasons as to why a great many patients, if not the vast majority, undergoing venous surgery in the world end up having recurrence due to the wrong veins being treated.

Traditionally, in medical schools, doctors are taught that varicose veins occur due to incompetence of valves in either the great or small saphenous veins. There is still a widespread belief following the original observations by Trendelenburg at the end of the nineteenth century that valves in these major truncal veins fail due to "pressure" from above. Hence, we still hear people talking about constipation, being overweight, pregnancy, pelvic tumours and other causes of intra-abdominal pressure being a cause of varicose veins. This has shown to be incorrect, and in 2001, we published our own evidence for the ascending progression of venous reflux [6]. However, even at that stage, this idea was not new, and many workers in the field interested in haemodynamics had suggested this already [7].

The difficulties that arise from this misunderstanding are twofold. Firstly, most doctors think that if the top of the great saphenous or small saphenous is competent, then that vein is not relevant to the venous reflux and formation of varicose veins. Hence, doctors frequently perform a "limited" Doppler or venous duplex examination, only looking at the top of the veins. They often erroneously deemed that the truncal vein is not involved in the varicose vein formation because the top is still competent.

The second problem with this old understanding of venous disease is that sources of venous reflux causing varicose veins are many and varied and not related only to the great and small saphenous vein. It is now readily recognised that significant varicose veins can be associated with venous reflux in anterior accessory saphenous veins [8], incompetent perforating veins [9, 10] and pelvic veins [11–13]. With so many sources of venous reflux, it is now inadequate to use handheld Doppler, and indeed, a cursory look at the truncal veins with venous duplex ultrasound scan is similarly inadequate, although a small improvement upon the older technology.

There has been a call in the venous world for patients to have, what is called in the USA, an "extended venous duplex ultrasound scan". However, in my own practice, we would regard this as the only appropriate investigation that patients should undergo to diagnose varicose veins, and anything less than this is inadequate. Therefore, rather than being an "extended" scan, it is actually a venous duplex ultrasound scan.

So, if we do not want varicose veins to recur due to our failure to treat the correct veins, we need to ensure that we perform an adequate venous duplex ultrasound scan on every patient that we wish to treat.

At The Whiteley Clinic, every patient presenting with varicose veins has a venous duplex ultrasound scan that includes examination in the erect position, ensuring that any venous reflux will be seen. Manual calf compression or distal manual compression is used as the stimulation. Any varicose veins are traced back to their source to identify exactly where they are arising from. The superficial venous trunks, great saphenous vein, small saphenous vein, anterior accessory saphenous vein and posterior accessory saphenous vein are all checked for patency and competence. The deep veins are all checked for patency and competency from the ankle to groin. In particular, posterior tibial, peroneal and popliteal veins are checked for patency and reflux. Above-knee, peri-knee and below-knee perforating veins are checked for competence, particularly if associated with varicosities or any inflammatory skin damage/ulceration.

If during this venous duplex ultrasonography venous reflux is found to be arising from veins coming from the pelvis, then pelvic vein imaging will be suggested. In women, this will be a transvaginal venous duplex ultrasound scan performed using the Holdstock protocol [14], with the patient positioned at 45°, and using Valsalva for venous stimulation. In females unable or unwilling to undergo this, and in men, an MRV is performed in the first instance understanding that venous diameter alone is not adequate to diagnose venous reflux [15].

By identifying all of the areas of venous reflux, a strategy can be tailored to each individual patient to ablate all incompetent veins and hence satisfy the requirement to stop all underlying superficial venous reflux. By following this strategy, we are able to overcome the first cause of recurrent varicose veins.

4.2 The Correct Veins Were Treated but Using Techniques that Allow Recurrent Reflux to Develop

One of the biggest errors that has been made in medical thinking relating to varicose veins surgery is mistaking the target vein to be an organ.

Surgeons traditionally remove organs or lesions and, once they are removed, are fairly safe in the knowledge that they are gone and will not come back. It would be very rare for a gallbladder to be removed, for instance, only to grow back at a later stage.

However, all surgeons instinctively know that the connective tissue that they cut through in open surgery to perform such procedures will "heal". They will understand that the skin, subcutaneous tissue, muscle and fascia will all heal post-operatively. Surgeons will also know that when they cut through scar tissue that has been left after previous operations, it is common to cut through veins that are embedded in the scar tissue but which bleed actively.

Hence, it is obvious that veins act as part of the connective tissue complex and regrow after division. This is well recognised in the wound healing literature stemming from development of the rabbit ear chamber model from the 1960s [16], and there are very clear descriptions in such models as to how veins heal after being divided. A divided vein produces a haematoma and thrombus within the end of the vein, preventing exsanguination. Provided the subject survives, endothelium buds out of the cut ends of the vein, producing solid cords of endothelial cells that branch into the haematoma. The haematoma appears to stimulate this process, and some studies have suggested that rather than the endothelial cells growing out of the ends of the damage vein, these endothelial cords may well arise from fibroblasts [17] or even bone marrow-derived stem cells in the haematoma itself [18].

When these solid cords meet, they start to form endothelial tubes, allowing the transmission of venous blood. What is interesting is that as these fine new vessels grow, they appear to coalesce to form larger veins and media cells appear in the vein wall. Of more interest to surgeons performing varicose vein treatments, these new veins do not show any valves and are therefore incompetent.

This process is well recognised by most surgeons as "healing", but when it comes to a surgeon who is trying to convince himself that he has removed a varicose vein, then suddenly this process is called "neovascularisation". For many years, surgeons refused to believe that this occurred.

When I started venous surgery at the end of the 1980s, neovascularisation was frowned upon by many general surgeons. With the advent of venous duplex ultrasonography and an increasing interest in venous surgery, neovascularisation has become more widely studied and is now generally accepted as a consequence of open venous surgery, particularly in the groin or popliteal fossa [19].

However, many advocates of stripping refused to accept that it is possible for a body to produce such a neovascular reaction to replace a whole great saphenous vein that has been stripped. The usual argument is that the stripped vein is "just too long" to allow such a process to occur. Of course, this is nonsense. Just because a surgeon does not wish a process to happen, it does not mean to say it does not.

When a great saphenous vein is stripped, there is haematoma between the saphenofemoral junction stump and the bottom end of the stripped vein. There is endothelium at both of these points that is free and quite able to be involved in the process of neovascularisation. However, what makes the process easier to occur is the fact that neovascularisation does not happen just between these two ends. Any surgeon who has ever harvested a great saphenous vein for bypass will know that there are any number of tributaries and perforators that have junctions with the great saphenous vein in the thigh. During the stripping process, all of these become contributing veins to the formation of the haematoma but also contributing points to the process of neovascularisation. However, when we talk about the regrowth of a stripped truncal vein, we tend to call it "strip tract revascularisation" rather than neovascularisation, keeping this latter word for the small serpiginous veins usually seen local to the site of the surgical incision.

In 2007, we published our observations of a follow-up study we had performed to see the recurrence rates after stripping [20]. The original study had been a randomised controlled study to see if the treatment of incompetent perforators reduces the risk of recurrent varicose veins. We randomised patients with varicose veins due to great saphenous vein reflux, and who also had incompetent perforating veins, into either high saphenous tie and stripping with phlebectomies alone or high saphenous tie and stripping, subfascial endoscopic perforating vein surgery (SEPS) and phlebectomies. The aim of the study was to see whether treating incompetent perforators as part of the anti-reflux strategy would reduce recurrence when compared to patients in which they were left untreated [21].

All patients underwent stripping of the vein in the usual manner, with intraoperative ultrasound being used to ensure the correct vein had been removed in its entirety. Patients were then followed up over several years.

Unfortunately, we were never able to find out whether the treatment of incompetent perforating veins reduced the risk of recurrence of varicose veins, as the recurrence from strip tract revascularisation and neovascularisation completely overshadowed any effect of the incompetent perforators. We were amazed to see, when patients were followed up with very precise ultrasound, that we could observe the veins growing back along the tract of the original vein, through what had originally been haematoma.

After 1 year, we observed some strip tract revascularisation in 23% of patients, with 5% of patients having total strip tract revascularisation. As stated above, all of these new veins were incompetent as none of them had any valves at all. It was fascinating to see how the early strip tract revascularisation was seen as several smaller channels, and with time, these coalesced into single or a few large-diameter incompetent veins.

We published this finding in the *British Journal of Surgery* but were not allowed to publish the most interesting finding of all. The duplex ultrasound that was used in the paper was of a patient who clearly had what looked like four incompetent veins, all closely related, within the saphenous fascia and following the route that would be normal for the great saphenous vein. This patient had allowed us to perform a biopsy of the vein mass and this had been done. The specimen was taken as an excision biopsy and it was sent off for histology.

I reviewed the histology with the consultant histopathologist the following week. This histopathologist was quite adamant that we had missed the area that we wanted to biopsy, as the wall of the vessel was completely normal histologically. He was able to see endothelium, media and adventitia although he was surprised about the amount of scar tissue surrounding the vein. It was only when I removed the slide from the microscope and held it up to the light that it was clear that there were four lumens rather than the one that would be expected. Hence, it was clear that histologically the strip tract revascularisation vessels are morphologically hard to distinguish from normal vein wall, although the macroscopic view is clearly very deformed.

The referees from the *British Journal of Surgery* allowed publication of the study but on the condition that the histology was not published. It was felt that it was too much to claim that veins could regenerate after stripping, particularly as arterial surgeons had spent considerable time and effort unsuccessfully trying to grow vessels for bypass in arterial patients.

We have subsequently studied this group of patients again, inviting as many as who would attend 5–8 years after their original treatment. We published this study in 2014 and, not surprisingly, the process had continued with strip tract revascularisation being seen in over 82% of legs and complete reflux of the whole vein length in 12.8% [22].

This study, the two published papers, and the unpublished histology, give a very good insight into recurrent varicose veins. It clearly shows that excising a vein does not mean to say it is permanently removed. The body will try to heal and, when it comes to a transected vein, the healing process is of regenerating the vein—albeit without valves. Therefore, the principles of varicose vein surgery should include the absence of haematoma and the avoidance of free endothelium.

When we started performing endovenous surgery with the original VNUS closure radiofrequency catheter in March 1999, we attempted to heat the vein wall to 85 °C. The aim at that time was that we would be able to "close" the vein by heating the collagen. At 85 °C, the collagen would contract and the vein would constrict and close [23, 24]. In the early days of endovenous surgery, there was not much thought about the living cells of the vein wall.

Initially, we told patients that the advantages of having endovenous surgery were that it was less painful, allowed an early return to work and had tiny scars and hence was therefore more cosmetic. Because we wanted to make sure that our results were good, we followed up all of our first 500 patients regularly for the first year. During this time, we realised that the "closed" vein slowly atrophied completely. Furthermore, the saphenofemoral junction closed and the stump of the great saphenous vein generally shrank [25]. Most importantly, there were absolutely no signs of any neovascular tissue in the groin and no sign whatsoever of any strip tract revascularisation [26].

It became clear that the major advantage of endovenous surgery was not of reduced pain, improved mobility and return to work, nor better cosmetic result but was actually a reduction in the risk of recurrence of the treated vein. Having understood how veins healed again by neovascularisation and strip tract revascularisation after stripping, endovenous thermoablation with radiofrequency was clearly causing a different healing process in the treated vein. I treated a segment of ex vivo great saphenous vein with a VNUS closure catheter so that I can see the effect that the radiofrequency ablation was having on the vein wall directly. The white vein with a mild pink hue from being freshly removed shrivelled and contracted on the VNUS Closure catheter, turning beige as the protein constricted and burned.

I sent a section of this off for histopathology along with a control section of the same vein that I had not treated. I published the comparison in the Charing Cross book chapter that I wrote with Judy Holdstock in 2004 [27]. It was clear that the thermal damage was not restricted to the endothelial but was truly transmural.

This became clear to me that successful thermal ablation of the truncal great saphenous vein required transmural thermal damage and indeed transmural death of the cells within the vein wall.

Was this assumption of cellular death deducible from the above information at the time?

There were several reasons why this became obvious.

Firstly, the presence of haematoma and endothelium clearly allows neovascularisation. This same process appears to occur when one has a thrombus within a vein lumen. No matter how successfully one might kill the endothelium at the point of thrombus, there will always be living endothelium at the end of the thrombus allowing the process of recanalisation within the lumen to occur.

If the media cells are still alive, this will act as a "vein skeleton" as I suggested in 2005 [28] and 2006 [29], directing the recanalisation. All doctors have experience of this when veins thrombose after intravenous cannulation for a "drip", forcing the doctor to cannlate another vein. However, weeks later, the "closed" vein has reopened and is patent once again.

The presence of living media and adventitia, surrounding thrombus, may lead to a "closed" vein after endovenous treatment on duplex ultrasound scanning, but this situation is likely to lead to reopening and not to the total atrophy of the vein that we find in successful endothermal ablation. Indeed, I would now regard any vein that is "closed" but not atrophied at 6 months or more after treatment to be at high risk of recanalisation in the future.

Therefore, when we are considering which endovenous treatments for varicose veins are likely to reduce recurrence in the future, we need to consider treatments that will lead to atrophy of the vein and not just "closure" by thrombus. Hence, from what we have learnt above, we are looking for endovenous techniques that cause transmural death of the vein wall. When we are looking at the causes of recurrent varicose veins due to the same vein reopening, we are looking at the reverse of this—techniques that have failed because of failure to cause transmural death of the vein wall.

Considering endovenous thermoablation first of all, there are some general principles that reach across all devices and techniques. The two most commonly used at present are radiofrequency ablation and endovenous laser ablation. Of course, these are not individual techniques as each has many subdivisions. Radiofrequency ablation devices now have segmental radiofrequency devices of fixed treatment length, bipolar and monopolar radiofrequency devices. Endovenous laser stretches across many wavelengths, many fibre diameters and many tips giving different distributions of the laser energy once inside the vein.

In addition, there are other devices using endovenous thermoablation including steam vein sclerosis that has been around for quite some time and the newer endovenous microwave devices. There are some new combination treatments using low-level laser, insufficient for thermal ablation combined with sclerotherapy such as LAFOS. I will discuss these later as these are not purely thermoablation devices.

I have discussed elsewhere the difference between the individual devices, but in principle, all of the thermoablation devices are currently catheter based and are placed within the vein lumen under ultrasound control. They all need some form of anaesthesia, whether in the form of tumescence directly around the vein or regional/general anaesthesia with or without compression such as an Esmarch bandage on the leg. In today's world, it is hard to justify anything but tumescence and a walk-in walk-out procedure. Some doctors still give sedation or other forms of anaesthesia for a variety of reasons ranging from funding through to traditional organised pathways of treatment, perceived patient preference and their own confidence (or lack of) in cannulating veins.

When considering the mechanism of action of endovenous devices, the biggest difference between radiofrequency ablation and endovenous laser is the need for vein wall contact. All of the radiofrequency devices work on the principle of contact between the electrodes or radiofrequency conducting coil and the vein wall itself. The heat is generated by the passage of electrons alternating in direction either in the vein wall or on the surface of the conductor, at radiofrequency rates, generating heat very close to the point of contact. The practical point is that radiofrequency ablation can fail if there is a lack of contact with the vein wall for any reason such as failure to empty the vein, large aneurysmal segments or the presence of thrombus within the vein lumen.

Conversely endovenous laser emits photons of electromagnetic radiation, either in the visible light range (some of the lasers that use haemoglobin as a chromophore) or in the microwave range (usually those lasers that use water as a chromophore). As with all electromagnetic radiation, these photons travel in straight lines until interacting with something, which is usually the chromophore in endovenous surgery, which then heats up by the interaction. The advantage of laser is that there is no need for direct contact between laser device and vein wall, allowing the treatment to be used even if the vein wall cannot be contacted directly at a certain point, such as in an aneurysmal sac or in the presence of thrombus.

The principles of endovenous thermoablation causing transmural death of the vein wall come down to the total energy used per unit of vein length (often measured as the linear endovenous energy density or LEED [30, 31]), the rate at which the energy is supplied and the absence of any blood or other fluid in the lumen that might reduce the thermal energy getting to the vein wall.

It is quite clear that for most truncal veins, a LEED over 60 J/cm is required to cause ablation (i.e. transmural death) [32]. "Closure" can be obtained at lower values, but this often leads to recanalisation in the future, as can be seen in reports where the success rate drops as the follow-up continues over the first year or two. Successful ablation should lead to atrophy and no chance of any reopening. There have been arguments from clinical practice that the microwave lasers that use water as a chromophore can reach the same clinical end-point at a lower LEED than the visible light lasers using haemoglobin as a chromophore. Our in vitro studies [33–35] have shown that there is certainly some evidence to support this view, although our review on the subject suggests that any LEED under 60 J/cm is likely to have a significant chance of recanalisation and keeping to the higher range of LEED is probably safer in terms of atrophy and permanent ablation of the vein [32].

However, a discussion of how much energy is used per centimetre of vein is clearly a simplified approach as veins have different sizes (diameters) and, more importantly, have different thicknesses of vein wall. It must be remembered that when we are talking about thermoablation and transmural death, it is the volume of the vein wall that is the target and not the size of the lumen of the vein—even though it is the diameter of the vein lumen that is usually measured on ultrasound and recorded in patient notes.

Furthermore, a discussion of energy per centimetre alone, without a discussion of what time (and hence at what power) the energy is delivered, is also overly simplified. To ensure transmural death of the vein wall from endovenous thermal ablation devices, it is necessary to supply the thermal energy to the inner aspect of the vein wall at a rate that does not cause carbonisation at the point of contact and allows thermal conduction throughout the wall of the vein [36]. Heating too quickly wastes energy by converting the intimal layer into carbon, preventing this energy from transmitting through the media and coagulating cells throughout the vein wall.

In 2015, we published an in vitro study showing how changing the power and time of pullback dramatically changes the efficacy of thermoablation [33]. The RFiTT device, initially produced by Celon and subsequently by Olympus Celon, is a bipolar radiofrequency ablation device that is a typical endovenous thermoablation catheter. In the mid-2000s, it was sold with the recommendation of using the device at 18 or 20 W to ablate veins. For purely theoretical reasons, it was clear to us that this power was too high and it was unlikely that an appropriate LEED would be reached due to carbonisation at the vein surface. Indeed, studies started appearing using this power, and many noted that the device got "stuck" and had to be removed and the carbon residue removed from the electrodes. Moreover, even reasonable ablation rates were only obtained when doctors with the worst results were excluded from the study [37].

In a series of 3 studies, we showed that if the power was reduced and the time of treatment was increased, the same LEED could be reached but with a better thermal spread through tissue and without carbonisation at the point of contact. Initially, we proved this point in an in vitro porcine liver model, checked our theory in ex vivo great saphenous vein and finally showed 100% success in closing great saphenous veins using a protocol derived from this work [33, 34, 38].

Finally, in the early days of endovenous surgery, I was often asked by some companies that I did consultancy work for to go and observe certain doctors who were not getting good ablation results despite using standardised protocols for energy power levels and pullback regimes. In virtually every case, the reason for the poor rates of closure was that the patient was not placed in the head down position and/or tumescence was inadequate. The thermoablation device was being activated correctly, but the heat generated was distributed both in the blood and the vein wall rather than in the vein wall alone. This not only led to a core of thrombus within the vein but also an inadequate heating of the vein wall. Of course, this led to a thrombus within a vein that had a living vein skeleton of media—and an ideal situation for recanalisation of the vein.

Hence, it is clear that to reduce the risk of recurrent varicose veins after endovenous thermoablation, it is not which device you use, but it is the understanding of the total energy that is reaching the vein wall and over what time period the energy is applied, ensuring that adequate penetration throughout the vein wall is achieved—which of course means ensuring transmural death of the vein wall.

When looking at the nonthermal endovenous techniques, the most commonly used is sclerotherapy. Nowadays, the trend to use foam sclerotherapy in medium to large veins has become the norm; liquid sclerotherapy tends to only be used for very small veins such as cosmetic telangiectasia. Foam sclerotherapy of course is not magical. The active ingredient of the foam is still the sclerosant. The sclerosant commonly used is a detergent (usually polidocanol or sodium tetradecyl sulphate or STS). The detergent works by binding protein or fat and emulsifying it with water—effectively destroying the endothelial cell wall and hence killing the endothelium [39]. However, recent studies have also shown that sclerosants can induce apoptosis in sub-lytic concentrations [40]. Mixing the sclerosant with gas to make foam reduces the concentration of sclerosant, but the physical presence of foam pushes blood out of the lumen of the vein to be treated, ensuring that the sclerosant gets to the vein wall [41].

Traditionally, sclerotherapy has been thought to damage the endothelial layer of the vein, allowing the vein to be "stuck" together after compression. However, this does not follow the principles of transmural death of the vein wall and also doesn't help us understand why sclerotherapy is so effective in small veins with thin walls but less effective in large veins with thick walls. This observation lends more credence to the idea that sclerotherapy also works by causing transmural death.

One group looking at the effect of detergent sclerosants in the vein wall suggested that the sclerosant can penetrate the vein wall itself [42]. However, we have recently published a study using immunohistochemistry that suggests very strongly that the effect of sclerotherapy is actually apoptosis, instigated by the action of sclerosant on the endothelium and the effect spreading into the media [43]. Using optimal conditions and 3% STS, we found the apoptotic effect could be identified up to about 200–250 μm into the vein wall with minimal effect deeper than that. This was matched with immunohistochemistry showing media cells dying in the inner part of the media, but those cells outside of the 250 μm zone showed no sign of disappearing.

We felt that this study shows that thin-walled veins are likely to be treated effectively by good sclerotherapy technique as it is possible to cause transmural death if the vein wall is 250 μm or less in thickness. However, thick-walled veins, such as truncal veins, are unlikely to undergo complete transmural death when treated with sclerotherapy, resulting in intraluminal thrombus and a living skeleton of media in the vein wall, an ideal situation for late recanalisation.

Hence, it is likely that this is the mechanism of failure in the current clinical studies showing high recanalisation rates after the treatment of truncal veins with foam sclerotherapy [44].

This failure of sclerotherapy in some truncal veins can be successfully addressed using mechanochemical ablation (MOCA). The ClariVein® catheter uses a rotating wire that emerges from the end of the endovenous catheter to damage the inside of the vein wall whilst sclerotherapy is infused simultaneously. Although some investigators have suggested a direct effect of the wire on the endothelium [45, 46], our own research has suggested that the mechanism is actually a shearing stress produced in the vein wall from the rotating wire, creating channels in the vein wall like a "Swiss cheese" which allows the sclerosant to penetrate the vein wall itself [47]. This allows sclerotherapy to enter the vein wall, allowing the effect of the sclerosant to penetrate deep inside the wall and achieving transmural death. Not surprisingly, the results of closure of a treated GSV from MOCA appear to be far higher than foam sclerotherapy alone in truncal veins at 1 year [48, 49].

We can now finally turn to some of the latest techniques that are being used without tumescence. The first are the cyanoacrylate glues and the second are a group of combination techniques using low-power laser with sclerotherapy.

The cyanoacrylate glue is a relatively new treatment that has not been available for the treatment of varicose veins as long as endovenous laser and radiofrequency, and so it has not been studied to the same extent. The mechanism of action on the vein wall has been studied in the swine superficial epigastric vein model which suggests that the lumen is filled with the adhesive, occluding it (occasionally mixing with the blood), and over 30 and 60 days, inflammatory processes affect the intima and project into the media of the vein [50, 51]. In addition, at 60 days, fibrous tissue was seen to project into the lumen [51].

Therefore, the early effect of cyanoacrylate glue appears to be purely adhesive with a foreign body inflammatory reaction occurring in the inner layers of the vein wall. There is no clear evidence of transmural death, and the clinical studies show a 1-year occlusion rate of between 75.7 and 92.9% [50–52]. As such, although there are clear advantages in terms of ease of use and lack of tumescence, long-term studies need to be done to show that the lack of transmural death of the vein wall doesn't result in failures and recanalisation.

Finally the recent appearance of combinations of sclerotherapy, usually as foam, and low-power endovenous laser are interesting but certainly not proven. Enthusiasts suggest that the low-power lasers can either cause constriction of the vein which they seem to think will help the action of the foamed sclerosant [53] or interact with the sclerosant making it more active [54].

These theories might be true. However, before they become widely accepted, they should be proven to cause transmural death of the vein wall in in vitro or ex vivo biological models and then, once the technique has been optimised, to show a clinical efficacy before they can be taken as serious contenders to the current endovenous techniques.

Following the above principles (choosing the optimal device and using a technique to ensure transmural death of the vein whilst preventing thrombus and exposure of endothelium outside of the vein), recurrence of varicose veins due to recanalisation of treated veins should reduce. However, it is clear that no one single technique can be used to treat all of the different incompetent veins in the network found in most patients suffering from varicose veins. Techniques and settings, such as power of thermoablation devices or concentrations and volumes of sclerosant, may need to be adjusted dependent upon the thickness of the vein wall to be treated.

4.3 "Recurrent Varicose Veins" due to De Novo Venous Reflux

Population studies have shown that the incidence of developing varicose veins in a population of adults who have a familial history of varicose veins is approximately 3.0–4.5% per year [55].

As all patients who present with varicose veins clearly already have a predisposition to the condition, then it can safely be assumed that they fall into this population. As such, if a patient had perfect treatment of their varicose veins, with complete ablation of all incompetent veins and removal of all varicosities, and their venous system in the affected leg was returned to as near-normal as possible, they would still have a 3.0–4.5% chance of developing new varicose veins in that leg per year. Such varicose veins would arise from veins that had previously been competent and had become incompetent during that year. This development of new varicose veins from previously normal veins is called “de novo” varicose veins.

It is interesting to note that the “de novo” rate of developing new varicose veins is the minimum recurrence rate that is possible, and to even achieve this, one has to completely overcome the risks of recurrent varicose veins that are discussed above. This has been the aim of The Whiteley Clinic over the last 18 years. Through the development of a rigid protocol of venous duplex ultrasound diagnosis and treatment of all venous incompetence, including incompetent perforators and pelvic vein incompetence, using techniques that we have shown to cause transmural death in the treated vein segments, our audited recurrence rate is consistently 3.3% per year. This recurrence rate, coupled with the identification of the source of any recurrent reflux and checking that it is always from a de novo source and not a previously targeted vein, allows us to be confident that our protocol—The Whiteley Protocol—is currently the optimal way to treat varicose veins.

References

1. Ruckley CV, Evans CJ, Allan PL, Lee AJ, Fowkes FG. Chronic venous insufficiency: clinical and duplex correlations. The Edinburgh Vein Study of venous disorders in the general population. J Vasc Surg. 2002;36(3):520–5.
2. Evans CJ, Fowkes FGR, Ruckley CV, Lee AJ. Prevalence of varicose veins and chronic venous insufficiency in men and women in the general population: Edinburgh Vein Study. J Epidemiol Community Health. 1999;53:149–53.
3. Maurins U, Hoffmann BH, Losch C. Distribution and prevalence of reflux in the superficial and deep venous system in the general population—results from the Bonn Vein Study, Germany. J Vasc Surg. 2008;48:680–7.
4. Pannier F, Rabe E. Progression in venous pathology. Phlebology. 2015;30(1 Suppl):95–7. https://doi.org/10.1177/0268355514568847.
5. Franceschi C. Ambulatory and hemodynamic treatment of venous insufficiency (CHIVA cure). J Mal Vasc. 1992;17(4):291–300.
6. Fassiadis N, Holdstock JM, Whiteley MS. The Saphenofemoral valve: gate keeper turned into rear guard. Phlebology. 2002;17:29–31.
7. Abu-Own A, Scurr JH, Coleridge Smith PD. Saphenous vein reflux without incompetence at the saphenofemoral junction. Br J Surg. 1994;81(10):1452–4.
8. Schul MW, Schloerke B, Gomes GM. The refluxing anterior accessory saphenous vein demonstrates similar clinical severity when compared to the refluxing great saphenous vein. Phlebology. 2016;31(9):654–9. https://doi.org/10.1177/0268355515604532.
9. Rutherford EE, Kianifard B, Cook SJ, Holdstock JM, Whiteley MS. Incompetent perforating veins are associated with recurrent varicose veins. Eur J Vasc Endovasc Surg. 2001;21(5):458–60.
10. Whiteley MS. Part One: for the motion. venous perforator surgery is proven and does reduce recurrences. Eur J Vasc Endovasc Surg. 2014;48(3):239–42. https://doi.org/10.1016/j.ejvs.2014.06.044.
11. Hobbs JT. Varicose veins arising from the pelvis due to ovarian vein incompetence. Int J Clin Pract. 2005;59(10):1195–203.
12. Giannoukas AD, Dacie JE, Lumley JS. Recurrent varicose veins of both lower limbs due to bilateral ovarian vein incompetence. Ann Vasc Surg. 2000;14(4):397–400.
13. Whiteley AM, Taylor DC, Dos Santos SJ, Whiteley MS. Pelvic venous reflux is a major contributory cause of recurrent varicose veins in more than a quarter of women. J Vasc Surg Venous Lymphat Disord. 2014;2(4):411–5. https://doi.org/10.1016/j.jvsv.2014.05.005.
14. Whiteley MS, Dos Santos SJ, Harrison CC, Holdstock JM, Lopez AJ. Transvaginal duplex ultrasonography appears to be the gold standard investigation for the haemodynamic evaluation of pelvic venous reflux in the ovarian and internal iliac veins in women. Phlebology. 2015;30(10):706–13. https://doi.org/10.1177/0268355514554638.
15. Dos Santos SJ, Holdstock JM, Harrison CC, Lopez AJ, Whiteley MS. Ovarian vein diameter cannot be used as an indicator of ovarian venous reflux. Eur J Vasc Endovasc Surg. 2015;49(1):90–4.
16. Asano M, Yoshida K, Tatai K. Observation of the behavior of microcirculation by rabbit ear chamber technique. I. Bull Inst Publ Health. 1963;12:34.
17. Kon K, Fujiwara T. Transformation of fibroblasts into endothelial cells during angiogenesis. Cell Tissue Res. 1994;278(3):625–8.
18. Asahara T, Masuda H, Takahashi T, Kalka C, Pastore C, Silver M, Kearne M, Magner M, Isner JM. Bone marrow origin of endothelial progenitor cells responsible for postnatal vasculogenesis in physiological and pathological neovascularization. Circ Res. 1999;85(3):221–8.
19. Jones L, Braithwaite BD, Selwyn D, Cooke S, Earnshaw JJ. Neovascularisation is the principal cause of varicose vein recurrence: results of a randomised trial of stripping the long saphenous vein. Eur J Vasc Endovasc Surg. 1996;12(4):442–5.
20. Munasinghe A, Smith C, Kianifard B, Price BA, Holdstock JM, Whiteley MS. Strip-track revascular-

ization after stripping of the great saphenous vein. Br J Surg. 2007;94(7):840–3.
21. Kianifard B, Holdstock J, Allen C, Smith C, Price B, Whiteley MS. Randomized clinical trial of the effect of adding subfascial endoscopic perforator surgery to standard great saphenous vein stripping. Br J Surg. 2007;94(9):1075–80.
22. Ostler AE, Holdstock JM, Harrison CC, Price BA, Whiteley MS. Strip-tract revascularization as a source of recurrent venous reflux following high saphenous tie and stripping: results at 5-8 years after surgery. Phlebology. 2015;30(8):569–72. https://doi.org/10.1177/0268355514535927.
23. Rautio T, Ohinmaa A, Perälä J, Ohtonen P, Heikkinen T, Wiik H, Karjalainen P, Haukipuro K, Juvonen T. Endovenous obliteration versus conventional stripping operation in the treatment of primary varicose veins: a randomized controlled trial with comparison of the costs. J Vasc Surg. 2002;35(5):958–65.
24. Fassiadis N, Kianifard B, Holdstock JM, Whiteley MS. A novel endoluminal technique for varicose vein management: the VNUS closure. Phlebology. 2002;16:145–8.
25. Fassiadis N, Kianifard B, Holdstock JM, Whiteley MS. Ultrasound changes at the saphenofemoral junction and in the long saphenous vein during the first year after VNUS closure. Int Angiol. 2002;21(3):272–4.
26. Kianifard B, Holdstock JM, Whiteley MS. Radiofrequency ablation (VNUS Closure®) does not cause neo-vascularisation at the groin at one year: results of a case controlled study. Surgeon. 2006;4(2):71–4.
27. Whiteley MS, Holdstock J. Percutaneous radiofrequency ablations of varicose veins (VNUS closure). In: Greenhalgh RM, editor. Vascular and endovascular challenges. London: Biba Publishing; 2004. p. 361–81.
28. Whiteley M. Varicose veins: endovascular options. In: Greenhalgh RM, editor. Towards vascular and endovascular consensus. London: Biba Publishing; 2005. p. 564–72.
29. Whiteley M. New methods of vein ablation. In: Davies AH, Lees T, Lane IF, editors. Venous disease simplified. London: Harley; 2006.
30. Proebstle TM, Krummenauer F, Gül D, Knop J. Nonocclusion and early reopening of the great saphenous vein after endovenous laser treatment is fluence dependent. Dermatol Surg. 2004;30(2 Pt 1):174–8.
31. Proebstle TM, Moehler T, Gül D, Herdemann S. Endovenous treatment of the great saphenous vein using a 1,320 nm Nd:YAG laser causes fewer side effects than using a 940 nm diode laser. Dermatol Surg. 2005;31(12):1678–83.
32. Cowpland CA, Cleese AL, Whiteley MS. Factors affecting optimal linear endovenous energy density for endovenous laser ablation in incompetent lower limb truncal veins - a review of the clinical evidence. Phlebology. 2017;32(5):299–306. https://doi.org/10.1177/0268355516648067.
33. Badham GE, Strong SM, Whiteley MS. An in vitro study to optimise treatment of varicose veins with radiofrequency-induced thermo therapy. Phlebology. 2015;30(1):17–23. https://doi.org/10.1177/0268355514552005.
34. Badham GE, Dos Santos SJ, Whiteley MS. Radiofrequency-induced thermotherapy (RFiTT) in a porcine liver model and ex vivo great saphenous vein. Minim Invasive Ther Allied Technol. 2017;26:200–6. https://doi.org/10.1080/13645706.2017.1282520.
35. Ashpitel H, Salguero F, La Ragione R, Whiteley M. Radial-firing endovenous laser penetrates deeper into the vein wall than forward-firing jacket-tipped fibers and reduces carbonization — an ex vivo study using histology and immunohistochemistry. J Vasc Surg Venous Lymphat Disord. 2017;5(1):147–8. https://doi.org/10.1016/j.jvsv.2016.10.016.
36. Whiteley MS. Endovenous thermal ablation of varicose veins and examination of the use and failings of linear endovenous energy density (LEED). In: Whiteley M, Dabbs E, editors. Advances in phlebology and venous surgery, vol. 1. Milton Keynes: Whiteley Publishing; 2017. p. 11–24.
37. Braithwaite B, Hnatek L, Zierau U, Camci M, Akkersdijk G, Nio D, Sarlija M, Ajduk M, Santoro P, Roche E. Radiofrequency-induced thermal therapy: results of a European multicentre study of resistive ablation of incompetent truncal varicose veins. Phlebology. 2013;28(1):38–46. https://doi.org/10.1258/phleb.2012.012013.
38. Badham GE, Dos Santos SJ, Lloyd LBA, Holdstock JM, Whiteley MS. One-year results of the use of endovenous radiofrequency ablation utilising an optimised radiofrequency-induced thermotherapy protocol for the treatment of truncal superficial venous reflux. Phlebology. 2017;33:298. https://doi.org/10.1177/0268355517696611.
39. Parsi K. Interaction of detergent sclerosants with cell membranes. Phlebology. 2015;30(5):306–15. https://doi.org/10.1177/0268355514534648.
40. Cooley-Andrade O, Cheung K, Chew AN, Connor DE, Parsi K. Detergent sclerosants at sub-lytic concentrations induce endothelial cell apoptosis through a caspase dependent pathway. Apoptosis. 2016;21(7):836–45. https://doi.org/10.1007/s10495-016-1252-3.
41. Wollmann JC. The history of sclerosing foams. Dermatol Surg. 2004;30(5):694–703.
42. Ikponmwosa A, Abbott C, Graham A, Homer-Vanniasinkam S, Gough MJ. The impact of different concentrations of sodium tetradecyl sulphate and initial balloon denudation on endothelial cell loss and tunica media injury in a model of foam sclerotherapy. Eur J Vasc Endovasc Surg. 2010;39(3):366–71. https://doi.org/10.1016/j.ejvs.2009.12.025.
43. Whiteley MS, Dos Santos SJ, Fernandez-Hart TJ, Lee CT, Li JM. Media damage following detergent sclerotherapy appears to be secondary to the induction of inflammation and apoptosis: an immunohistochemical study elucidating previous histological observations. Eur J Vasc Endovasc Surg. 2016;51(3):421–8. https://doi.org/10.1016/j.ejvs.2015.11.011.

44. Lam YL, Lawson JA, Toonder IM, Shadid NH, Sommer A, Veenstra M, et al. Eight-year follow-up of a randomized clinical trial comparing ultrasound-guided foam sclerotherapy with surgical stripping of the great saphenous vein. British Journal of Surgery. 2018;105(6):692–8.
45. Kendler M, Averbeck M, Simon JC, Ziemer M. Histology of saphenous veins after treatment with the ClariVein® device - an ex-vivo experiment. J Dtsch Dermatol Ges. 2013;11(4):348–52. https://doi.org/10.1111/ddg.12022.
46. Boersma D, van Haelst ST, van Eekeren RR, Vink A, Reijnen MM, de Vries JP, de Borst GJ. Macroscopic and histologic analysis of vessel wall reaction after mechanochemical endovenous ablation using the clarivein OC device in an animal model. Eur J Vasc Endovasc Surg. 2017;53(2):290–8. https://doi.org/10.1016/j.ejvs.2016.11.024.
47. Whiteley MS, Dos Santos SJ, Lee CT, Li JM. Mechanochemical ablation causes endothelial and medial damage to the vein wall resulting in deeper penetration of sclerosant compared with sclerotherapy alone in extrafascial great saphenous vein using an ex vivo model. J Vasc Surg Venous Lymphat Disord. 2017;5(3):370–7. https://doi.org/10.1016/j.jvsv.2016.12.009.
48. Boersma D, van Eekeren RR, Werson DA, van der Waal RI, Reijnen MM, de Vries JP. Mechanochemical endovenous ablation of small saphenous vein insufficiency using the ClariVein(®) device: one-year results of a prospective series. Eur J Vasc Endovasc Surg. 2013;45(3):299–303. https://doi.org/10.1016/j.ejvs.2012.12.004.
49. Todd KL, Wright D, Orfe E. The durability of polidocanol endovenous microfoam treatment effect on varicose vein symptoms and appearance in patients with saphenofemoral junction incompetence: one-year results from the VANISH-2 study. J Vasc Surg Venous Lymphat Disord. 2014;2(1):112. https://doi.org/10.1016/j.jvsv.2013.10.027.
50. Chan YC, Law Y, Cheung GC, Cheng SW. Predictors of recanalization for incompetent great saphenous veins treated with cyanoacrylate glue. J Vasc Interv Radiol. 2017;28(5):665–71. https://doi.org/10.1016/j.jvir.2017.01.011.
51. Chan YC, Law Y, Cheung GC, Ting AC, Cheng SW. Cyanoacrylate glue used to treat great saphenous reflux: measures of outcome. Phlebology. 2017;32(2):99–106. https://doi.org/10.1177/0268355516638200.
52. Proebstle TM, Alm J, Dimitri S, Rasmussen L, Whiteley M, Lawson J, Cher D, Davies A. The European multicenter cohort study on cyanoacrylate embolization of refluxing great saphenous veins. J Vasc Surg Venous Lymphat Disord. 2015;3(1):2–7. https://doi.org/10.1016/j.jvsv.2014.09.001.
53. Frullini A, Fortuna D. Laser assisted foam sclerotherapy (LAFOS): a new approach to the treatment of incompetent saphenous veins. Phlebologie. 2013;66(1):51–4.
54. Smarandache A. Laser beams interaction with polidocanol foam: molecular background. Photomed Laser Surg. 2012;30(5):262–7. https://doi.org/10.1089/pho.2011.3187.
55. Brand FN, Dannenberg AL, Abbott RD, Kannel WB. The epidemiology of varicose veins: the Framingham Study. Am J Prev Med. 1988;4(2):96–101.

5 Relevance of Wavelength in Laser Treatment of Varicose Veins

Harinder Singh Bedi and Yudhishtar Singh Bedi

Endovenous laser therapy (EVLT) or endovenous laser ablation (EVLA) was introduced as a minimally invasive treatment for varicose veins. Lasers work by producing endovenous thermal damage and hence obliteration of the diseased vein. The short- and long-term efficacy and extent of ablative damage and also the complications of pain, phlebitis, etc. are dependent to some extent on the wavelength of the laser. There are continuous modifications in the wavelength used with the aim of minimizing side effects and improving efficiency. Different laser systems as well as varying application strategies are under study. Investigational research and close analysis have helped in a better understanding of the relationship between the clinical efficacy and the physical aspects of the laser with a continuous refinement of treatment.

Endovenous thermal ablation of varicose veins came into vogue because of the need for reducing the morbidity associated with the open stripping technique and to reduce the hospitalization and pain and need for general anaesthesia and so hasten patient recovery. Early clinical results of endovenous laser therapy (ELT) were published by Navarro and Bone [1].

The laser system introduces the laser light into the vein lumen by a malleable optical fibre. Laser energy is absorbed and transformed into heat energy. Depending on the absorption characteristics of the target molecules in the tissue (e.g. water or haemoglobin) and on the laser wavelength used, there are cellular damage and destruction and collagen shrinkage leading to occlusion of the vein. The laser light energy is carried in a fibre of diameter of up to 600 μm. The fibre is inserted into the vein via a catheter system. Systems emitting laser light of wavelengths in the near-infrared spectral field (810, 940, 980, 1064, 1320 and 1470 nm) are used in clinical practice.

Using these techniques, the thermal damage of the vein results in occlusion. One characteristic of ELT is the different varieties of treatment protocols using different laser systems. A critical analysis of clinical results and research have elucidated on the connection between different types of laser application and efficacy of clinical results. This has led to a continuous refinement and development of ELT. The following article outlines the basics of endovenous laser and research for improving this minimally invasive procedure.

H. S. Bedi (✉)
Cardiovascular Sciences of Ludhiana Mediways Hospital, Ludhiana, Punjab, India

Y. S. Bedi
USC, Los Angeles, CA, USA

A. K. Khanna, R. Jindal (eds.), *Venous Disorders*, https://doi.org/10.1007/978-981-13-1108-6_5

5.1 Simple Basics of a Laser

5.1.1 Spontaneous and Stimulated Emission

By nature most atoms exist in a low-energy (ground) state [2, 3]. They can be excited to a higher-energy state when they absorb thermal, optical or electrical energy. An electron in a higher-energy orbit is unstable. On returning to the original state, it releases its defined energy as a photon (particle of light). This is known as spontaneous emission. The amount of energy released determines the wavelength or colour of the light emitted. If an electron already in an excited state encounters a photon of the proper energy, the electrons drop to a lower orbit and emit a photon. The stimulating photon is not absorbed but continues on its way, resulting in two identical energy or wavelength photons. Einstein called this stimulated emission. For stimulated emission to occur in a majority, it is necessary for more electrons to be in the upper energy level. This is known as population inversion. It is created by pumping electrical or light energy into the population of atoms (the gain medium) to move them to higher-energy levels. When the laser is switched on, the gain medium is pumped, population inversion occurs and individual atoms in the population undergo spontaneous emission, emitting photons in random directions. A photon will pass by an atom with electrons in the upper level and cause it to emit a second photon travelling in the same direction, phase and wavelength. There are now two photons; each can cause stimulated emission and give four photons and so on. In order for photons to continuously amplify, the gain medium is placed between two mirrors. One of these emitted photons, purely by accident, is in the axis of the two mirrors and is reflected back into the gain medium, continuing the amplification. Each photon reflected back causes stimulated emission, and photon numbers go on increasing. This produces an avalanche of coherent light. One of the mirrors is designed to allow some of the light through—the output beam. The beam is monochromatic, collimated and coherent.

5.1.2 Laser Construction

There are three components making up a laser system: an energy source or a pump, a gain medium and two mirrors that form an optical resonator [2, 3]. The pump source which provides energy to the laser system includes electrical discharges, flash lamps, light from another laser and even chemical reactions. The type of pump source used principally depends on the gain medium. The gain medium is the major determining factor of wavelength and energy, and it can be a gas, liquid, solid or semiconductor (diode laser) (Fig. 5.1). In this gain medium, spontaneous or stimulated emission of photons takes place. The optical resonator, or optical cavity, in its simplest form is two mirrors at each end of the gain medium. Light from the medium, produced by spontaneous emission, is reflected back into the medium many hundreds of times amplifying the beam. Thus we have LASER: Light Amplified by Stimulated Emission of Radiation.

5.2 Radiation

Radiation is a form of energy that travels at the speed of light and spreads out or radiates [2, 3]. It includes visible light, infrared, ultraviolet, radio waves, microwaves and X-rays. Energy and momentum get imparted when the radiation interacts with matter.

The electromagnetic spectrum is a complete range of electromagnetic waves (waves with both electric and magnetic components) ranging from those with low frequency and energy levels along with correspondingly long wavelengths to those with high-frequency and high-energy levels with correspondingly short wavelengths (Fig. 5.2). This relationship is explained by the formula:

Wavelength = speed of light/frequency; and
energy = Planks constant (h)
× frequency.

Lasers produce nonionizing radiation at frequencies in the infrared, visible or ultraviolet region of the electromagnetic spectrum.

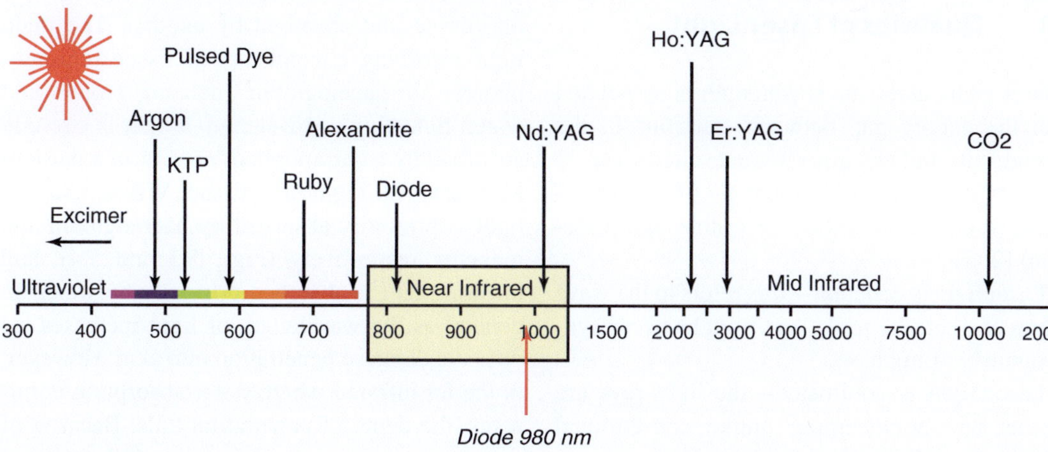

Fig. 5.1 The types of lasers

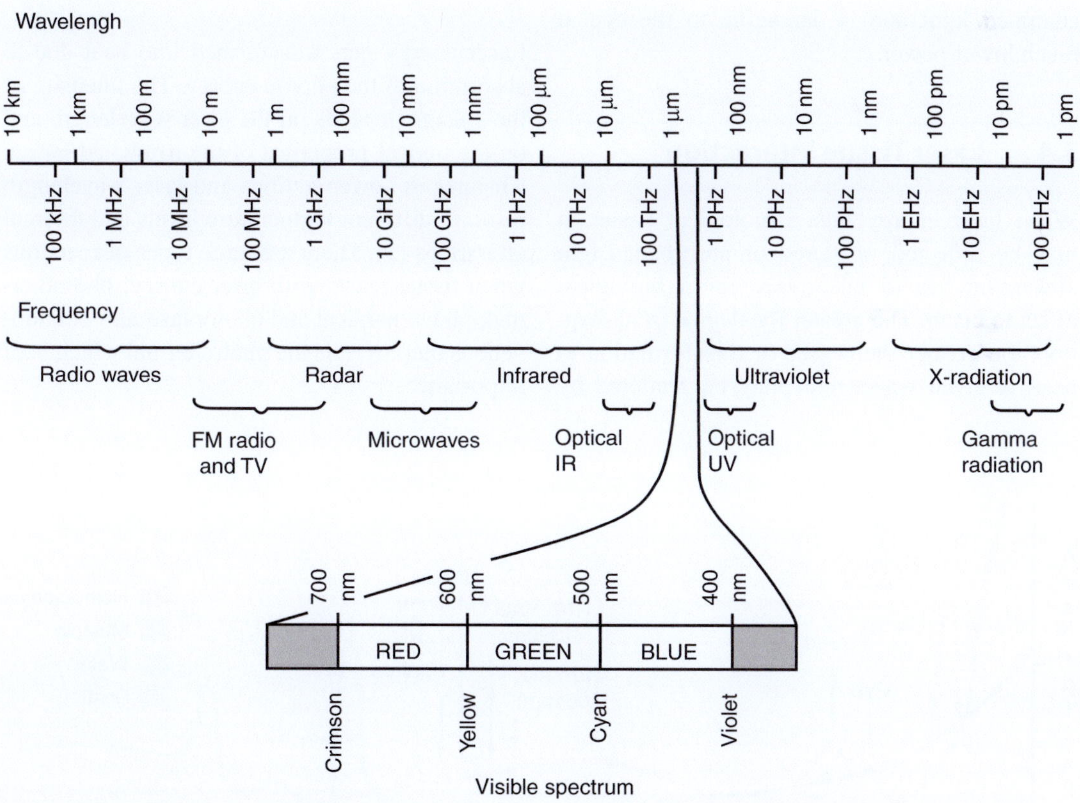

Fig. 5.2 The electromagnetic spectrum

5.3 Qualities of Laser Light

A laser's characteristic wavelength is associated with the energy gap between electrons in the ground state and electrons in the excited state.

Laser light is monochromatic—of one wavelength or colour (if within the visible light spectrum) [2, 3].

Laser light is coherent—this refers to the wave nature of light; the peaks and troughs occur synchronously or in phase.

Laser light is collimated—the light rays are parallel and nondiverging unlike conventional light sources that emit light in all directions. A laser is more powerful than ordinary light of the same power. If light from a 60 W bulb enters the eye, it would not damage the retina. A collimated laser beam on the other hand is a focused, concentrated light and is damaging to the eye at much lower power.

5.4 Laser Tissue Interaction

When laser energy hits a biological tissue, it may be reflected, scattered or absorbed. Light absorption has to take place for a biological effect to occur. The greater the degree of absorption, the greater the degree of transformation to heat. A given wavelength may be scattered by one tissue and absorbed by another. The main light-absorbing components of tissue (chromophores) are haemoglobin, melanin, protein and water. Selecting a wavelength which is strongly absorbed by a chromophore present in a particular tissue will target that tissue. Visible and UV light is primarily absorbed by haemoglobin and melanin, respectively (Figs. 5.3 and 5.4), and infrared light is absorbed primarily by water. In general as the wavelength of light increases, so does the depth of penetration into skin. However, in the far infrared where water absorption dominates, the depth of penetration falls. Because of the strong absorption of water at 418, 542 and 577 nm, depth of penetration is attenuated [4, 5].

5.5 Biological Effects of Lasers

Laser energy gets transformed into heat due to absorption of the photon energy. The intensity of the change depends on the laser wavelength and on the optical properties of the irradiated tissue. Changes in power settings and laser wavelength result in different temperature levels and thermal alterations [3]. There are three types of reactions when tissue reacts with laser energy: photothermal, photochemical and photoplasmal. For endovenous therapy, it is the photothermal which is of importance.

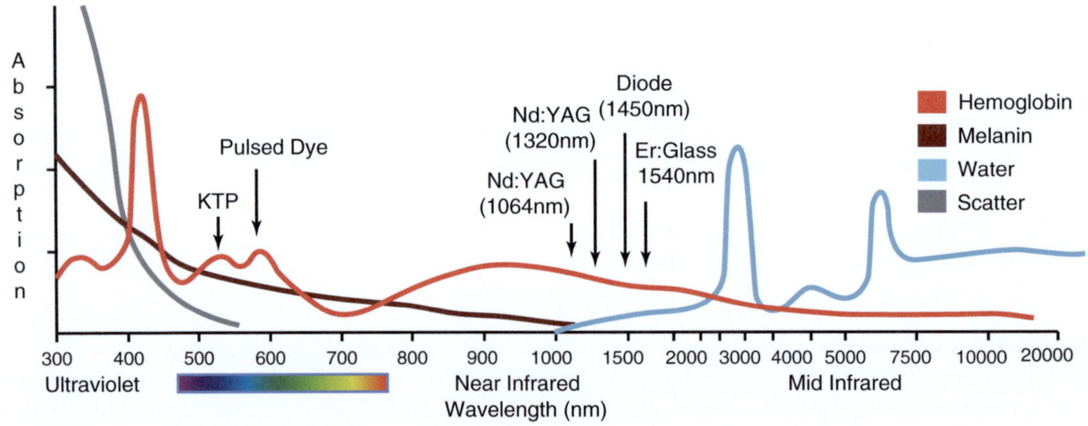

Fig. 5.3 The relationship of absorption vs wavelength for various lasers

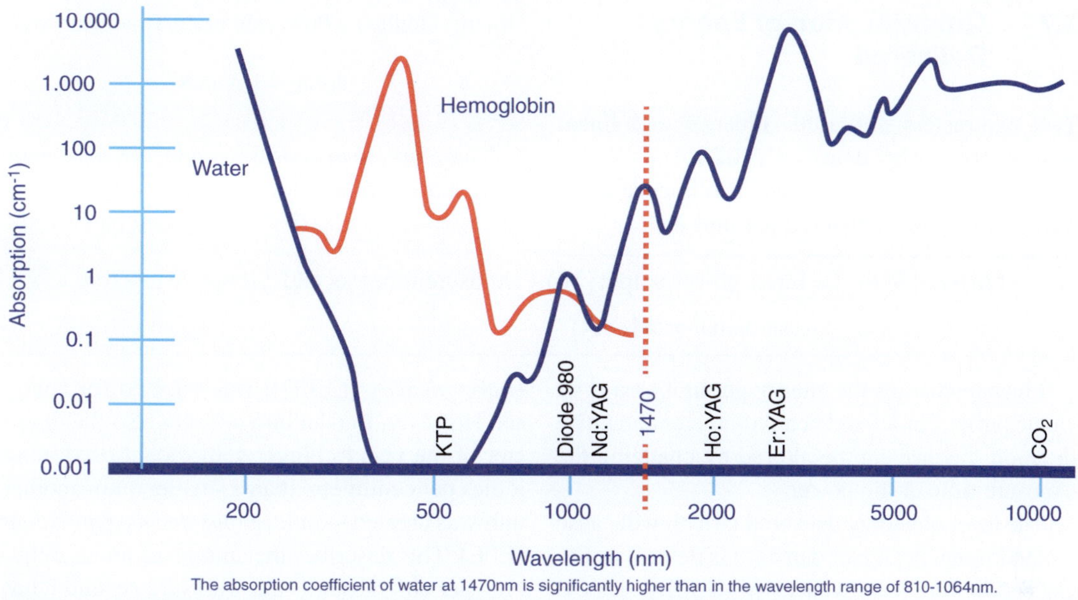

Fig. 5.4 The absorption coefficient of water and water in relation to wavelength

5.5.1 Photothermal

Tissue chromophores absorb laser light and heat is generated. Depending on the duration and peak value of the temperature achieved, different effects like coagulation, vaporization, carbonization and melting may occur.

At tissue temperatures of 42–50 °C (hyperthermia), bond destruction and membrane alteration occur ending in necrosis if the hyperthermia lasts for several minutes. Beyond 50 °C, enzyme activity is reduced, cell immobility occurs and cell repair mechanisms are disabled. At 60 °C, there is denaturation of proteins and collagen leading to coagulation of tissue and necrosis of cells. At >80 °C, membrane permeability is increased. At 100 °C, there is vaporization of water molecules. Gas bubbles are formed inducing mechanical cell rupture and thermal decomposition (photoablation). At temperatures exceeding 100 °C, carbonization occurs; beyond 300 °C, melting can occur [3].

In general, the exact temperature for the onset of cell necrosis varies and is dependent on the temperature achieved and also on the duration. Quite often, several thermal effects are induced depending on laser parameters; in most applications, however, only one specific effect is aimed at and a precise biological target can be thermally damaged [2].

5.6 Wavelength

Wavelength determines to some extent the effect of light energy on tissue. Erythema, hyperpigmentation and cutaneous cancer can be caused by light in the UV region (100–400 nm) which is invisible to the human eye. Light energy in the visible spectrum (380–700 nm) is mostly innocuous but can be absorbed and cause thermal damage when delivered to the skin at high intensity. Light in the near-infrared (IR) region of the spectrum (780–3000 nm), invisible to the human eye, causes skin and retinal injury [6].

The degree of absorption and its thermal effect on tissue vary with the amount and type of chromophores present. Different chromophores have different absorption coefficients. As laser is monochromatic and has narrow bandwidth, it permits selective targeting of chromophores [6].

5.7 Quantification of Energy Delivered

Two parameters are used: Fluence and linear endovenous energy density (LEED).

Fluence is a unit of energy. The fluence is the energy (in Joules) delivered per unit area.

$$\text{Energy (Joules)} = \text{Power (Watts)} \times \text{Time (seconds)}$$

$$\text{Joule} = 1\,\text{Watt/s}$$

Therefore, fluence is the product of irradiance and exposure time:

$$\text{Fluence}\left(\text{J/cm}^2\right) = \text{Laser power output}\left(\text{W}\right) \times \text{exposure time}\left(\text{seconds}\right)/\text{laser beam cross} - \text{sectional area}\left(\text{cm}^2\right)$$

Fluence denotes the energy per unit area for a single pulse. For a fixed beam diameter and pulse duration, fluence can be altered by changing the exposure time or the power.

The level of energy delivered (which will cause a proportional degree of damage) is defined as linear endovenous energy density (LEED). This is measured in reference to the length and diameter of the vein segment to be treated and is described in Joule per cm of vein [7]. The laser energy applied in relation to the irradiated surface is described as endovenous fluence equivalent (EFE) given in Joule/cm^2. For this parameter a cylindrical model of the vein segment is used, calculating the inner vein surface according to $F = 2 \times r \times p \times 1$, where r is the vein radius and l the length of the treated vein segment. Hence, it is important to note the following parameters for every treatment: vein diameter d (cm), length of the treated vein segment l (cm), laser wavelength λ (nm), laser power P (Watt), irradiation time t (s) or pull-back speed v (mm/s) for continuous pull-back. Only then will we be able to compare clinical results with different regimes.

Inappropriate results like non-occlusion or recanalization after ELT treatment are observed less when sufficiently high-energy density is used—compared to lower LEED or EFE [8–15].

On the other hand, energy densities above a certain level can lead to side effects such as transmural ablation, perforations and alteration of perivenous tissue [16, 17].

5.8 Thermal Ablation: Energy Dosing

Earlier a unit with the dimension of joules per centimetre of vein length (called *linear endovenous energy density* [LEED]) was selected for analysis. However, to take into account also the diameter of the vein (a bigger vein should need more joules per centimetre than a smaller one), another unit was created—*endovenous fluence equivalent* (EFE). This describes the amount of joules delivered per cm^2 of inner vein wall surface, and it has proven to be the unit that is statistically linked to a sustained GSV occlusion or an early recanalization after laser ablation [8].

Calculation of the inner surface of the GSV is done by a cylindrical approximation using the biggest diameter of the GSV measured while the patient is lying down. Testing of this unit was performed in a prospective series of GSV diode laser ablations, and it was found that a 100% occlusion rate and a recanalization rate of not more than 1% was possible during a 1-year follow- up period if an EFE of more than 20 J/cm^2 is delivered [10].

Even now it has not been possible to establish generally valid recommendations for appropriate energy density. Table 5.1 gives an overview of recommendations from a number of authors.

A recent trend has been observed towards recommendations for higher-energy density.

Table 5.1 Recommendations for appropriate energy density for endovenous lasers

Author	Wavelength (nm)	LEED (J/cm)	EFE (J/cm^2)
Proebstle et al. [7]	940	23.6	13.0
Timperman et al. [9]	810/940	>80	n.d.
Proebstle et al. [10]	940	n.d.	20.0
Kim [11]	980	32.7	9.82
Desmyttère et al. [12]	980	50–120	29–41
Kontothanassis et al. [13]	980	45–60	n.d.
Vuylsteke et al. [14]	980	n.d.	52.0
Elmore et al. [15]	810	109.6	46.6

5.9 Pulse Duration (Pulse Width)

This is the time during which the laser power remains continuously above half its maximum value. Pulsed laser systems may be either long-pulsed such as PDL (pulsed dye laser) with pulse durations ranging from 450 to 40 ms or very short-pulsed (5–100 ns) such as the quality-switched lasers. The pulse duration controls the spatial confinement of heat and should match the thermal relaxation time of the target. The thermal relaxation time is a measure of the cooling time of the target and is the time taken for the target to dissipate half of the incident thermal energy. Cooling time is related to the physical size of the target: the larger the target, the longer the thermal relaxation time. A pulse duration equal to or less than the thermal relaxation time of the target makes for reduced unwanted heat diffusion to adjacent tissue [18]. Extended pulse durations allow the delivery of higher fluences of energy in a more gentle fashion. Greater fluences enable treatment of veins that are larger and deeper in location. Also, the ability to deliver higher fluences in the management of lower extremity vessels has produced more consistent and complete destruction of vessels, leading to more consistent results [2].

5.10 Pulse Repetition Rate

This is the number of emitted pulses per second (Hz). After one pulse, if the second comes before sufficient thermal diffusion into the surrounding tissues occurs, a pronounced temperature rise and thermal damage can occur. Even ultrashort laser pulses with pulse durations shorter than 100 ps, each of them having no thermal effect, may add up to a measurable increase in temperature if applied at repetition rates higher than about 10–20 Hz [18].

5.11 Diode Lasers

Diode lasers generate coherent monochromatic light through excitation of small diodes.

5.12 Nd:YAG Laser (1064 nm)

A longer wavelength (e.g. the 1064-nm Nd:YAG laser) translates to a better penetration and a better absorption in deoxyhaemoglobin and the greater the sparing of the epidermis and a decreased melanin coefficient absorption.

5.13 Mode of Action of Lasers

The mechanism of action of lasers is still not fully understood. Vein wall injury is mediated both by direct effect and indirectly via laser-induced steam generated by heating small amounts of blood within the vein. Proebstle et al. [19] showed that intravascular blood plays a key role for this evenly distributed thermal damage to the inner vein wall during EVLA. Microscopic studies showed that in saline-filled veins, EVLA-induced vessel wall injury was confined to the site of direct laser impact. In contrast, blood-filled veins exhibited thermal damage in more remote areas including the vein wall opposite to the laser impact. Lasers generate steam bubbles in blood and not in normal saline or plasma. Thus the thermal damage is caused by direct absorption of the laser light and also by indirect heating of the vein wall by endovenous steam bubble formation, causing occlusion of the vessel [20]. Many researchers however believe that the combined effects of vein spasm, compression by perivenous tumescent anaesthesia and ablation in the Trendelenburg position result in an 'empty' vein and direct thermal damage to the vein wall. Several histological studies show that intimal damage combined with discrete full-thickness perforations and relatively 'normal' intervening veins [21, 22] occurs along with direct damage of the vein wall structures due to direct contact between the laser tip and the vein wall [23].

Occlusion is completed by collagen remodelling and proliferation of fibroblasts involved in the restructuring and repair processes [17, 24]. Initial energy absorption by the small amount of residual blood (the chromophore) in the target vein occurs and then this sets off a chain of events that leads to carbonization along the vein wall [25].

At a wavelength of 1320 nm (Nd:YAG laser) and 1470 nm (diode laser), the dominant chromophore is water, and the absorption is limited to water that is present in the endothelial cells. As biological tissue is mostly composed of water, deeper penetration and thermal effect can be achieved at lower power settings, typically 5 W. This protocol has not been complicated by postoperative pain or ecchymosis, as occurs with lower laser wavelengths [26, 27].

The level of thermal energy delivered at a specific vein segment is related to both temperature and duration. Denaturation of almost all the collagen fibres followed by the wound healing processes causes a complete and durable occlusion of the vein. High energy levels would guarantee a higher rate of occlusion but also a higher incidence of side effects.

808–1320-nm wavelength lasers have been used for EVLA. New modifications in laser technology are being analysed. A 1470-nm diode laser (absorption wavelength of water) is now being used, and data indicate that optimum occlusion rates are achieved with minimum laser energy of 60 J/cm [28].

But still there seems to be no clear agreement as to the optimum treatment protocol for EVLA. There is a considerable variation not only in the laser system used but also in patient selection, adjunctive procedures used (phlebectomies or sclerotherapy [foam or liquid]), compression following treatment, thromboprophylaxis, analgesia, anaesthesia and patient follow-up. Uniformity of EVLA technique, continued evaluation of different laser systems and their mode of action and of course long-term follow-up are needed to further define the role of laser. The author has studied the histopathological changes of radio frequency ablation on a human greater saphenous vein [29] and is currently undertaking a similar study using laser on a human vein.

5.14 Specificity of Lasers

Endovenous ablation lasers can be classified into haemoglobin-specific laser wavelengths (HSLWs) and water-specific laser wavelengths (WSLWs). The three HSLWs currently available, in order of increasing haemoglobin affinity, are 810, 940 and 980 nm. A 1320-nm and a 1470-nm WSLW are currently available.

Satisfactory vein ablation results have been noted with all HSLWs. Postoperative discomfort and bruising are often seen with HSLWs, which act by causing boiling blood to injure, and sometimes perforate, the vein wall. The 1320-nm WSLW was developed to minimize perforation by directly targeting the interstitial water in the vein wall [28].

The current stress is on reducing the side effects of bruising and pain. While higher energy is required for efficacy of vein closure, but with increased energy delivery, pain and bruising are increased. There is evidence [3, 17] that longer-wavelength lasers produce fewer side effects at comparable linear energy delivery. For laser wavelengths of 810 and 940 nm, recent data indicated a relationship between increased delivered LEED and improved closure rates [8, 9].

60 J–100 J/cm of LEED is required for effective vein closure. But, it has been reported that treatment with less energy causes less pain and bruising. Proebstle described a lower rate of side effects with 5 W than 8 W laser for a 1320-nm endovenous occlusion [30]. Kabnick [30] compared two HSLWs to determine if there were differences between the 810-nm laser and the 980-nm laser and showed that both the 810 and 980-nm wavelengths were effective in closing the GSV, but ecchymosis and superficial phlebitis were more often present with the 810-nm laser.

Significantly less pain was shown in patients treated with the 1320-nm laser when compared to the 940-nm laser (50% with 1320 nm/8 W vs 81% with 940 nm/30 W or 940 nm/15 W) [30]. Also, significantly reduced ecchymosis was noticed with the 1320-nm laser (61% with 1320 nm/8 W vs 81% with 940 nm/30 W and 78% with 940 nm/15 W). Among the three most studied HSLWs (810, 940 and 980 nm), higher wavelength has trended towards reduced side effects. The 1320-nm WSLW laser shows a trend towards fewer side effects than HSLW. Commercially available lasers for EVLA are most frequently diode lasers (810, 940 and 980 nm) or

Nd:YAG lasers (1064, 1320 nm). More recently, the 1470–1500-nm diode laser has been introduced. Whereas haemoglobin and to a lesser extent myoglobin in vein wall smooth muscle components are the main chromophores at the lower end of this range, at the 1320-nm and higher wavelengths, the absorption is limited to water that is present within the endothelial cells [21, 27]. The occlusion rate for the vessel wall (and for blood) at using lasers with wavelengths of 1470–1500 nm is at least five times higher than with the 980–810-nm lasers [31], which means that greater selectivity of the vein wall can be obtained with less energy [32].

In terms of volume, when comparing lasers delivering the same ranges of wavelengths, the energy deposited per unit volume is increased by a factor of 43; therefore, the same energy acts on a volume 43 times smaller, creating a risk of overdose and thus perforation [33, 34].

Pannier et al. [26, 35] reported the first results with the 1470-nm diode laser and found a high-occlusion rate of 100% 1 year after treatment. The same authors also suggest using LEED lower than 100 J/cm, as the incidence of paraesthesia significantly increased with LEED above 100 J/cm, likely due to thermal damage of perivascular skin nerves, whereas the occlusion rate remained the same for both groups.

Proebstle et al. [7] showed less bruising, less pain and lesser need for analgesics with the 1320-nm Nd:YAG laser than the 940-nm diode laser. Schwartz et al. [36] and Doganci et al. [37] showed less bruising with the 1470-nm diode laser.

In the early days of laser use for endovenous ablation, mostly diode lasers ranging from 810 to 980-nm wavelengths were used, causing more side effects than radio frequency (RF) closure.

5.15 Recent and Future Developments

An effective EVLA needs a sufficient intravascular heating to cause irreversible occlusion and subsequent fibrosis of the vein without undue damage to the adjacent tissue [25]. However at present the exact and optimal energy dose and treatment parameters for persistent vein closure with minimal side effects are still unknown.

With higher wavelength lasers, energy is preferably absorbed by water instead of haemoglobin, and perforations are much less frequent. The complication effects of a 1320-nm laser are observed less frequently and are observed for shorter durations. In general, the 1320-nm laser behaves more like radio frequency (RF) closure. An additional diode laser system with another water-absorbed wavelength of 1470 nm is now available. Further refinements are laser fibres with covered tips that may further reduce the risk of perforation (AngioDynamics, Inc., Queensbury, NY; Vascular Solutions, Inc., Minneapolis, MN). Another modification is a new fibre type delivering the laser beam in a radial fashion to the vein wall (Biolitec, Inc., East Longmeadow, MA).

There is a definite relationship between increased delivered LEED and improved closure rates [8, 9]. Between 60 and 100 J/cm of LEED is required for effective ablation. In contrast, it has been reported that treatment with less energy causes less pain and bruising. Proebstle described that the use of 5 W demonstrated a lower rate of side effects than 8 W for a 1320-nm endovenous occlusion [30].

Kabnick [38] compared two HSLWs (the 810-nm laser and the 980-nm laser) in a randomized and single-blinded fashion. Overall, the results of the study showed that both the 810-nm and 980-nm wavelengths were effective in closing the GSV. Few untoward events resulted with either device; no deep vein thrombosis, pulmonary embolism, skin burns or paraesthesia was reported. Ecchymosis and superficial phlebitis were more often present when the 810-nm laser was used.

Proestle et al. [7] in a study of endovenous ablative procedures performed at comparable LEED with either the 940-nm laser or the 1320-nm laser, showed significantly less pain in patients treated with the 1320-nm laser (50% with 1320 nm/8 W vs 81% with 940 nm/30 W or 940 nm/15 W). Again, significantly reduced ecchymosis was noticed with the 1320-nm laser

(61% with 1320 nm/8 W vs 81% with 940 nm/30 W and 78% with 940 nm/15 W). They found that lasers using water-specific wavelengths (1320 nm, 1470 nm) permitted the use of a lower laser fluence for equal efficacy.

Thus wavelength holds an important place in efficacy of ablation and also in reducing the incidence of side effects. Further research in this field will definitely go a long way in improving results.

References

1. Navarro L, Min RJ, Bone C. Endovenous laser: a new minimally invasive method of treatment for varicose veins--preliminary observations using an 810 nm diode laser. Dermatol Surg. 2001;27(2):117–22.
2. De Felice E. Shedding light: laser physics and mechanism of action. Phlebology. 2010;25:11–28.
3. Sroka R, Weick K, Sadeghi-Azandaryani M, Steckmeier B, Schmedt CG. Endovenous laser therapy – application studies and latest investigations. J Biophotonics. 2010;3:269–76.
4. Neimz MH. Laser tissue interactions. Fundamentals and applications. 3rd ed. Berlin: Springer; 2003.
5. Welch AJ, Torres JH, Cheong W-F. Laser physics and laser tissue interaction. Tex Heart Inst J. 1989;16:141–9.
6. Carruth JAS, McKenzie AL. Medical lasers. Science and clinical practice. Bristol: Adam Hilger; 1986.
7. Proebstle TM, Moehler T, Gül D, Herdemann S. Endovenous treatment of the great saphenous vein using a 1,320 nm nd: Yag laser causes fewer side effects than using a 940 nm d: Yag laser causes fewer side effects than using a 940 nm diode laser. Dermatol Surg. 2005;31:1678–84.
8. Proebstle TM, Krummenauer F, Gu¨l D, Knop J. Nonocclusion and early reopening of the great saphenous vein after endovenous laser treatment is fluence dependent. Dermatol Surg. 2004;30:174–8.
9. Timperman TE, Sichlau M, Ryu RK. Greater energy delivery improves treatment success of endovenous laser treatment of incompetent saphenous veins. J Vasc Interv Radiol. 2004;15(10):1061–3.
10. Proebstle TM, Moehler T, Herdemann SJ. Reduced recanalization rates of the great saphenous vein after endovenous laser treatment with increased energy dosing: definition of a threshold for the endovenous fluence equivalent. J Vasc Surg. 2006;44(4):834–9.
11. Kim HS, Nwankwo IJ, Hong K, McElgunn PS. Lower energy endovenous laser ablation of the great saphenous vein with 980 nm diode laser in continuous mode. Cardiovasc Intervent Radiol. 2006;29(1):64–9.
12. Desmyttère J, Grard C, Wassmer B, Mordon S. Endovenous 980-nm laser treatment of saphenous veins in a series of 500 patients. J Vasc Surg. 2007; 46(6):1242–7.
13. Kontothanassis D, Di Mitri R, Ruffino SF, Ugliola M, Labropoulos N. Endovenous thermal ablation. Standardization of laser energy: literature review and personal experience. Int Angiol. 2007;26(2):183–8.
14. Vuylsteke M, Liekens K, Moons P, Mordon S. Endovenous laser treatment of saphenous vein reflux: how much energy do we need to prevent recanalizations? Vasc Endovasc Surg. 2008;42:141–9.
15. Elmore FA, Lackey D. Effectiveness of endovenous laser treatment in eliminating superficial venous reflux. Phlebology. 2008;23:21–31.
16. Chang CJ, Chua JJ. Endovenous laser photocoagulation (EVLP) for varicose veins. Lasers Surg Med. 2002;31(4):257–62.
17. Schmedt CG, Sroka R, Steckmeier S, Meissner OA, Babaryka G, Hunger K, Ruppert V, Sadeghi-Azandaryani M, Steckmeier BM. Investigation on radiofrequency and laser (980 nm) effects after endoluminal treatment of saphenous vein insufficiency in an ex-vivo model. Eur J VascEndovasc Surg. 2006;32(3):318–25.
18. Anderson RR, Parrish JA. Selective photothermolysis: precise microsurgery by selective absorption of pulsed radiation science. Science. 1983;220:524–7.
19. Proebstle TM, Sandhofer M, Kargl A, et al. Thermal damage of the inner vein wall during endovenous laser treatment: key role of energy absorption by intravascular blood. Dermatol Surg. 2002;28:596–600.
20. Proebstle TM, Lehr HA, Kargl A, Espinola-Klein C, Rother W, Bethge S, Knop J. Endovenous treatment of the greater saphenous vein with a 940-nm diode laser: thrombotic occlusion after endoluminal thermal damage by laser-generated steam bubbles. J Vasc Surg. 2002;35:729–36.
21. Fan C-M, Rox-Anderson R. Endovenous laser ablation: mechanism of action. Phlebology. 2008;23:206–13.
22. Corcos L, Dini S, De A, et al. The immediate effects of endovenous diode 808-nm laser in the greater saphenous vein: morphologic study and clinical implications. J Vasc Surg. 2005;41:1018–24.
23. Min RJ, Khilnani NM. Endovenous laser ablation of varicose veins. J Cardiovasc Surg. 2005;46(4):395–405.
24. Manfrini S, Gasbarro V, Danielsson G, Norgren L, Chandler JG, Lennox AF, et al. Endovenous management of saphenous vein reflux. Endovenous Reflux Management Study Group. J Vasc Surg. 2000;32:330–42.
25. Diessehf BC, Rem AI, Verdaasdonk RM, Kinderen DJ, Moll FL. Endovenous laser ablation: an experimental study on the mechanism of action. Phlebology. 2008;23:69–76.
26. Pannier F, Rabe E, Maurins U. First results with a new 1470-nm diode laser for endovenous ablation of incompetent saphenous veins. Phlebology. 2009;24:26–30.

27. Goldman MP, Mauricio M, Rao J. Intravascular 1320-nm laser closure of the great saphenous vein: a six to 12-month follow-up study. Dermatol Surg. 2004;30:1380–5.
28. Theivacumar N, Beale R, Mavor A, Gough M. Factors influencing the effectiveness of endovenous laser treatment (EVLT) for varicose veins due to saphenofemoral (SF) and long saphenous (LSV) reflux. Eur J Vasc Endovasc Surg. 2008;35:119–23.
29. Bedi HS, Calton N, Kwatra KS, Tewarson V. Histopathological findings of the human great saphenous vein treated with endoluminal radio frequency ablation. Int Surg J. 2014;1(1):3–5.
30. Proebstle T, Moehler T, Gul D, et al. Endovenous treatment of the great saphenous vein using a 1,320 nm Nd:YAG laser causes fewer side effects than using a 940 nm diode laser. Dermatol Surg. 2005;31:1678–83.
31. Kuenstner JT, Norris KH. Spectrophotometry of human hemoglobin in the near infrared region from 1000 to 2500 nm. J Near Infrared Spectrosc. 1994;2:59–65.
32. Vuylsteke ME, Vandekerckhove PJ, De Bo T. Use of a new endovenous laser device: results of the 1,500 nm laser. Ann Vasc Surg. 2010;24:205–11.
33. Vuylsteke ME, Mordon SR. Endovenous laser ablation: a review of mechanism of action. Ann Vasc Surg. 2012;26(3):424–33.
34. Vuylsteke ME, Martinelli TH, VanDorpe J, et al. Endovenous laser ablation: the role of the intraluminal blood. Eur J Vasc Endovasc Surg. 2011;42: 120–6.
35. Pannier F, Rabe E, Rits J, Kadiss A, Maurins U. Endovenous laser ablation of great saphenous veins using a 1470 nm diode laser and the radial fibre-follow-up after 6 months. Phlebology. 2011;26: 35–9.
36. Schwartz T, von Hodenberg E, Furtwangler C, Rastan A, Zeller T, Neumann FJ. Endovenous laser ablation of varicose veins with the 1470 nm diode laser. J Vasc Surg. 2010;51:1474–8.
37. Doganci S, Demirkilic U. Comparison Of 980 nm laser and bare tip fibre with 1470 nm laser and radial fibre in the treatment of great saphenous vein varicosities: a prospective randomized clinical trial. Eur J Vasc Endovasc Surg. 2010;40:254–9.
38. Kabnick L. Outcome of different endovenous laser wavelengths for great saphenous vein ablation. J Vasc Surg. 2006;43:88–93.

Sclerotherapy for Varicose Veins

6

Tarun Grover

6.1 Introduction

Sclerotherapy is the term used to describe the process of injecting sclerosant into varicose veins to cause obliteration of its endothelium, thus resulting in closure of veins. Sclerotherapy aims to achieve endoluminal damage and cause vein wall fibrosis [1–5].

Wallois and Tournay are considered the first ones to start using liquid agent for sclerotherapy [6, 7]. In liquid sclerotherapy, small amount of special chemical is injected for closing small reticular veins and spider veins, mainly the ones which are 2–3 mm in size. The technique gained significant popularity in 1995 after Cabrera et al. started using foam prepared by mixing air with the detergent polidocanol for effectively causing obstruction of larger veins [8]. Guided Duplex ultrasound for foam sclerotherapy has been increasingly used for the management of primary as well as recurrent varicose veins now [9].

6.2 Method

During sclerotherapy, the patient is maintained in Trendelenburg position to empty out the veins being treated, and the foam is injected into the diseased vein [6]. The complete procedure is performed in the outpatient clinic. Mostly these procedures require 20–30 min depending on the size and number of veins being treated in one sitting. Usually the total amount of foam is restricted to 8 cc per leg. The procedure is followed by tight compression bandage. Good compression avoids formation of hard nodules over the injected area. Compression is usually maintained for 3–4 weeks.

6.3 Sclerosing Agents

Sclerosing chemicals result in fibrotic obstruction of veins by denaturation of endothelial wall which results in exposing the underneath collagen fibres. Endothelial damage is directly proportional to concentration of the solution used.

6.3.1 Osmotic Agents

Hyperosmolar sclerosing agents like hypertonic saline cause osmosis-mediated endothelial cell dehydration and death. Generally a concentration of 23.4% of sodium chloride is used.

6.3.2 Detergents

Detergents act by denaturation of proteins in the cell surface leading to endothelium

T. Grover
Division of Vascular and Endovascular Surgery,
Medanta Medicity Hospital, Gurugram, Haryana, India

A. K. Khanna, R. Jindal (eds.), *Venous Disorders*, https://doi.org/10.1007/978-981-13-1108-6_6

destruction. Sodium tetradecyl sulphate (STS) is a detergent with a long-chain fatty alcohol chemical structure. STS solution when injected is safe and painless. Polidocanol is a detergent which is very commonly used as a sclerotherapy agent, which also when injected is safe and painless. When used in low concentrations, it has a minimal risk of tissue necrosis. Though hyperpigmentation can occur, other complications like allergic or anaphylactic reactions occur rarely.

6.3.3 Alcohol Agents

Alcohol-based sclerosants are weak, and they damage the endothelium through contact and which is irreversible.

6.3.4 Liquid Sclerotherapy

Chemicals used for sclerotherapy have to be diluted before using them. While performing sclerotherapy of small veins like telangiectasia, the solution used must be of the lowest concentration. The concentrations of STS and polidocanol recommended are listed in Table 6.1.

While performing liquid sclerotherapy, one must use small-gauge needles (26G). One should start treating the larger varicose veins first followed by reticular veins and telangiectasias. The sequence of treating should begin in the proximal part of the limb followed by the distal limb. It is recommended that not more than 1 mL of the chemical is to be injected at one site. Also in each individual session, one should perform a maximum of 10–20 injections. Extravasation can cause severe pain while injecting at which time one should avoid any more injection [10].

Table 6.1 Indications and concentrations of sclerosing agents

Indications	Polidocanol	STS (sodium tetradecyl sulphate)
Varicosities <7–8 mm	1–3%	0.5–3.0%
Spider/reticular veins 2–4 mm	0.6–1.0%	0.25–0.5%
Telangiectasias 0.1–2.0 mm	0.25–0.6%	0.125–0.25%

6.3.5 Foam Sclerotherapy

Foam sclerotherapy is one of the minimally invasive techniques used for endovenous ablation of the saphenous vein. The report from the European Consensus Meetings on Foam Sclerotherapy showed that foam was a safe and effective minimally invasive endovenous procedure for varicose veins treatment and the complication rate is low [11, 12].

The method introduced by Tessari et al. has become very popular today, which uses a three-way which is connected to two syringes. It is recommended that the ratio of STS/polidocanol solution to air should be 1:4/5 [13, 14]. To create a bubble size of approximately 100 μm, the drug should be mixed from one syringe to another 20 times (Fig. 6.1).

The passage of foam through the veins can be monitored with the help of Duplex. Firstly, one should inject the saphenous trunk and subsequently the varicose veins and/or the perforators to be injected if required. The limb should

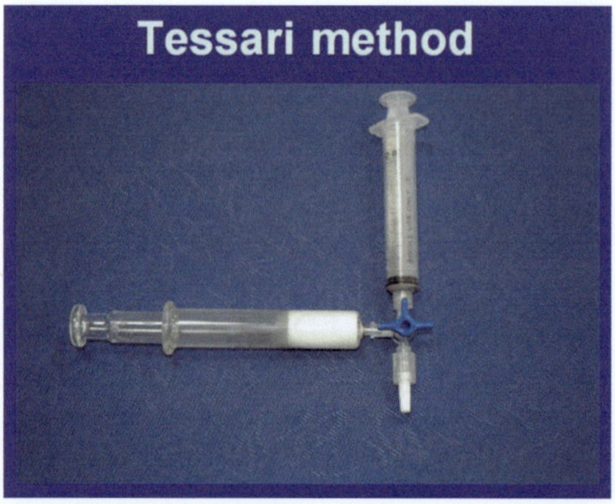

Fig. 6.1 Tessari method of preparation of foam sclerotherapy

be elevated for 10–15 min after injection as recommended by Bergan [14]. This minimises the amount of foam that enters the systemic circulation. It is recommended to apply a stretch bandage or 30–40 mmHg graduated compression stockings (or both) over the limb at the end of the procedure.

6.4 Patient Selection: Indications and Contraindications

Patient should be selected for foam sclerotherapy after studying the venous anatomy and based on the treatment aim. Most patients who have clinically significant varicosities can be treated with foam sclerotherapy, including elderly, obese, frail and ill patients. Obliterated deep veins and severe allergy are the only absolute contraindications. Table 6.2 lists some routine relative and absolute contraindications to foam sclerotherapy.

Table 6.2 Relative and absolute contraindications to foam sclerotherapy

Adverse patient factors (relative contraindications to treatment)
• Morbidly obese patients (BMI > 30)
• Patients of extreme age or frail
• Severe co-morbid diseases (malignancy, cardiovascular, respiratory)
• Known case of thrombophilia or history of prior DVT
• Patients with phobia to needles or those who prefer treatment under general anaesthesia
• Very thin patients may be left with lumps where the veins were obliterated following sclerotherapy and are less suitable for treatment
Adverse venous anatomy (relative contraindications to treatment)
• Severe post-thrombotic damage in the deep veins (little advantage of treating VVs)
• Very large varices (more complications of skin pigmentation and lumps following treatment)
• The lesion is an arteriovenous malformation (more difficult to treat)
Absolute contraindications to treatment
• Severe allergy to sclerosants
• Obliteration of deep vein system (e.g. following extensive previous DVT with no recanalization of deep veins)

6.5 Patient Consent

It's of utmost importance that the patients should be made aware of all treatment details and the complications associated with it. They should be informed about thrombophlebitis which may cause lumps. Skin pigmentation and the rare possibility of injection site ulceration should be informed. The consent should also include the occasional occurrence of visual disturbance, chest tightness and coughing. Though very uncommon, DVT and severe allergy should also be mentioned in the consent.

6.6 Treatment: Injecting the Foam

Using a scalp vein 21 g needle, superficial varicosities are injected first with 1% sclerosant foam. 1 mL is given per injection. Post injection, the Duplex linear probe can be used for gently massaging the injected area for uniform distribution of the foam through the varices. Foam is injected in all the previously placed butterflies, working from the calf towards the groin. Empty vein can be achieved by maintaining Trendelenburg's position or by lifting the leg well above the chest.

Passive dorsiflexion should be maintained to avoid the sclerosant entering the deep veins; postinjection patient should be encouraged to continue active dorsiflexion so that whatever foam has reached the deep veins can be washed away. Extravasation and the amount of foam entering the deep venous system can be monitored by ultrasound.

6.6.1 Compression Following Sclerotherapy

Crepe bandages or compression stockings are used over the treated leg for 2–3 weeks. Focal compression over the targeted area can be increased by placing a roller bandage between the layers of crepe. After each treatment session, the compression regimen should be repeated. Retained thrombus leading to hard nodular swelling and thrombophlebitis can result if the combination of crepe bandages is not used with compression stockings. One should encourage immediate mobilisation and resumption of day-to-day activity. Usually post procedure, no bed rest is warranted. All patients should be accompanied by some attendants to assist them travel safely back home.

6.6.2 Follow-Up Sessions

Post therapy, a 2-week interval is recommended for follow-up injections. Adverse consequences such as thrombophlebitis are best managed at this time. Duplex ultrasonography is performed of the treated leg to look for any thrombus in the femoral and popliteal veins. Foam sclerotherapy can be used for any residual segment of vein, which should be re-bandaged.

6.6.3 Treatment of Recurrent Varicose Veins After Surgery

Recurrent or residual varicosities are the ones which are clinically evident from the surgical incision proximally to popliteal fossa distally or even extending on to the lower leg. In such a situation, extensive surgical re-exploration and excision is not indicated. With more limited disease, ambulatory phlebectomy is suitable. Treating these recurrences of varicose veins after surgery is best performed with ultrasound-guided foam sclerotherapy. To avoid any nerve damage, this is the ideal treatment of choice since it avoids any unnecessary dissection in the popliteal fossa [15–17].

6.6.4 Treatment of Non-saphenous Reflux

Less than 10% of venous reflux is constituted by non-saphenous reflux, which commonly involves posterolateral thigh-buttock and occasionally perineum.

They form approximately 10% of venous disease. The tortuous and complex varicosities tend to be more symptomatic and painful [18]. Ultrasound-guided foam sclerotherapy is very useful in the management of aberrant varicosities or more commonly called non-saphenous vein reflux in the vaginal or pudendal and gluteal region [19]. Whenever reflux is observed from multiple sites, there is a high possibility of these patients having pelvic vein reflux. This would mandate further investigation to rule out ovarian vein incompetence. Rarely non-saphenous reflux could be caused by conditions that obstruct the venous flow back to the heart. May–Thurner syndrome (right common iliac artery compressing the left common iliac vein) and Nutcracker syndrome (compression of the left renal vein), along with some retroperitoneal tumours and iliac vein thrombosis, are some of the pathologies that impede the venous return.

6.7 Complications

Minor complications that are common include pain, pigmentation, allergy, skin urticaria and matting. The likelihood of hyperpigmentation is higher when higher concentration of the agent is used. Hyperpigmentation is a minor complication noted in up to 30% of the cases [20]. After 1 year of therapy, 70–95% of the pigmentations resolve [21]. Severe complications such as anaphylactic reaction, large areas of skin necrosis, pulmonary emboli, stroke and death are very rare (0.01%) [22]. Inadvertent arterial injection of the solution, deep vein thrombosis and nerve damage (saphenous, sural) are rare but severe complications [23]. Seen more frequently in patients with a patent foramen ovale, transient neurologic adverse effects can occur. These include visual disturbance, migraine-like headache, or confusional state [24]. In view of possible, but rare, allergic reactions and anaphylaxis after injection of a sclerosing solution, it is ideal to have an emergency protocol, oxygen, resuscitation equipments and drugs like steroids, cimetidine, epinephrine and diphenhydramine available.

6.8 Results

Liquid sclerosants have shown good early results for both reticular and varicose veins, but the status of the axial reflux decides the long-term efficacy of the same. The highest rate of recurrence was seen in those with untreated incompetent saphenous veins [25, 26]. Kern et al. reported the results of liquid sclerosants in 96 patients with telangiectasia and reticular veins. Elastic stockings for 3 weeks post treatment showed an early success rate of 76% [27].

Goldman compared the efficacy of polidocanol and STS, the liquid sclerosants used to treat telangiectasia and varicose veins and reported an average improvement by 70, and 70–72% in all vein categories were satisfied with the treatment with either solution [28].

Results of foam sclerotherapy are more encouraging than liquid sclerotherapy for the treatment of incompetent GSV. Rabe et al. reported the better efficacy and equal safety of 3% polidocanol foam over the 3% liquid sclerosant for the treatment of incompetent GSV in a multicentre RCT to evaluate the efficacy and safety of GSV sclerotherapy with standardized polidocanol foam [29].

A Cochrane review on sclerotherapy published in 2006 by Tisi et al. supported the current place of sclerotherapy in the modern clinical practice, which is usually limited to treat thread veins and recurrences after surgery [30].

6.8.1 Surgery vs Sclerotherapy

A Cochrane review done in 2004 by Rigby et al. to examine the results of surgery vs sclerotherapy for the treatment of varicose veins, reviewed 2306 references that included 61 comparative studies and 9 RCTs and observed that sclerotherapy was better at 1 year and surgery had a better outcome at 3–5 years. The meta-analysis concluded that there was insufficient evidence to preferentially recommend sclerotherapy for treatment of varicose veins over surgical treatment [31].

6.8.2 Surgery vs Endothermal Ablations vs Foam Sclerotherapy

In 2008, Luebke and Brunkwell carried out meta-analysis of endovenous laser ablation and radiofrequency ablation along with foam sclerotherapy for primary saphenous vein reflux [32]. The outcomes were analysed, and the results were compared to conventional open technique of high ligation and stripping. This meta-analysis involved 32 RFA, 29 EVLA and 22 sclerotherapy trials. Endovenous laser ablation and foam sclerotherapy established its superiority to radiofrequency ablation when compared to side effects like phlebitis, DVT and paraesthesia. Even the saphenous occlusion rate was better with endovenous laser ablation and foam sclerotherapy. Finally, the best occlusion rate among the three modalities was achieved by endovenous laser ablation with least chances of recurrent varicosities in patients having junctional incompetence of saphenofemoral and saphenopopliteal junctions. The conclusion made from this study has been that the short- and mid-term outcome of endovenous laser ablation, radiofrequency and foam sclerotherapy are good. In the future, large good-quality randomised control trial would be required to establish endovenous therapy as the standard of care for primary saphenous vein reflux disease.

Combination of endovenous laser therapy (EVLA) with foam sclerotherapy (FL) and without sclerotherapy was compared on 418 patients with 542 legs. Except for ecchymosis, incidence of other complications was not significantly different between both groups at 6 months. The EVLA/FS group exhibited more significant improvement in both AVVQ and EQ-5D scales than the EVLA group at 6 months while exhibiting poor improvement at 4 weeks. The EVLA/FS group had a significantly lower rate of residual varicosities than the EVLA group, thus reducing the need for the staged FS [33].

Conclusion

Sclerotherapy can be used in treating venous disease at every stage. Many sclerosants have unique properties, utilities and side effects. One should be aware of the differences between agents, accounting for disease presentation, vein characteristics and patient comorbidities when selecting the appropriate sclerosing agents.

Successful outcomes rely on proper patient evaluation and assessment for contraindications to sclerotherapy. Thorough patient education regarding realistic expectations with sclerotherapy in terms of symptoms relief, recurrence and improvement in appearance is of chief importance. Without any doubt, the technique of foam sclerotherapy is very effective and safe in the management of saphenous and non-saphenous vein reflux. There is adequate evidence in the published literature that sclerotherapy can be offered as a suitable treatment option for primary varicosities, recurrent varicose veins and patients with isolated perforator incompetence leading to lipodermatosclerosis. At present, most of the published data is supported by a limited follow-up to maximum of 3 years; hence, long-term clinical outcome at the end of 5 years remains uncertain.

References

1. McPheeters HO. Treatment of varicose veins; a twenty-five year reflection. Minn Med. 1956;39:271–5.
2. Sigg K, Zelikovski A. "Quick treatment": a modified method of sclerotherapy of varicose veins. Vasa. 1975;4:73–8.
3. Sigg K. Treatment of varicose veins and their complications. Dermatologica. 1950;100:315–20.
4. Fegan WG, Fitzgerald DE, Beesley WH. A modern approach to the injection treatment of varicose veins and its applications in pregnant patients. Am Heart J. 1964;68:757–64.
5. Fegan WG. Continuous compression technique of injecting varicose veins. Lancet. 1963;2:109–12.
6. Tournay R. Indications for a single sclerosing therapy or diphasic combined surgery-sclerosing therapy in varicose veins. Zentralbl Phlebol. 1965;87:133–42.
7. Wallois P. Incidents and accidents in the sclerosing treatment of varicose veins and their prevention. Phlebologie. 1971;24:217.
8. Cabrera Garido JR, Cabrera Garcia Olmedo JR, Olmedo DG. Nuevo metododel de esclerosis en las varices tronculares. Patol Vasculares. 1995;4:55–73.
9. Cabrera J, Redondo P, Becerra A, Garrido C, Cabrera J Jr, García-Olmedo MA, et al. Ultrasound-guided injection of polidocanol microfoam in the management of venous leg ulcers. Arch Dermatol. 2004;140:667–73.
10. Rabe E, Pannier-Fischer F, Gerlach H, Breu FX, Guggenbichler S, Zabel M, et al. Guidelines for sclerotherapy of varicose veins (ICD 10: I83.0, I83.1, I83.2, and I83.9). Dermatol Surg. 2004;30:687–93.
11. Breu FX, Guggenbichler S, Wollmann JC. European Consensus Meeting on Foam Sclerotherapy 2006, Tegernsee, Germany. Vasa. 2008;37(suppl 71):1–29.
12. Breu FX, Guggenbichler S. European Consensus Meeting on Foam Sclerotherapy, April 4–6, 2003, Tegernsee, Germany. Dermatol Surg. 2004;30:709–17.
13. Tessari L, Cavezzi A, Frullini A. Preliminary experience with a new sclerosing foam in the treatment of varicose veins. Dermatol Surg. 2001;27:58–60.
14. Bergan J. Sclerotherapy: a truly minimally invasive technique. Perspect Vasc Surg Endovasc Ther. 2008;20:70–2.
15. Perrin M, Gillet J-L. Management of recurrent varices at the popliteal fossa after surgical treatment. Phlebology. 2008;23(2):64–8.
16. Perrin MR, Guex JJ, Ruckley CV, et al. Recurrent varices after surgery (REVAS), a consensus document. Cardiovasc Surg. 2000;8(4):233–45.
17. Malgor RD, Labropoulos N. Pattern and types of non-saphenous vein reflux. Phlebology. 2013;28(Suppl 1):51–4.
18. Darvall KA, Bate GR, Adam DJ, Silverman SH, Bradbury AW. Duplex ultrasound outcomes following ultrasound-guided foam sclerotherapy of symptomatic recurrent great saphenous varicose veins. Eur J Vasc Endovasc Surg. 2011;42(1):107–14.
19. Paraskevas P. Successful ultrasound-guided foam sclerotherapy for vulval and leg varicosties secondary to ovarian vein reflux: a case study. Phlebology. 2011;26(1):29–31.
20. Munavalli GS, Weiss RA. Complications of sclerotherapy. Semin Cutan Med Surg. 2007;26:22–8.
21. Goldman MP, Sadick NS, Weiss RA. Cutaneous necrosis, telangiectatic matting, and hyperpigmentation following sclerotherapy: etiology, prevention, and treatment. Dermatol Surg. 1995;21:19–29.
22. Guex JJ. Complications and side-effects of foam sclerotherapy. Phlebology. 2009;24:270–4.
23. Bergan JJ, Weiss RA, Goldman MP. Extensive tissue necrosis following high-concentration sclerotherapy for varicose veins. Dermatol Surg. 2000;26:535–41.
24. Ceulen RP, Sommer A, Vernooy K. Microembolism during foam sclerotherapy of varicose veins. N Engl J Med. 2008;358:1525–6.

25. Hobbs JT. The treatment of varicose veins: a random trial of injection- compression therapy versus surgery. Br J Surg. 1968;55:777–80.
26. Chant AD, Jones HO, Weddell JM. Varicose veins: a comparison of surgery and injection-compression sclerotherapy. Lancet. 1972;2:1188–91.
27. Kern P, Ramelet AA, Wütschert R, Hayoz D. Compression after sclerotherapy for telangiectasias and reticular leg veins: a randomized controlled study. J Vasc Surg. 2007;45:1212–6.
28. Goldman MP. Treatment of varicose and telangiectatic leg veins: double-blind prospective comparative trial between aethoxyskerol and sotradecol. Dermatol Surg. 2002;28:52–5.
29. Rabe E, Otto J, Schliephake D, Pannier F. Efficacy and safety of great saphenous vein sclerotherapy using standardised polidocanol foam (ESAF): a randomised controlled multicentre clinical trial. Eur J Vasc Endovasc Surg. 2008;35:238–45.
30. Tisi PV, Beverley C, Rees A. Injection sclerotherapy for varicose veins. Cochrane Database Syst Rev. 2006;18(4):CD001732.
31. Rigby KA, Palfreyman SJ, Beverley C, Michaels JA. Surgery versus sclerotherapy for the treatment of varicose veins. Cochrane Database Syst Rev. 2004;18(4):CD004980.
32. Luebke T, Brunkwall J. Systematic review and meta-analysis of endovenous radiofrequency obliteration, endovenous laser therapy, and foam sclerotherapy for primary varicosis. J Cadiovasc Surg. 2008;49: 213–33.
33. Wang JC, Li Y, Li GY, Xiao Y, Li WM, Ma Q, Liu JL, Lu SY. A comparison of concomitant tributary laser ablation and foam sclerotherapy in patients undergoing truncal endovenous laser ablation for lower limb varicose veins. J Vasc Interv Radiol. 2018;29(6):781–9. https://doi.org/10.1016/j.jvir.2018.01.774. [Epub ahead of print].

Nerve Injury due to Endovenous Thermal Ablation for Varicose Veins

7

Shoaib F. Padaria

7.1 Introduction

Superficial venous insufficiency of the lower limbs is a common condition, involving up to 35% of women and 15% of men [1]. Ligation and stripping of the great saphenous vein (GSV) and small saphenous vein (SSV) at their junctions has been the standard of care for many decades. Surgery performed under general, spinal, epidural or, occasionally, regional anaesthesia was associated with a high recurrence rate of up to 40% at 5 years [2]. Nerve damage with patient complaints of post-operative pain was commonly reported in between 7 and 40% but was of clinical relevance in a smaller number of patients [3].

In the last two decades, less invasive methods such as endovenous laser ablation (EVLA) [4], radio frequency ablation (RFA) [5] and ultrasound-guided foam sclerotherapy [6] have been widely used with a view to reduce complications, costs and post-operative recovery period.

In the endovenous thermal ablation techniques, there is generation of heat energy inside the lumen of the vein, which serves to damage the endothelium and cause vein spasm, leading to permanent closure of the refluxing vein lumen.

The endovenous thermal procedure carries a small risk of peripheral nerve injury. The nerves which can be injured include the saphenous nerve, the sural nerve, the peroneal nerve, the tibial nerve and smaller branches. Neurological problems are usually obvious in the post-operative period and can be responsible for significant symptoms in some patients.

One of the commonest causes of litigation following VV surgery is due to alleged injury to various nerves [7].

The actual incidence and the natural history of nerve injuries are poorly described in literature. Certain questions need to be addressed.

a. Should nerve injury be regarded as unavoidable consequence of varicose vein treatment that can occur even with the most experienced operators?
b. What is the true incidence of nerve injury after varicose vein treatment?
c. Why do only a small percentage of patients with documented nerve injury develop symptoms of pain and dysesthesia, whilst the majority of them are asymptomatic?
d. What sort of specific treatment is required for nerve injury?
e. What are the steps to be taken to minimize the risk of nerve injury [8]?

S. F. Padaria
Department of Vascular Sciences, Jaslok Hospital and Research Centre, Mumbai, India

A. K. Khanna, R. Jindal (eds.), *Venous Disorders*, https://doi.org/10.1007/978-981-13-1108-6_7

7.2 Long Saphenous Vein and Saphenous Nerve Injury

7.2.1 Anatomy of the Saphenous Nerve

The saphenous nerve (L3, 4) descends along with the superficial femoral artery, and in the lower part of the adductor canal it lies deep to the sartorius muscle. An infrapatellar branch of the saphenous nerve innervates the skin medial to the knee and distal to the patellar. The main saphenous nerve pierces the deep fascia just above the knee and becomes superficial at the level of the knee between sartorius and gracilis muscles. In this area, the nerve lies deep and posterior to the long saphenous vein, separated from it by subcutaneous fat. Below this the saphenous nerve gets progressively more superficial and anterior and eventually lies adjacent to the long saphenous vein. This usually occurs about 2–3 cm below and medial to the tibial tuberosity, at the level of the Boyd perforator. Below this level the nerve and its branches are often wrapped around the long saphenous vein and its tributaries (Fig. 7.1).

A study by Murakami et al. [9] demonstrated that in the thigh the long saphenous vein rarely ran close to the saphenous vein. In the leg however, the long saphenous vein frequently ran close to the saphenous nerve, 59.5% in the middle third of the leg and in 83.1% of cases in the lower third of the leg. Furthermore, in the latter in 50% of cases, there was an adhesive association between the epineurium of the nerve and the adventitia of the LSV.

The saphenous nerve innervates the skin of the medial surface of the calf and the medial surface of the foot. Damage to the saphenous nerve usually causes sensory loss on the medial aspect of the calf, above the medial malleolus (Fig. 7.2).

Since the saphenous nerve runs adjacent to the long saphenous vein only in the calf, surgical stripping of the long saphenous vein to just below the knee has been historically performed, with minimal risk of nerve injury [10]. Endovenous thermal ablation of the long saphenous vein is therefore also usually performed up to just below the level of the knee joint.

Some patients will have significant reflux in the below-knee long saphenous vein and its major tributaries. Leaving such reflux alone leads to persistent incompetence in medial calf perforators [11, 12]. Therefore in those patients where there is demonstrable reflux in the below-knee long saphenous vein, endovenous thermal ablation may be performed up to the ankle.

7.2.2 Radio Frequency Ablation (RFA)

Radio frequency energy is used to close the long saphenous vein by heating the vessel wall to 120 °C [13].

Data has demonstrated lesser incidence of paraesthesia when the procedure is done up to the knee rather than up to the ankle [14]. This data was collected from 31 sites worldwide, and the assessment methods were not specified.

Paraesthesia incidence	12-month follow-up (%)	24-month follow-up (%)
Overall	3.9	5.6
VNUS up to knee	2.8	4.5
VNUS up to ankle	7.5	9.7

Goldman reported no paraesthesia in a series of 41 legs [5]; Weiss a prevalence of 8.5% (12/140) [13] and Fassiadis a prevalence of 33% (6/18) in limbs treated for recurrent long saphenous vein reflux [15]. Since details of the assessment methods are not described, the actual number of true saphenous nerve injury cases is not clear.

In summary, there is no evidence as yet to suggest that radio frequency ablation significantly reduces the incidence of saphenous nerve injury as compared to surgery. However since the thermal energy is confined to the vessel wall, it is likely that the injury to the nerves is less than compared to surgery in which there may be shear damage to the nerve, especially in the below-knee segments.

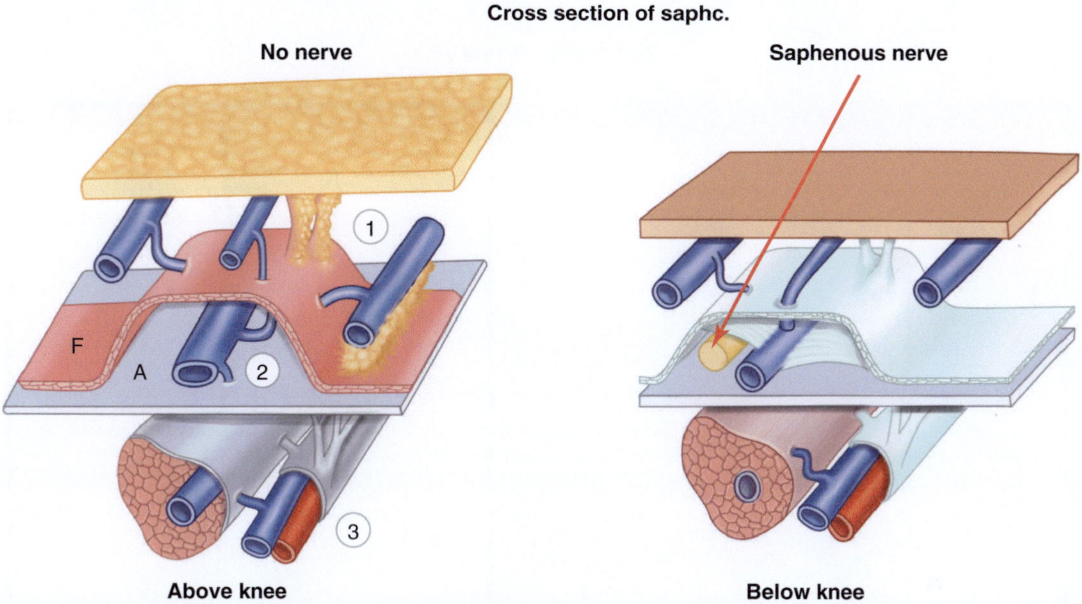

Fig. 7.1 Relation of long saphenous vein to saphenous nerve

7.2.3 Endovenous Laser Thermal Ablation (EVLT)

Endovenous laser ablation uses pulsed light energy to obliterate the long saphenous vein.

A study by Beale was performed [16] to demonstrate the safety of heat energy generated by laser within the vein. Twelve patients underwent treatment of the long saphenous vein using laser. Thermocouples were placed at distances of 3, 5 and 10 mm away from the long saphenous vein, which was then treated by laser after injection of adequate amount of tumescent anaesthesia. In experimental models, an intravascular temperature of up to 1334 °C was recorded. In this study, the median temperatures in the surrounding tissues were 34.5, 33.7 and 31.1 °C at 3, 5 and 10 mm away from the long saphenous vein. This study therefore confirmed that heat energy was not transmitted away from the vein lumen in significant amount to be responsible for any soft tissue or neural damage.

Proebstle treated 31 legs with long saphenous vein reflux and did not have any case of nerve injury [17]. In a series of 90 legs, treated by Min et al. there was a single case of paraesthesia involving the medial calf, which resolved completely at 6 weeks [18].

7.3 Small Saphenous Vein and the Sural Nerve

It has been shown that up to 20% of patients of varicose veins have reflux in the small saphenous vein [19].

Study results of thermal ablation of the long saphenous vein may not be applicable to the small saphenous vein since there are anatomical differences between the sapheno-femoral junction and the sapheno-popliteal junction, as well as the proximity of the sural nerve to the small saphenous vein.

There are three anatomic patterns of the small saphenous vein [20].

Type A: Sapheno-popliteal junction with no significant branches of the small saphenous vein.

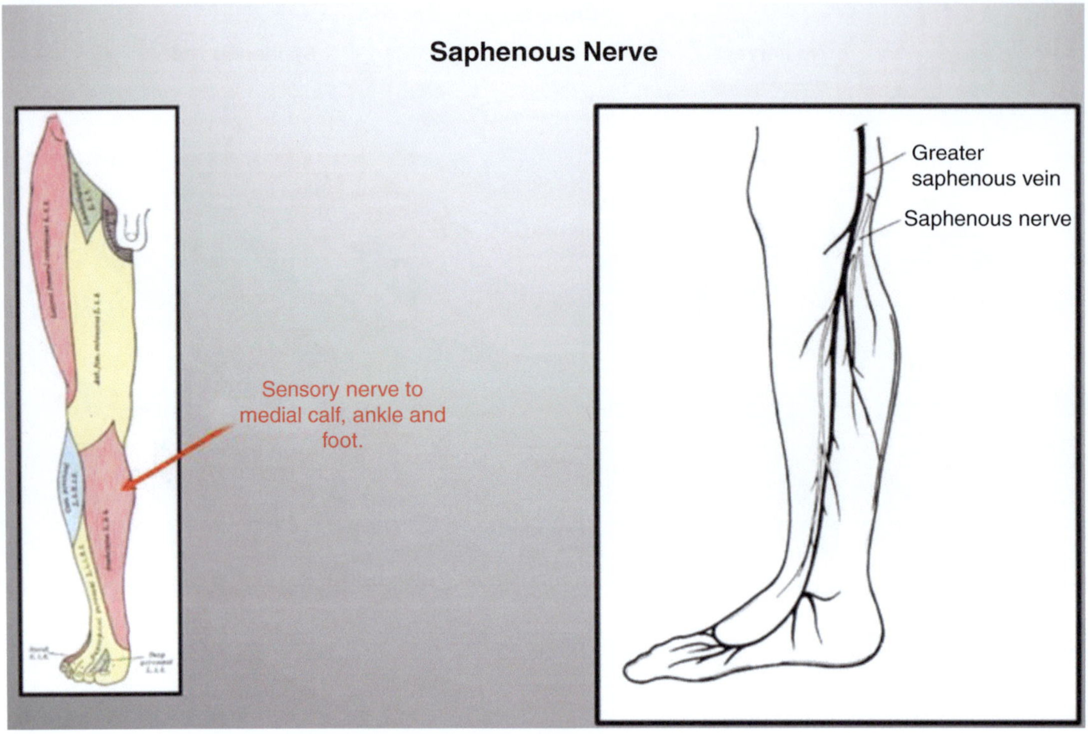

Fig. 7.2 Relation of saphenous nerve to long saphenous nerve

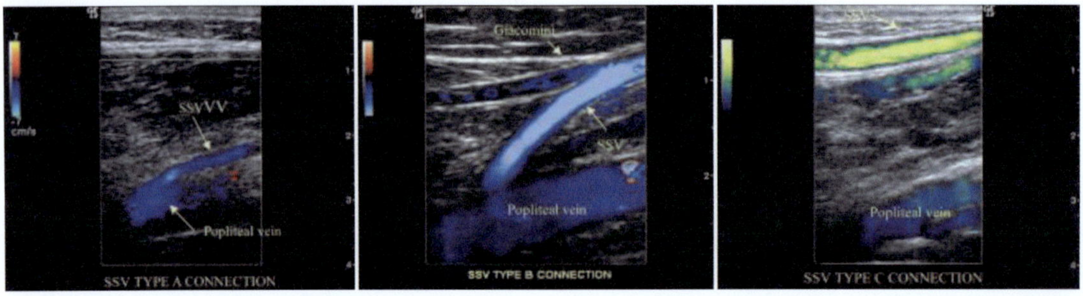

Fig. 7.3 Anatomical pattern of short saphenous vein

Type B: Sapheno-popliteal junction with a large cranial extension of the small saphenous vein—Giacomini vein.

Type C: No direct termination of the small saphenous vein into a deep vein (sapheno-popliteal or sapheno-femoral junction), and the small saphenous vein continues as a Giacomini vein above the popliteal fossa (Fig. 7.3).

7.3.1 Anatomy of the Sural Nerve

The sural nerve arises from the tibial nerve in the popliteal fossa, and then travels in the back of the leg to the posterior surface of the lateral malleolus.

The sural nerve lies below the deep fascia on the lateral head of gastrocnemius and then travels caudally to lie in the groove between

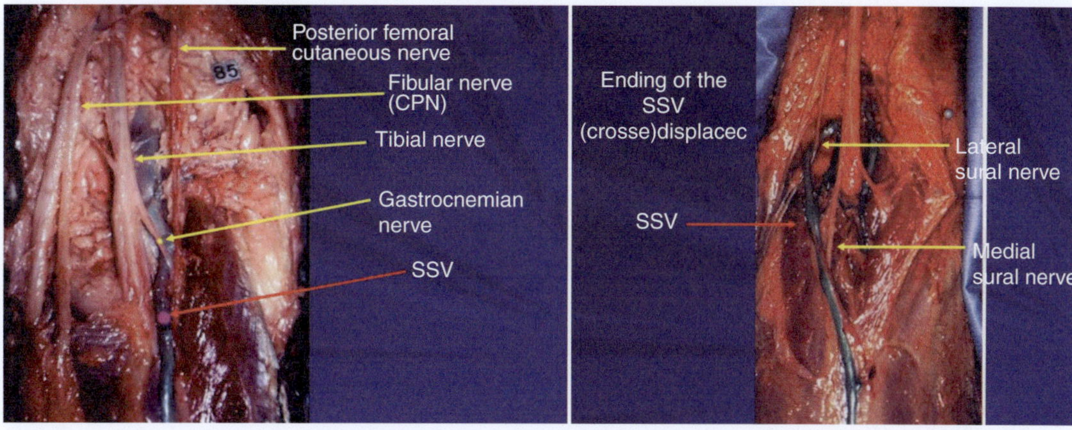

Fig. 7.4 Relation of nerves to short saphenous vein

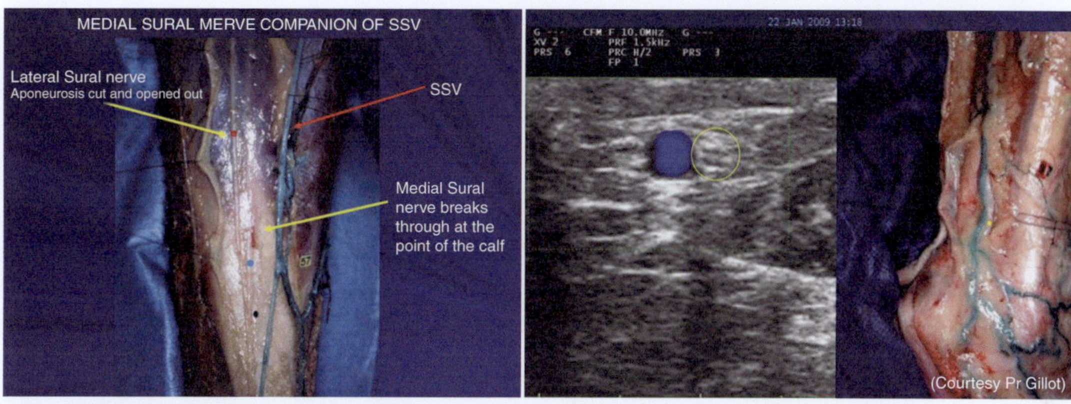

Relationship of Medial Sural Nerve to SSV

Sural nerve at the lateral malleolus (stuck to the SSV)

Fig. 7.5 Relation of sural nerves to short saphenous vein

the two heads of gastrocnemius, lateral to the small saphenous vein. In the middle third of the calf, it pierces the deep fascia after it joined by a branch of the peroneal nerve and lies superficially. The sural nerve lies close to and lateral to the small saphenous vein throughout its length especially in the lower third. The sural nerve innervates the skin of the lower half of the posterior aspect of the leg, the lateral part of the dorsum of the foot and the lateral side of the little toe (Figs. 7.4 and 7.5).

Damage to the sural nerve due to thermal ablation can cause troublesome numbness or it can cause significant burning and pain in the heel and lateral aspect of the foot (Figs. 7.6 and 7.7).

There are some concerns about usage of thermal ablation in the treatment of small saphenous vein reflux, due to the proximity of the sural nerve to the small saphenous vein as well as concern about popliteal vein thrombosis. Only 1.6% of patients in Gibson's study of endovenous laser treatment of the small saphenous vein complained of numbness at the 6-week follow-up. Of these, only in one patient could EVLT alone be implicated in causing numbness. In all the patients, the numbness was not of any significant discomfort. Gibson also demonstrated that a substantial fascial sheath surrounds the small saphenous vein, which eases the creation of adequate tumescence of the small saphenous vein, separating the sural

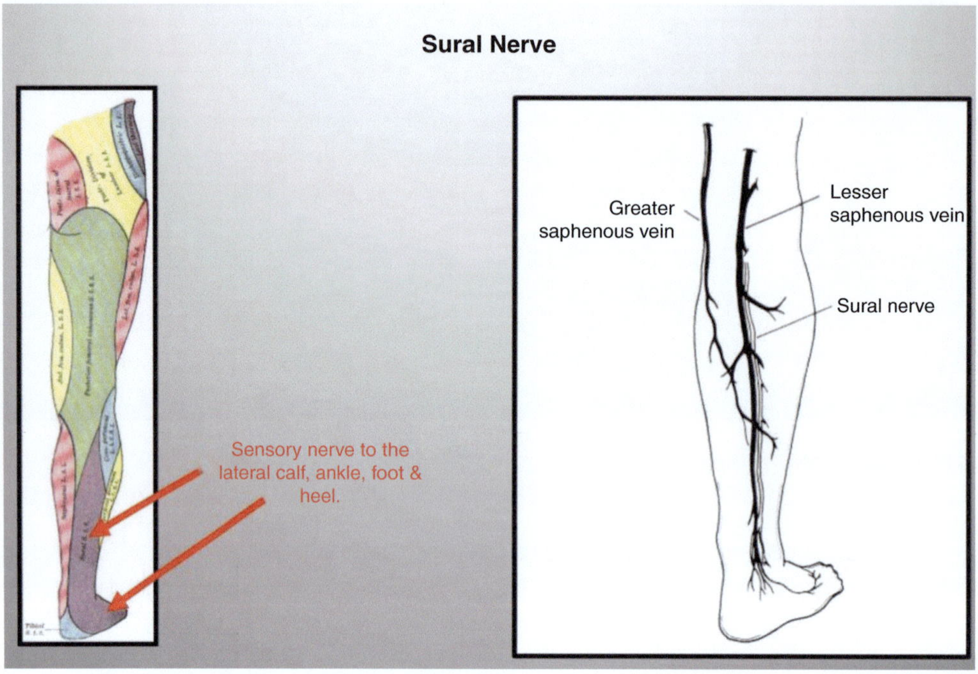

Fig. 7.6 Relation of sural nerve to short saphenous vein

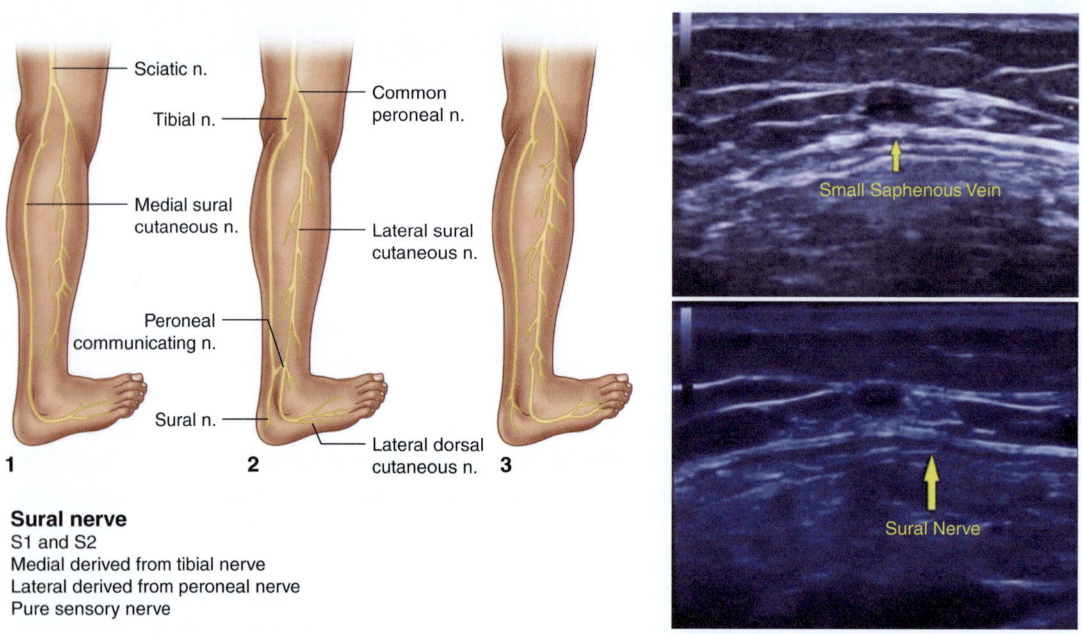

Fig. 7.7 Sural nerve

nerve from the small saphenous vein. This is the likely reason why the incidence of sural nerve injury was low in this study.

Proebstle et al. [21] reported paraesthesia in 11% of 33 patients who had small saphenous vein treatment with EVLT. The duration of paraesthesia ranged from 3 to 8 weeks, with a mean duration of 6.5 weeks.

There are 15 specific studies of nerve injury due to laser treatment of small saphenous vein with values ranging from 1.6 to 11%, with an average of 4%. In the vast majority of these cases, there is a sensory loss due to involvement of the sural nerve.

	Patients	F-U	Occlusion (%)	Paraesthesia	DVT
Roopram 2013	118EVLA	6 W	91/67	6.7/31%	1
Samuel 2013	53 EVLA	12 M	96.2	7.5%	
Doganol 2011	60 (68) 30Mal/30Mid-calf	6 M	100	20% malleolus 3.5% mid-calf (2 W)	0 0
D'Othée 2009	67 (63)		100	2%	4 (4%)
Desmyterre 2009	128 (147)	3 Y	97	40% (2 W)	0
Huismans 2008	150	3 M	98	1.3%	0
Trip-Hoving 2009	52 (49)	6.5 M	100	6%	1
Kontothanassis 2008	204 (229)	16 M	98.7	2.25%	3
Park 2008	84 (96)	12 M	96	4.2%	0
Nwaejike 2008	66	14 M	100	0%	0
Park 2008	108 (390)	12 M	94	2.6%	0
Gibson 2007	120 (210)	4 M	96	1.6%	12
Theivacumar 2006	48 (68)	6 M	100	4.4%	0
Ravi 2006	37 (101)	3Y	84		
Proebstle 2003	35 (41)	3 M	100	11% (4–8 w)	1

7.3.2 Common Peroneal Nerve and Tibial Nerve

The commonest nerve injury, accounting for about 50% of cases following varicose vein surgery, is to the common peroneal nerve. It is usually damaged just before or, as it crosses the neck of the fibula. The common peroneal nerve can be involved in 2–4.7% of cases of small saphenous vein surgery [22]. Common peroneal nerve injury can produce serious disability as it contains both motor and sensory fibres and can lead to permanent foot drop (Fig. 7.8).

Proximal to the knee joint, the sciatic nerve divides into the tibial and common peroneal nerves. Above the knee, the common peroneal nerve leaves the tibial nerve and travels obliquely along the lateral side of the popliteal fossa to the fibular head. It curves lateral to the fibular neck and divides into superficial and deep peroneal nerves. The common peroneal nerve is relatively superficial and remains unprotected as it traverses the lateral aspect of the head of the fibula, and it is easily compressed at this site. Thermal ablation of superficial varicosities in the region of the head of the fibula may lead to damage to the common peroneal nerve, although it is very rarely seen.

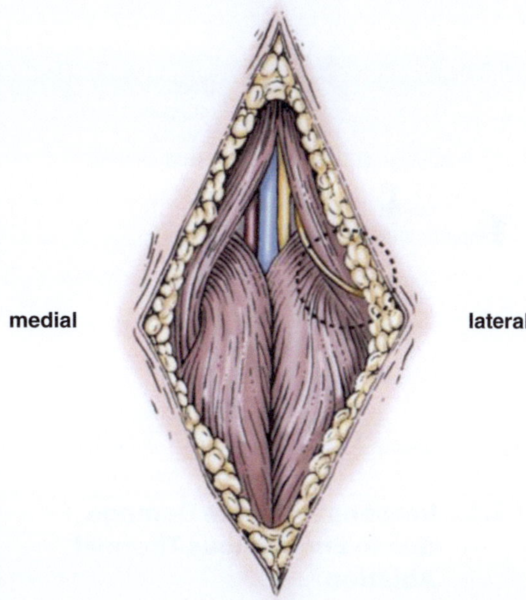

Fig. 7.8 Course of the common peroneal nerve in the popliteal fossa. Dotted area shows maximum place of injury

The higher the termination of the small saphenous vein, the closer is the tibial nerve. In such situations, it is imperative to be very careful when performing thermal ablation of the small saphenous vein (Figs. 7.9 and 7.10).

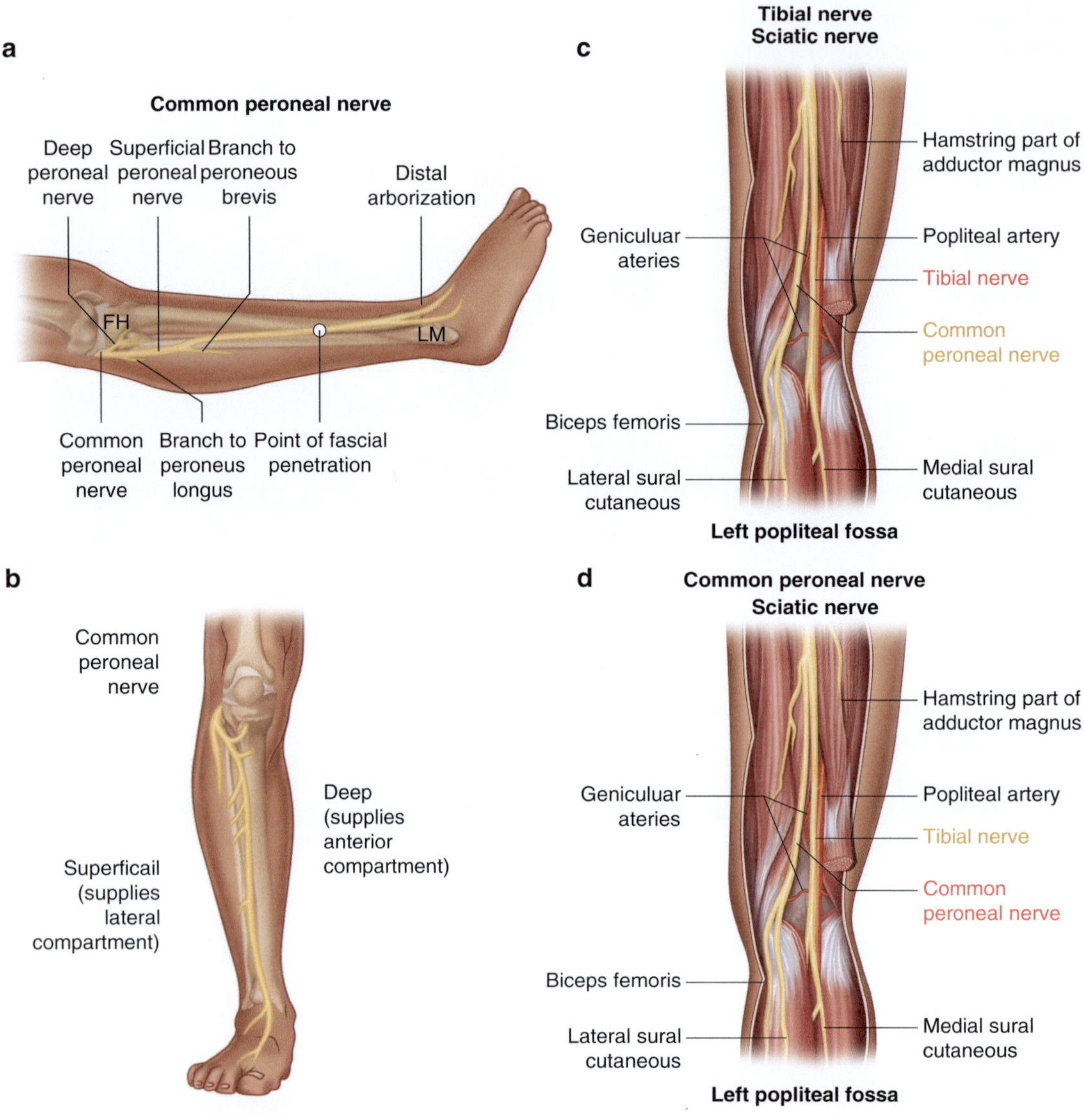

Fig. 7.9 Anatomy of common peroneal and tibial nerve

7.3.3 Reasons for Nerve Damage due to Endovenous Thermal Ablation

There are three main reasons why damage can occur to nerves during endovenous thermal ablation procedure.

1. Needle stick injury during vein cannulation
2. Needle stick injury during administration of tumescent anaesthesia
3. Heat transfer during endovenous thermal ablation.

7.3.4 Strategies to Prevent Nerve Injury

1. Know the anatomic lie of the veins and nerves—determine level of vein entry.
   - In case of the long saphenous vein, it is preferable to cannulate it just below the knee joint. In cases where the reflux is demonstrable to a lower level, entry may be even above the ankle; at this level a smaller gauge needle is used for initial cannulation.
   - For the small saphenous vein, it is preferable to cannulate the vein at the mid-calf

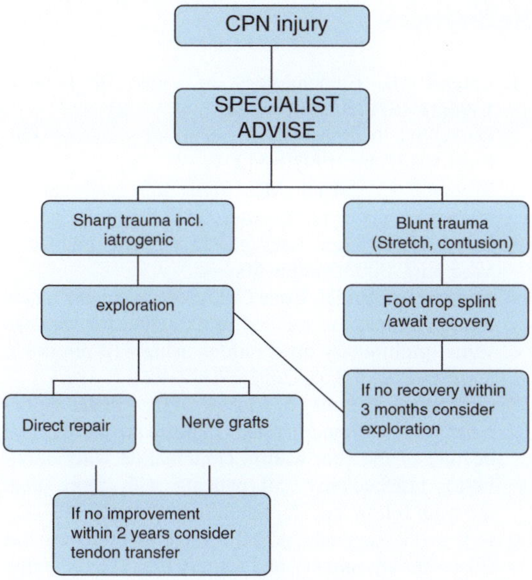

Fig. 7.10 Management of common peroneal nerve injury. Eur J Vasc Endovasc Surg Vol 31, April 2006

level. If the vein below this level is dilated, then foam sclerotherapy may be used to ablate the lower segment of the vein.

2. Observe the vein and nerve by ultrasound, during cannulation and delivery of anaesthetic.
   - A higher-frequency ultrasound probe is very useful in adequately identifying the veins and nerves, especially the sural nerve in the calf. Accurate identification of the vein aids cannulation as well as delivery of tumescent anaesthesia into the saphenous sheaths.
3. Withdraw the needle immediately if patient has sharp pain.
   - Pain usually denotes that the needle has touched the nerve fibres. In such cases, either the level of cannulation is changed or the vein is approached from a different angle in order to avoid the nerve.
4. Adequate amount of delivery of tumescent to separate the nerves from the vein.
   - Adequate amount of delivery of tumescent anaesthesia around the vein to be ablated is the key to successful outcome of the treatment, as well as avoidance of nerve damage.

7.4 The Natural History and Prognosis of Nerve Damage

In most patients the area of paraesthesia due to nerve injury improves over time. A small number of patients however develop a disturbing syndrome, sometimes called saphenous and sural neuritis.

7.5 Treatment of Symptoms due to Nerve Injury

In the vast majority of cases, the symptoms due to injury to the saphenous or sural nerve are sensory in origin, usually in the form of altered sensation to the affected area, or, in a smaller group of patients, pain. Most of the symptoms tend to ablate within a few days or weeks, although in a small number they tend to persist for few months and are quite disturbing. Application of ice pack to the affected area helps significantly. Medications may need to be prescribed in a few patients for relief.

Choosing which pain medication is applicable depends on whether the pain is caused by inflammation (nociceptive pain) or a disorder of the nerve tissue (neuropathic pain). Moreover, the choice of pain medication is also dependent on other factors that can negatively influence pain, such as fear and depression.

7.5.1 Medications for Nociceptive Pain

In the acute phase (first 3 months):

- NSAIDs
- Paracetamol
- COX-2-inhibitors

In the chronic phase (more than 3 months):

- Tricyclic anti-depressive drugs
- Weak opioids
- Opioids

7.5.2 Medications for Neuropathic Pain

Depending on the findings of the neurological examination for neuropathic pain, various kinds of medication can be prescribed.

- Anticonvulsive drugs
- Antiarrhythmic drugs
- Tricyclic anti-depressive drugs
- Topical anaesthetics
- Baclofen
- Opioids
- Clonidine
- NMDA antagonists

In severe cases, local anaesthetic nerve blocks may be used, especially in cases of sural nerve injury which causes pain and difficulty in walking.

Conclusion

1. Cutaneous nerve injury during endovenous thermal ablation of varicose veins occurs in a small number of patients, even with experienced operators. In the vast majority of cases, it is a sensory affection, and patients should be made aware of this possible complication. It is a small but disturbing problem.
2. Thermal ablation of the long saphenous vein to just below the level of the knee offers the optimum balance between undertaking an effective treatment and minimizing the risk of saphenous nerve injury.
3. Thermal ablation of the small saphenous vein can be safely performed up to the level of the mid-calf. Below this level, there is a real chance of injury to the sural nerve, and excellent and accurate ultrasound visualization of the vein and nerve is required for safe treatment.
4. None of the newer, minimally invasive, thermal techniques appear to afford significant protection against cutaneous nerve injury as compared to routine surgery.
5. The natural history of saphenous nerve and sural nerve injury following endovenous thermal ablation of varicose veins is unknown.

References

1. Callam MJ. Epidemiology of veins. Br J Surg. 1994;81:167–73.
2. Darke SG. Morphology of recurrent varicose vein. Eur J Vasc Surg. 1992;6:512–7.
3. Morrison C, Dalsing MC. Signs and symptoms of saphenous nerve injury after GSV stripping, prevalence, severity and relevance to modern practice. J Vasc Surg. 2003;38:886–90.
4. Navarro L, Min RJ, Boné C. Endovenous laser a new minimally invasive method of treatment for varicose veins- preliminary observations using 810 nm diode laser. Dermatol Surg. 2001;27:117–22.
5. Goldman MP, Amiry S. Closure of the greater saphenous vein with endoluminal radiofrequency thermal heating of the vein wall in combination with ambulatory phlebectomy: 50 patients with more than 6-month follow-up. Dermatol Surg. 2002;28:29–31.
6. Belcaro G, Nicolaides AN, Ricci A, et al. Endovascular sclerotherapy, surgery and surgery plus sclerotherapy in superficial venous incompetence: a randomized, 10 year follow up trial- final results. Angiology. 2000;51:529–34.
7. Campbell WB, France F, Goodwin HM. Medicolegal claims in vascular surgery. Ann R Coll Surg Engl. 2002;84:181–4.
8. Sam RC, et al. Eur J Vasc Endovasc Surg. 2004;27:113–20.
9. Murakami G, Negishi N, et al. Okajimas Folia Anat Jpn. 1994;71(1):21–33.
10. Lees TA, Beard JD, Ridler BMF, Szymanska T. A survey of the current management of varicose veins by members of the Vascular Surgical Society. Ann R Coll Surg Engl. 1999;81:407–17.
11. MacKenzie RK, Paisley A, Allan PL, Lee AJ, Ruckley CV, Bradbury AW. The effect of long saphenous vein stripping on quality of life. J Vasc Surg. 2002;35:1197–203.
12. Stuart WP, Adam DJ, Allan PL, Ruckley CV, Bradbury AW. Saphenous surgery does not correct perforator incompetence in the presence of deep venous reflux. J Vasc Surg. 1998;28:834–8.
13. Weiss RA, Weiss MA. Controlled radiofrequency endovenous occlusion using a unique radiofrequency catheter under duplex guidance to eliminate saphenous varicose vein reflux: a 2-year follow-up. Dermatol Surg. 2002;28(1):38–42.
14. Merchant RF, dePalma RG, Kabnick LS. Endovascular obliteration of saphenous reflux: a multicentre study. J Vasc Surg. 2002;35:1190–6.
15. Fassiadis N, Kianifard B, Holdstock JM, Whiteley MS. A novel approach to the treatment of recurrent varicose veins. Int Angiol. 2002;21:275–6.
16. Beale RJ, Mavor AID, Gough MJ. Heat dissipation during endovenous laser treatment of varicose veins: is there a risk of nerve injury? Phlebology. 2006;21:32–51.
17. Proebstle TM, Lehr HA, Kargl A, Espinola-Klein C, Rother W, Bethge S, et al. Endovenous treatment of the greater saphenous vein with a 940-nm diode laser:

thrombotic occlusion after endoluminal thermal damage by laser-generated steam bubbles. J Vasc Surg. 2002;35:729–36.
18. Min RJ, Zimmet SE, Isaacs MN, Forrestal MD. Endovenous laser treatment of the incompetent greater saphenous vein. J Vasc Interv Radiol. 2001;12:1167–71.
19. Englehorn CA, Englehorn AL, Cassou MF, Salles-Cunha SX. Patterns of saphenous reflux in women with varicose veins. J Vasc Surg. 2005;41:645–51.
20. Gibson KD, et al. Endovenous laser treatment of the short saphenous vein: efficacy and complications. J Vasc Surg. 2007;45(4):795.
21. Proebstle TM, Gul D, Karg l A, Knop J. Endovenous laser treatment of the lesser saphenous vein with a 940 nm diode laser: early results. Dermatol Surg. 2003;29:357–61.
22. Lucerni G, et al. Injury to the CPN during surgery of the SSV. Phlebology. 1999;14:26–8.

Endothermal Heat-Induced Thrombosis

8

Vijay Thakore, Hiral Varnami, and Karan Thakore

8.1 Introduction/Overview

Superficial venous insufficiency of lower extremity is one of the common vascular problems most of the vascular specialists come across in clinical practice. Recently, endovenous ablation (EVA) of the saphenous vein is the mainstay of treatment in symptomatic varicose veins due to its noninvasiveness, faster recovery time, fewer complications, and improved quality of life [1].

Due to recent advances in ultrasound, radiofrequency, and laser technology, EVA has become an attractive alternative to traditional surgery. However, EVA has its own complications such as ecchymosis, bruising, thrombophlebitis, nerve injury, deep venous thrombosis, and pulmonary embolism. Endothermal heat-induced thrombosis (EHIT) of GSV is an expected outcome of EVA, but its extension to deep venous system causing deep vein thrombosis (DVT) is unclear. The incidence reported in literature varies from 0 to 16% [2]. Though physicians are aware about EHIT, there is no clear verdict about the clinical outcome and consequences of the same. As etiology and natural history are different from that of unprovoked DVT, various aspects of EHIT of deep veins like incidence, risk factors, role of post-procedure Doppler ultrasound, timing of EHIT, and treatment guidelines are not well established.

In EVA, the heat caused by reaction, together with the steam bubbles, destroys the endothelial lining of vein wall causing an inflammatory reaction. A subsequent thrombotic occlusion closes off the vein and leads to eventual fibrosis. Various wavelengths of laser work on different segments such as 810 nm is specific for hemoglobin, and 980 nm is specific for hemoglobin and water, whereas 1470 nm is specific for water. Different variables of laser like wavelength, power, energy, different mode of energy delivery, type of laser fiber (bare-tip or radial), etc. are also not studied so far to with regard to EHIT.

Due to relatively short learning curve and excellent patient satisfaction, EVA has become very appealing to patients and physicians, both. The safety and efficacy of these procedures is also either equal to or better than traditional surgery [3]. Despite the encouraging results of EVA, there is a concern by physicians over the incidence of DVT and the potential risk of pulmonary embolism following these procedures. EHIT of the GSV is an expected outcome following EVA; what remains unclear is the clinical consequences of EHIT at or near saphenofemoral junction. There are reports in the literature about the progression of de novo superficial venous thrombophlebitis of GSV into deep venous system and

V. Thakore (✉) · H. Varnami
Angiocare VINS Hospital, Baroda, Gujarat, India

K. Thakore
Department of Surgery, Karamsad Medical College, Baroda, Gujarat, India

A. K. Khanna, R. Jindal (eds.), *Venous Disorders*, https://doi.org/10.1007/978-981-13-1108-6_8

potential risk of pulmonary embolism [4]. This has prompted a debate regarding the treatment of superficial vein thrombosis.

8.2 Our Experience

From January 2016 to December 2016, we examined 178 consecutive patients prospectively for the occurrence and outcome of EHIT. All the patients were from C4 to C6 group. In our study, 68% were males and 32% were females. Mean age of all patient is 45.7 years. Eighty-eight percent of patients underwent endoablation for GSV and 12% of patients for SSV. Seventy-seven percent of patients underwent laser ablation, and 23% of patients underwent radiofrequency ablation. Eight-nine percent of patients were given femoral nerve block with tumescent anesthesia. Eleven percent of patients were given spinal anesthesia. Eighty percent of patients had adjuvant hook phlebectomies and 95% adjuvant foam sclerotherapy.

Most of the patients underwent either laser ablation with 1470 nm laser with radial fiber with the machine settings being signal mode, 8 W of power, and 80 J of energy per cm of vein. In most of the patients, the distance between the tip of laser fiber/RFA fiber and the saphenofemoral junction was between 2.0 and 2.5 cm. Tumescent anesthesia was given to all patients.

All patients were examined by duplex ultrasound after 10 and 30 days of the procedure. We found total incidence of EHIT in our study was 3/178 patients.

One patient with EHIT class 4 was treated with oral anticoagulation (rivaroxaban) and compression stockings for 6 months. A duplex ultrasound performed at 6 months showed complete resolution of DVT. Another patient presented very late, i.e., 2 months after the procedure with iliofemoral DVT. She underwent catheter-directed thrombolysis with endovenectomy followed by oral anticoagulation (rivaroxaban) for 6 months.

8.3 Discussion

To certain extent, EHIT can be compared to superficial vein thrombophlebitis. SVT is relatively a benign disease which can be treated with analgesics, anti-inflammatory medications, and ice/gel application, whereas some people have reported 11–33% incidence of progression of SVT to DVT and pulmonary embolism prompting them to treat with anticoagulation [5, 6]. Based on these studies, treatment of GSV thrombophlebitis is recommended with anticoagulation and/or SF J ligation, when it is in proximity to the SF junction.

With paradigm shift in the treatment of varicose veins by endoablation, thrombus formation into the common femoral vein secondary to thermal injury has become reality. Various groups have reported the incidence of EHIT from 0 to 16% [7, 8]. Meta-analysis from 13 randomized trials have shown overall incidence of DVT 0.85%; however, occurrence of EHIT-DVT is 3.5 times more frequent than non-EHIT-DVT [7].

Kabnick et al. have developed and defined the classification of EHIT which is as follows.

Class 1. Venous thrombosis to the superficial-deep vein junction (i.e., saphenofemoral junction or saphenous-popliteal junction, but not extending into the deep system)

Class 2. Nonocclusive venous thrombosis with an extension into the deep system of a cross-sectional area of less than 50%

Class 3. Nonocclusive venous thrombosis into deep venous system with an extension into the deep system of a cross-sectional area of more than 50%

Class 4. Occlusive deep vein thrombosis of the common femoral vein [9]

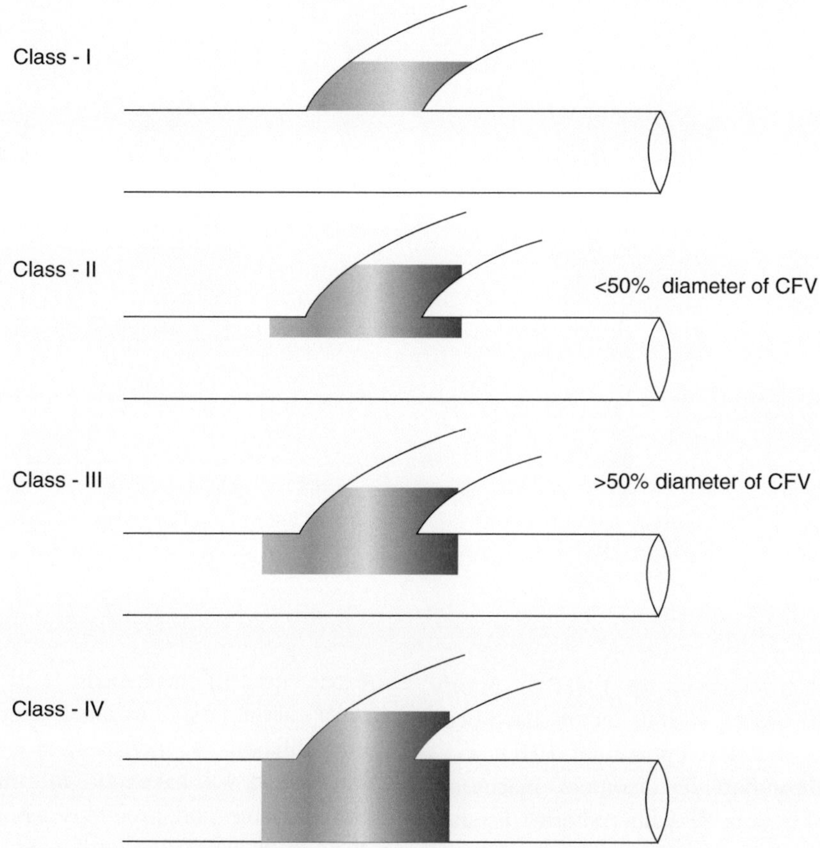

The thrombus produced by thermal injury has a different echogenicity than de novo DVT. EHIT clots are more echogenic as compared to de novo clots. Moreover, EHIT clots are more stable and do regress or disappear completely.

Based on this classification, treatment algorithm is suggested which is as follows. Duplex ultrasound is recommended after 1 week of the procedure, and if EHIT is found in class 1, the patient is advised serial duplex ultrasound every month until clot regresses. If EHIT 2 is found, LMWH is advised for 2 weeks, and duplex ultrasound is done after 2 weeks. If clot regression is found, LMWH treatment is discontinued. If clot still persists, LMWH is continued till clot disappears on duplex ultrasound which is performed every week. IF EHIT 3 and EHIT 4 are found, it should be treated like any other provoked DVT as per guidelines with full anticoagulation [10, 11].

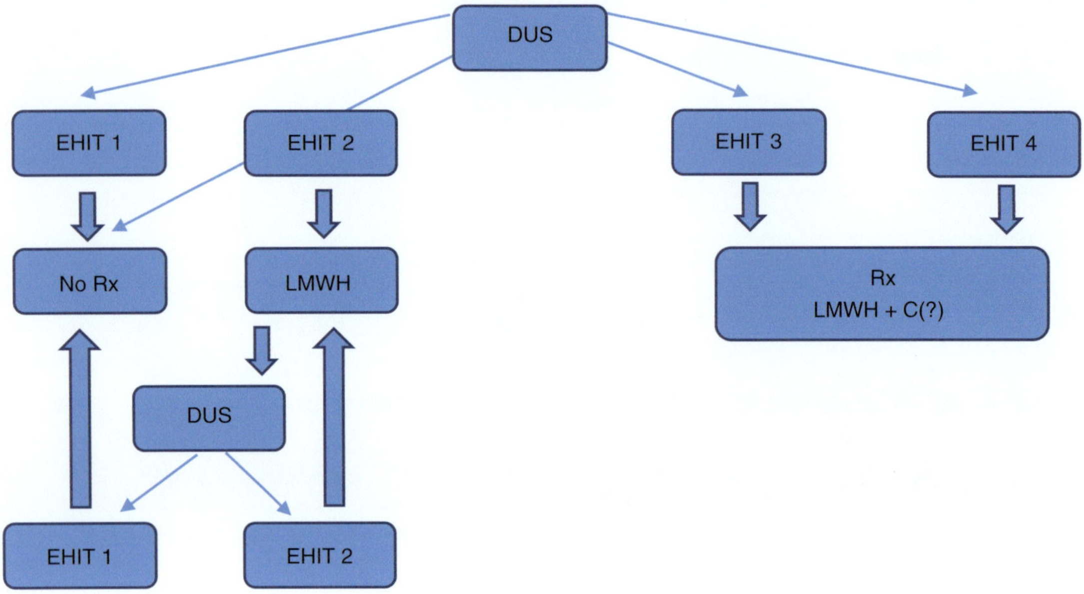

The exact mechanism for EHIT is poorly understood. However, various factors have been suggested for the development of EHIT, viz., preexisting thrombophilia disorders, inaccurate positioning of laser or RFA fiber, shorter distance from SF junction, use of general/epidural/spinal anesthesia, large diameter of vein, adjuvant hook phlebectomies, etc. [8, 12]. To reduce the incidence of EHIT, people have suggested administration of LMWH before or after endoablation. Knipp et al. did not show any significant reduction of EHIT with prophylactic heparin administration [13]. Some people have also recommended placement of laser fiber or RFA fiber little more than 2 cm, i.e., 2.5 cm away from SF junction to reduce the incidence of EHIT.

Still there are few unanswered questions about EHIT like whether the thrombus resolves, retracts, or embolizes which remain to be determined. Though we know theoretically EHIT does occur, its clinical significance is unknown.

Conclusion

Thrombosis due to thermal injury behaves completely different than de novo thrombosis. It also has a different ultrasonic echogenicity. There is a classification to categorize the extent of thrombosis. As we do not know the exact cause of mechanism [12], we are not clear about the treatment guidelines. As endoablation is increasing by heaps and bounds, we will have more information about the outcome and problems associated with that. With larger and systematic experience, we should be able to make clear recommendations about treatment options.

References

1. Kundu S, Lurie F, Millward SF, Padberg F Jr, Vedantham S, Elias S, et al. Recommended reporting standards for endovenous ablation for the treatment of venous insufficiency: joint statement of the American Venous Forum and The Society of Interventional Radiology. J Vasc Surg. 2007;46:582–9.
2. Berland TL, Hakaim AG, Oldenburg WA, et al. Thrombus extension into common femoral vein following endovenous ablation of great saphenous vein for the treatment of venous insufficiency. J Vasc Ultrasound. 2006;30(3):129–31.
3. Puggioni A, Kalra M, Carmo M, Mozes G, Gloviczki P. Endovenous laser therapy and radiofrequency ablation of great saphenous vein: analysis of early efficacy and complications. J Vasc Surg. 2005;42(3): 488–93.
4. Jorgensen JO, Hanel KC, Morgan AM, Hunt JM. The incidence of deep venous thrombosis in patients with superficial thrombophlebitis of the lower limbs. J Vasc Surg. 1999;24(5):745–9.

5. Chengelis DL, Bendick PJ, Golver JL, Brown OW, Ranval TJ. Progression of superficial venous thrombosis to deep vein thrombosis. J Vasc Surg. 1996;24(5):745–9.
6. Gale SS, Dosick SM, Seiwert AJ, Comerota AJ. Regarding "Deep venous thrombosis after radiofrequency ablation of greater saphenous vein". J Vasc Surg. 2005;41(2):374.
7. Subromonia S, Lees T. Regarding deep vein thrombosis after radiofrequency ablation of greater saphenous vein: a word of caution. J Vasc Surg. 2005;41: 915–6.
8. Kane K, Fisher T, Bennett M, Shutz W Jr, Hicks T, Grimsley B. The incidence and outcome of endothermal heat induced thrombosis after endovenous laser ablation. Ann Vasc Surg. 2014;28:1744–50.
9. Kabnick L, Bernland T. Endothermal heat-induced thrombosis. Paper presented at: 38th Annual Vascular and Endovascular issues, Techniques and Horizons (VEITH symposium). 2011; pp. 16–20.
10. Hirsh J, Guyatt G, Albers GW, Harrington R, Schunemann HJ. Executive summary: American College of Chest Physicians Evidence-Based Clinical Practice Guidelines (8th edition). Chest. 2008;133(6 Suppl):715–1095.
11. Harlander-Locke M, Jimenez JC, Lawrence PF, Derubertis BG, Rigberg DA, Gelabert HA. Management of endovenous heat induced thrombus using a classification system and treatment algorithm following segmental thermal ablation of the small saphenous vein. J Vasc Surg. 2013;58:427–31.
12. Rhee SJ, Cantelmo NL, Conrad MF, Stoughton J. Factors influencing the incidence of endovenous heat –induced thrombosis. Vasc Endovasc Surg. 2013;28:1744–50.
13. Knipp BS, Blackburn SA, Bloom JR, Felow E, Laforge W, Pfeifer JR, et al. Endovenous laser ablation: venous outcomes and thrombotic complications are independent of the presence of deep venous insufficiency. J Vasc Surg. 2008;48(6):1538–45.

Deep Vein Thrombosis: The Disease

9

Devendra Dekiwadia

9.1 Introduction

Deep vein thrombosis (DVT) is a complex set of diseases. Nowhere else in the vascular network does such a challenging 'easy to find and difficult to treat' situation occur. The large-volume low-flow venous system in humans is affected by gravity in the erect posture, and the blood within the entire system reacts differentially to various stimuli according to flow mechanics, physiologic stress, endocrinal effects, and genetic predisposition [1].

9.2 Normal Venous Vasoregulation and Venous Biomechanics

The venous system has excellent bio adaptation. Veins are large-volume capacitance vessels with tonal regulation. Sixty to eighty percent of the circulating blood is stored in/passes through the veins at any given time. This capacitance system maintains the filling pressure of the heart, and compensates for orthostatic changes. The average pressure in foot veins is approximately 100 mmHg. Ambulation and the recumbent position significantly drop this pressure [2]. During ambulation the muscular pump evacuates/pushes blood towards the heart. In the recumbent posture, owing to the loss of gravitational pull, the pressure drops and more 'static' blood remains in the capacitance vessels [3].

Unlike arteries, the veins lack an extensive elastic lamina, resulting in greater distensibility. These vein mechanics form an integral part of vessel wall imaging in the understanding of venous thromboembolism. Active vasoregulation is provided by smooth muscle cells acting through sympathetic nerves; body temperature; blood volume; and physiologic stress [4]. Circulating vasoactive mediators, such as the hormones noradrenalin and epinephrine, cause contraction, while acetylcholine causes relaxation. Vasodilatation is mediated through nitric oxide (NO) relaxing factor. Muscarinic activation and thrombin and alpha adrenergic agents stimulate NO production. Prostaglandin synthesis in the vein wall is stimulated by numerous substances promoting vasodilatation. Local factor endothelin-1 causes contraction, while vasoactive prostanoid, which alters venous tone, is produced both intraluminally and extraluminally.

9.3 Natural Anticoagulants

In normal life, micro coagulation is regulated by the body mechanism of natural anticoagulation, called natural systemic anticoagulation. The basic molecule required for coagulation is thrombin.

D. Dekiwadia
Dekiwadia Hospital, Rajkot, Gujarat, India

A. K. Khanna, R. Jindal (eds.), *Venous Disorders*, https://doi.org/10.1007/978-981-13-1108-6_9

Thrombin formation is inhibited chiefly by antithrombin (AT), a central anticoagulant protein that binds to thrombin. AT itself also interferes with coagulation, preventing the removal of fibrinopeptide A (fPA) and fPB from the blood. During natural anticoagulation, there is an unavailability of thrombin for factors V and VIII activation. Platelet aggregation and activation are inhibited by AT. AT also inhibits factors VIIIa, IXa, Xa, XIa, and XIIa [5–9]. Patients with genetic AT deficiency are at a higher risk of venous thromboembolism (VTE). In the presence of natural heparin, accelerated inhibition of thrombin by AT results in systemic anticoagulation. Activated protein C (APC) and cofactor S inhibit factors Va and VIIIa. Despite the anticoagulation mechanism in the body, in normal day-to-day life, micro or minor coagulations do occur, and these events are regulated by physiologic thrombolysis.

9.4 Physiologic Thrombolysis

Physiologic thrombolysis is a continuous process that prevents pathologic intravascular thrombosis. The basic building block of a thrombus consists of fibrin threads, and these fibrin threads must be destroyed to prevent thrombus formation. For this purpose a fibrinolytic substance, in enzyme form, circulates in the blood. This fibrinolytic enzyme is plasmin, which is generated by the pro-enzyme plasminogen. Plasmin acts on fibrin, fibrinogen, and other factors.

9.5 How Does Plasminogen Activation Occur?

Plasminogen is activated in four ways:

1. Vascular endothelial cells produce thrombin. Activated thrombin results in the formation of fibrin, in which the platelets are trapped and onto which they adhere. Circulating tissue plasminogen activator (tPA) and alpha-2 antiplasmin are incorporated into this fibrin clot. Plasminogen is activated by fibrin-bound tPA. The treatment termed intra-thrombus catheter-directed thrombolysis (CDT) is based on this process.
2. Plasmin produced by tPA activates urokinase plasminogen activator (u-PA), which is an endogenous activator of plasminogen. This cycle augments further fibrinolysis.
3. A contact activation system activates the third mechanism of plasminogen activation, which consists of activated factors XIII and XI.
4. Activated protein C inactivates a specific type-I plasminogen activator inhibitor that is present in the circulation, thus promoting plasminogen activation.

Degradation of fibrin by plasmin produces fragments E and D, the latter being released as a covalently linked dimer—the D dimer. The ongoing risk of recurrent VTE can be predicted by the detection of D-dimer in the circulation. Thus, D-dimer works as a marker for detecting an ongoing thrombotic metabolism.

Within the vein wall, the fibrinolytic system has a significantly lower resting state in the area of the valve cusps. The areas of lowest fibrinolytic activity in the veins are in the veins of the lower limb, in the soleus venous sinuses, popliteal veins, and the femoral vein region. This observation accounts for the popular hypothesis that DVT most commonly originates in the lower limbs. But in vivo real-time imaging has not shown how and where DVT forms.

9.6 Plasminogen Inhibitors and Thrombosis

The primary inhibitor of plasminogen activation in plasma is plasminogen activator inhibitor-1 (PAI-1), which is stored in the alpha granules of platelets. PAI-1 levels are higher in people with hyperlipidemia and factor-5 Leiden genetic abnormalities.

9.7 Changes in the Endothelium

Thrombosis and thrombolysis occur in juxtaposition in the endothelium. Under normal conditions, endothelial cells maintain a vasodilatory and local fibrinolytic state. After endothelial injury, a prothrombotic and pro-inflammatory state sets in. The production of Von Willebrand factor (vWF), tissue factor (TF), and PAI-1 is promoted by the release of endothelin-1, a process that augments thrombosis. tPA is less common in the venous endothelium than in the arterial endothelium and therefore this may explain why venous thrombosis is more common than arterial thrombosis.

9.8 Inflammation

Inflammation increases TF, membrane phospholipids, and fibrinogen, as well as increasing platelet reactivity (Fig. 9.1).

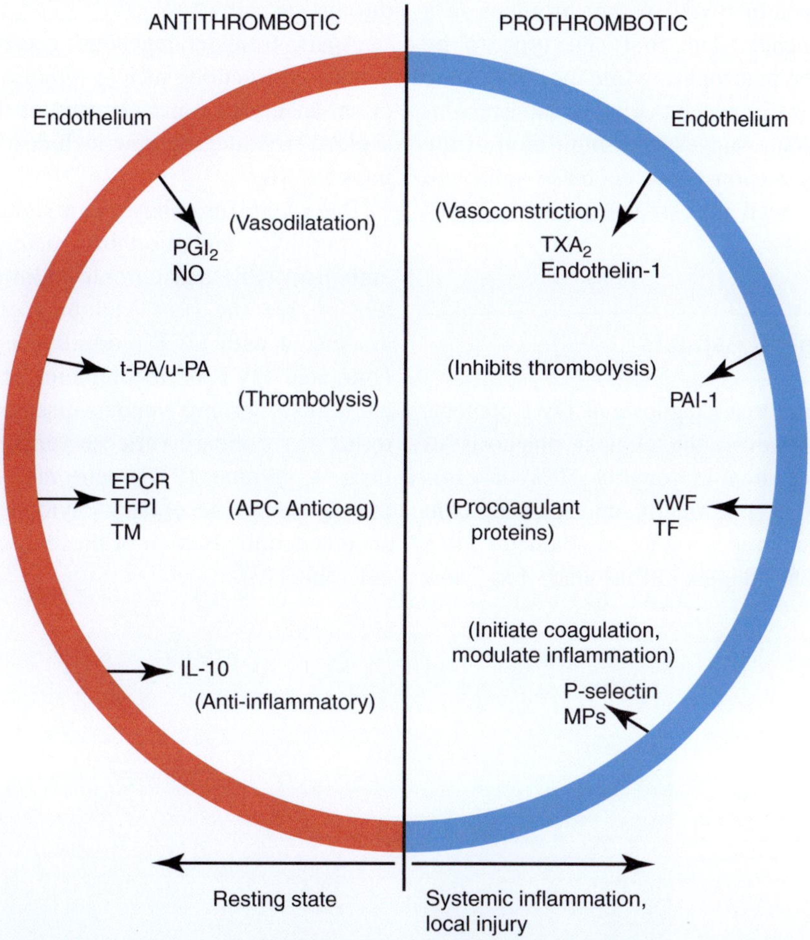

Fig. 9.1 A balance between the antithrombotic and prothrombotic milieux exists at the endothelial level. Prostacyclin and nitric oxide (NO) are antithrombotic mediators. Tissue plasminogen activator (t-PA) and urokinase plasminogen activator (u-PA) confer local thrombolysis. Endothelial receptor for protein C (ERPC), tissue factor pathway inhibitor (TFPI), and thrombomodulin (TM) inhibit thrombosis. Interleukin-10 (IL-10) is an anti-inflammatory cytokine. On the prothrombotic side, thromboxane (TXA_2) and endothelin-1 promote vasoconstriction. Plasmogen activator inhibitor-1 (PAI-1) inhibits thrombolysis, and both Von Willebrand factor (vWF) and tissue factor (TF) are procoagulant proteins. Finally, P-selectin and microparticles (MPs) initiate coagulation, as well as modulating inflammation. *APC* Activated protein C, *PGI_2* prostaglandin I_2

9.9 Thrombus Resolution and Vein Wall Remodeling

The thrombus resolution process is complex and its mechanism is not fully understood. Natural fibrinolysis breaks thrombi at variable rates. The thrombus resolution process, which involves pro-fibrotic growth factor, the deposition of collagen, and the activation of matrix metalloproteinases, resembles wound healing. Leucocytes are involved in the thrombus in a specific sequence. The first cell type to be involved is the neutrophil, while monocytes are one of the most important cells for later resolution. Recent data suggest that inhibition of the inflammatory response can decrease vein wall fibrosis. Vein wall fibrosis can promote recurrent thrombosis.

9.10 Clinical Aspects

Prompt and accurate diagnosis of DVT prevents morbidity. However, the clinical diagnosis of DVT is misleading in roughly 50% of cases (Fig. 9.2) [10, 11]. Formerly, an ascending contrast venogram was the gold standard for DVT diagnosis, but duplex ultrasound has now replaced venography. The availability, non-invasive nature, and relative ease of use of ultrasound has increasingly led to its use in providing early and accurate diagnosis [12].

Virchow's DVT triad of: stasis, changes in vessel walls, and thrombogenic changes in blood is now thought of differently. Stasis may not be a direct cause of DVT. Recent thinking shows a shift in the causal balance toward systemic infection and systemic inflammation promoting thrombotic pathways.

Apart from endogenous causes, extrinsic venous obstructions such as tumors, hematomas, cysts, aneurysms, and changes in the musculoskeletal structure are now included in the thinking on stasis.

Deep vein thrombosis is a significant cause of morbidity and mortality; acute pulmonary embolism (PE) and chronic pulmonary hypertension are the best examples of conditions associated with DVT morbidity and mortality. Untreated DVT or incompletely treated DVT can cause chronic venous disease, mainly in terms of secondary varicose veins, post-thrombotic syndrome (PTS), chronic stasis ulcerations, and secondary lymphedema; the socioeconomic burden of these diseases is considerable [13].

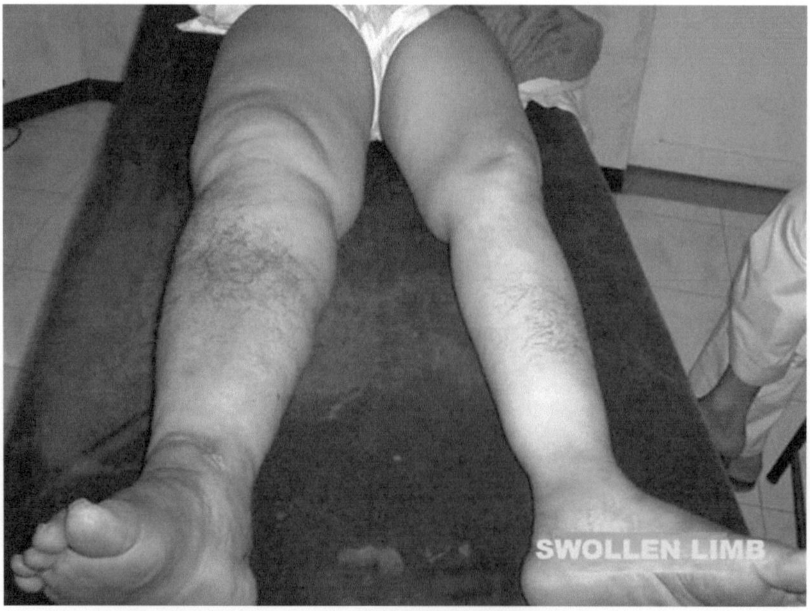

Fig. 9.2 Swollen limb

High risk factors for DVT are age above 40 years; a past history of DVT; orthopedic surgery; and the presence of malignancy, trauma, spinal cord injury, or a hypercoaguable state (thrombophilia).

9.11 Clinical Examination

Acute pain and swelling of the limb that is uniformly spread from groin to toes or from knee to toes is the primary observation. Tender calf and tender femoral vein in the inguinal region are important signs. Mild cyanosis of the toes may be present. Many signs and maneuvers described earlier do not have proven clinical accuracy [14–16].

In the event of associated infection, the extreme peripheral venules can be seen to be thrombosed, with the surrounding tissue showing signs of acute inflammation.

Extreme swelling may be seen in phlegmasia cerulea dolens or phlegmasia alba dolens. If the limb is enlarged and associated with varicose veins or spider veins and acute pain, recurrent DVT with chronic venous insufficiency should be suspected. The varicosity in the vein can be primary or secondary, owing to previous DVT [17].

9.12 Doppler Ultrasound Examination

Doppler ultrasound is the mainstay of DVT diagnosis. During ultrasound examination, the salient features of suspected unilateral DVT are observed, along with the features of a normal limb. A normal vein is compressible with an ultrasound probe, while a thrombosed vein is not compressible. Careful examination may demonstrate a thrombus head. The vein should be traced from the tibial vein up to the inferior vena cava (IVC). The iliac vein and IVC require a convex probe and the compressibility test may be difficult; however, color flow imaging and compression of the opposite normal side help to secure the diagnosis (Fig. 9.3).

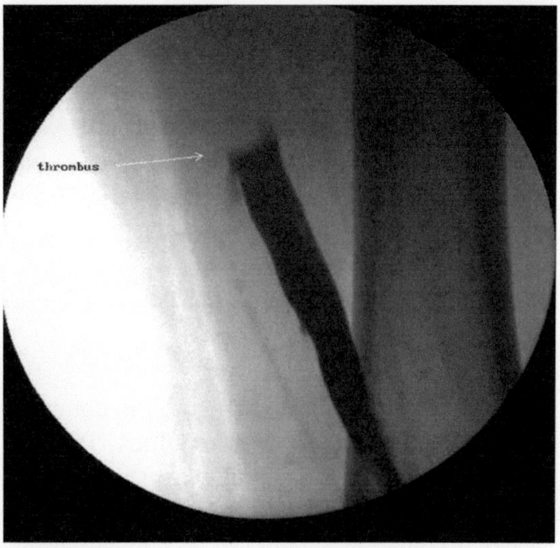

Fig. 9.3 Thrombus on venography

9.13 Acute Versus Chronic Thrombus

An acute (fresh) thrombus seen in a dilated vein is hypoechoic, homogenous, and slightly compressible and may sometimes be floating. In color mode, a gentle proximal compression may show some color flow between the thrombus and the vein wall. The vein wall is thin, smooth, and echolucent.

A chronic thrombus is hyperechoic, heterogeneous, non-compressible, and firmly adherent to the vein wall. The vein wall is thick and irregular. In color mode, multiple intra-thrombus channels may be seen. The channels may be refluxing. There may be dilated, collateral, or multiple refluxing tributaries, particularly in the inguinal region.

9.14 Superficial Vein Thrombosis

Superficial vein thrombosis, also known as superficial vein phlebitis, can occur in any vein of the extremities. In the current era of medical practice the presence of peripheral and central lines can cause thrombosis owing to sensitivity to infused drugs. Cracks in the feet may carry infection and cause thrombophlebitis. Recurrent fleeting thrombophlebitis may indicate a hidden malignancy. Varicose veins can become thrombosed. Coagulation abnormalities in the form of a hypercoagulable state can promote superficial vein thrombosis. Superficial vein thrombosis can progress to the deep veins, resulting in DVT and even in PE [18].

9.15 Upper Extremity DVT

Upper extremity DVT is uncommon in comparison to that in the lower extremities. Primary upper extremity DVT, or spontaneous thrombosis of the axillary subclavian vein, accounts for up to 24% of all upper extremity DVTs. Upper extremity DVTs are mostly associated with unusual hyperabduction activity such as that occurring during painting. Other factors associated with the occurrence of these DVTs are venous thoracic outlet syndrome, chronic atriovenous fistula created for dialysis, axillary lymph node dissection (postoperatively), the use of crutches in lower limb amputees, traumatic fracture of the clavicle, and effort thrombosis. Upper extremity DVTs caused by effort thrombosis tend to affect young healthy adults who participate in sporting activities.

9.16 Thrombosis at Other Sites

Thrombosis can occur at other sites, such as cavernous sinus thrombosis (intracranial), mesenteric and portal vein thrombosis, thrombosis of the dorsal vein of the penis, and isolated renal vein thrombosis. Superior vena cava (SVC) thrombosis can occur in patients on renal dialysis that is carried out via upper extremity vessels. Radiation over the chest and intrathoracic tumors causing external compression can also cause thrombosis. Inferior vena cava (IVC) thrombosis may be a result of retroperitoneal fibrosis. While the thrombosis in the hepatic-renal- atrial valves could also be a cause of IVC thrombosis.

9.17 Acute DVT: Pathophysiology and Natural History

A complication of acute DVT, VTE, is the most common and most preventable cause of sudden death owing to DVT. Improvements in our understanding of the coagulation and fibrinolytic systems, of the vascular endothelium in thrombosis and hemostasis, and of newly identified prethrombotic conditions, have changed the scenario. A new area of investigation is the tissue response to prothrombosis and how this response leads to thrombus augmentation. This tissue response occurs through the convergence of several risk factors against the background of an imbalance between coagulation and fibrinolysis. Non-invasive diagnostic methods have been an asset in recognizing and observing the progress of treatment [5].

9.17.1 Epidemiology

Whites have a lower incidence of VTE than do African Americans (104 versus 141 per 100,000) and the inhabitants of all the Asian Pacific islands (104 versus 21 per 100,000); in the year [19], the total number of new VTE cases in the United States was more than 275,000.

9.17.2 Population Affected

Individuals at risk for DVT have been less well studied. The incidence of VTE is directly related to and the use of thromboprophylaxis, the intensity of screening, and the accuracy of the diagnostic test used. For example, in acute spinal cord injury patients who were studied with venography, DVT was demonstrated in 81%. However, DVT was diagnosed in 64% of these patients after discharge from the intensive care unit (ICU). Thirty percent of these patients experienced recurrence in a 10-year time span. In another study, there was a 1% incidence of PE and a 0.36% incidence of death from PE in all hospitalized patients.

9.18 Risk Factors for DVT

In patients with DVT with an absence of risk factors the condition is termed primary or idiopathic. Some investigators have found the risk of acute DVT to be significantly higher only for those with three or more independent risk factors.

9.19 Independent Risk Factors for VTE

9.19.1 Age

A population-based study [20] has shown the incidence of VTE to increase exponentially with age. The relative risk increases by 1.9 for each 10-year increase between the age groups of 20 and 80 years. Changes in the venous system associated with increased stasis and increased levels of thrombin activation markers, leading to an acquired prothrombotic state, are some of the multiple factors associated with age.

VTE in children is almost always associated with recognizable thrombotic risk factors. Multiple risk factors are often required to precipitate thrombosis. The risk factors are hospitalization, hospitalization in the ICU, spinal cord injury, and prolonged immobilization owing to orthopedic procedures . DVT may occur in as many as 3.7% of pediatric patients immobilized in halo-femoral traction for the preoperative treatment of scoliosis [21]. Local infection with trauma; an inherited hypercoagulable state; the use of femoral venous catheters; and the presence of concomitant severe respiratory, oncological, and infectious diseases are precipitating causes of DVT.

9.19.2 Geographic Differences

The postoperative incidence of DVT is reported to be higher in Europeans than in Asians. The presence of genetic risk factors such as blood group and factor V Leiden mutation varies in geographic areas and this could be associated with the incidence of DVT [22–25].

9.19.3 Immobilization

Stasis in the soleal veins and behind the valve cusps is exacerbated by advancing age and inactivity of the calf muscle pump. In autopsy studies DVT was found to have paralleled the duration of bed rest, with an increase during the first 3 days of confinement and a rapid rise to very high levels after 2 weeks [26–28].

The incidence of lower extremity thrombosis prior to prophylaxis use was noted to increase within 3 days of bed rest. Also, the incidence rapidly rose to 15%, 77%, and 94% after 1, 2, and 4 weeks of confinement, respectively. Bilateral thrombosis is frequent following bed rest, whereas unilateral thrombosis is associated with stroke confined to the paralyzed limb.

9.19.4 Travel

DVT has also been called "economy class syndrome". After a meeting in 2001, the World Health Organization published a consensus statement [29], in which it was observed that, over a period of 8 years, 56 of 135.3 million airline passengers had severe PE. The frequency in those who traveled more than 5000 km was 150 times higher than the frequency in those who traveled less than 5000 km. A history of previous VTE, recent trauma, the presence of varicose veins, obesity, immobility during flight, and cardiac disease were predisposing risk factors.

9.19.5 Recurrent Thromboembolism

Recurrent thromboembolism develops in 1 of every 11–50 persons with a previous episode of thromboembolism. Recurrent thromboembolism occurs as a result of disordered venous hemodynamics and the resultant damage. Heterozygous factor V Leiden and impaired fibrinolysis are correlated in recurrent thromboembolism. A higher incidence of thromboembolism was noted in patients with irreversible thrombotic risk factors than in those with idiopathic DVT [30, 31].

9.19.6 Malignancy

The hypercoagulable state in malignancy has been well studied and is multifactorial. Venous compression secondary to tumor growth, cancer-associated thrombocytosis, an indwelling central line, chemotherapy, and radiotherapy are causes of primary importance in the development of VTE.

However, the systemic prothrombotic response seen in malignancy is mediated by cytokines, inhibitors of fibrinolysis, and procoagulants. These cytokines initiate hemostasis through the expression of TF. Normally TF is not expressed on the resting vascular endothelium; its expression is induced by chemicals and mediated during times of inflammation or vessel damage. This will bind to factors VII and VIIa and activate factor X. It has been detected in 81% of cancer patients. The platelet adhesion molecules glycoprotein Ib and glycoprotein IIb/IIIa have also been identified on tumor cells. Cytokines such as vascular endothelial growth factor, tumor necrosis factor-alpha, and IL-1 contribute to the prothrombotic potential and their action is mediated through the induction of TF on the vascular endothelium, monocytes, and leukocytes is classically associated with mucinous gastrointestinal tumors. In other malignancies and carcinoma of the lung may be associated with DVT in 19–30% of cases. Of all patients presenting with idiopathic thrombosis, 3–23% develop a malignancy within 2 years, probably owing to the activation of coagulation, mediated by TF, cancer procoagulants, and macrophage-associated cytokines.

9.19.7 Protein C

An increase in thrombotic risk is associated with an acquired or an inherited reduction in protein C activity. Autosomal-dominant inherited deficiency of protein C is classified as type I protein C deficiency, and is characterized by a reduction in both antigenic and functional levels, while in type II protein C deficiency, antigen levels are normal. In a study conducted on VTE, 3.2% of 2132 patients were found to have protein C deficiency [32]. In addition to VTE, neonatal purpura fulminans and warfarin skin necrosis are also associated with protein C deficiency. Patients with conditions associated with acute thrombotic events, such as liver disease, renal disease, disseminated intravascular coagulation, hemolytic-uremic syndrome, chemotherapy with L-asparaginase, thrombotic thrombocytopenic purpura, and acute infection, can also have an acquired protein C deficiency.

9.19.8 Protein S

Protein S is a vitamin K-dependent cofactor for the protein C-mediated inactivation of factor Va and factor VIIIa. Deficiency of protein S—which is autosomal dominant in nature—is more common than protein C deficiency. The incidence of protein S-associated VTE has been reported to be 5–7%, with the prevalence in the general population being 0.13%. There are more than 130 types of protein S mutation and these can be grouped into three categories. Type I deficiency is quantitative, type II deficiency is qualitative, and type III deficiency is caused by a mutation that increases the affinity of protein S for C4b-binding protein [33].

9.19.9 Antithrombin

The incidence of VTE associated with antithrombin deficiency has been reported to be 0.5–3%, with a prevalence of 0.2% in the general population.

9.19.10 Other Inherited Thrombophilias

Dysfibrinogenemia, manifested by elevated levels of factors VIII, IX, and XI, has been demonstrated to be an independent risk factor for VTE.

9.19.11 Pregnancy

The incidence of VTE in the pregnant population is six to ten times greater than that in non-pregnant controls. The occurrence of thrombosis is equally distributed throughout all three trimesters.

Impaired venous outflow occurs secondary to uterine compression, and up to 97% of reported thromboses have been isolated to the left leg. There is a transient hypercoagulable state because of increases in the levels of fibrinogen; vWF; and factors II, VII, VIII, and X. Additionally, the development of acquired functional resistance to APC is seen in pregnant patients. Furthermore, protein S levels are decreased by 50–60% early in pregnancy. The fibrinolytic system is also altered in pregnancy, with decreased levels of tPA and increased levels of PAI-1 and PAI-2. Inherited thrombophilia is an additional risk factor.

Worldwide, VTE is the second most common cause of death associated with pregnancy, the most common being abortion [34]. An acquired pre-thrombotic state impairs venous outflow. The incidence of VTE worldwide is 0.75 per 1000 deliveries. Factor V Leiden mutation and suppression of lactation tend to be two to three times higher in patients with postpartum DVT than in those with no DVT.

9.19.12 Oral Contraceptives and Hormonal Therapy

Estrogen in pharmacological doses is associated with alterations in the coagulation system that may contribute to VTE. Such alterations include decreases in PAI-1 and increases in blood viscosity, fibrinogen, plasma levels of factors VII and X, and platelet adhesion and aggregation. Increases in factor VIIa levels, as well as depressed AT and protein S activity, are associated with pharmacological doses of estrogen. The calculated absolute risk of VTE is approximately 3.3 per 1000 regular users of oral contraceptives [35].

9.19.13 Blood Group

The prevalence of DVT is higher in people with blood group A.

9.19.14 Inflammatory Bowel Disease

DVT may complicate inflammatory bowel disease in 1.2–7.1% of cases [36, 37]. Thromboses occur in young patients, and are more common in those with active disease and in areas such as the cerebral veins. Active inflammation is associated with the activation of coagulation, possibly mediated by endotoxin-induced monocyte activation.

9.19.15 Systemic Lupus Erythematosus (SLE)

SLE may be complicated with an underlying syndrome of arterial and venous thrombosis, recurrent abortion, thrombocytopenia, and neurological disease and by the presence of anti-phospholipid antibodies. Patients with SLE who have lupus anticoagulant have a sixfold higher risk of VTE.

9.20 Anatomic Risk Factors

VTE and anatomic anomalies or syndromes are congenital risk factors for DVT.

9.20.1 Iliac Vein Compression

May-Thurner syndrome is a classical example of venous compression by surrounding structures. In this syndrome the right common iliac artery compresses the left iliac vein against the sacral promontory. Whether the condition is congenital or acquired is a matter of debate, but clinical observations show that DVT occurs more commonly on the left side.

9.20.2 Popliteal Vein Entrapment

Popliteal vein entrapment occurs because of anatomic anomalies of the medial head of the gastrocnemius; it occurs either alone or together with the artery in 10% of cases of DVT. Venous entrapment has been reported to occur almost 70% of the time in females with DVT [38].

9.20.3 Inferior Vena Caval Anomalies

Congenital hypoplasia or absence of the IVC presents another anatomic risk factor for DVT.

9.20.4 Surgery

Risk factors causing DVT are preoperative immobilization, activated coagulation, and transient depression of fibrinolysis; increases in thrombin activation, as well as elevated levels of PAI-1, are also risk factors for DVT.

9.20.5 Trauma

Blood transfusion; surgery; fracture of the pelvis, femur, or tibia; spinal cord injury; and femoral venous catheters are all risk factors for DVT. Virchow's triad and all its components are also regarded as risk factors in trauma.

9.21 Primary Hypercoagulable State

Certain thrombophilic conditions form a genetic basis for DVT. Recently described abnormalities are substantially more common than those previously described [39]. In 20% of DVT cases factor V Leiden mutation is present. In approximately 6% of those with DVT and this mutation, the condition is associated with a point mutation in the 3'region of the prothrombin gene, at nucleotide position 20,210; this is associated with increased plasma levels of prothrombin. Hyperhomocysteinemia is another inherited hypercoagulable state that is an independent risk factor.

9.22 Other Risk Factors

Obesity, cardiac disease, systemic hypercoagulability, and congestive heart failure are other important risk factors for DVT [7, 8].

However, thrombotic risk is not uniformly distributed in the population. The associated risk factors provide insight into the underlying pathophysiology, blood flow abnormalities, and vessel wall injury. Abnormalities of blood coagulation and fibrinolysis result in imbalances within the coagulation and fibrinolytic systems.

9.23 Newer Thinking in Venous Thrombogenesis

There is little evidence that either microscopic or gross endothelial injury plays a significant role in venous thrombogenesis, exceptions being direct venous trauma, hip arthroplasty, and the presence of a central venous catheter. It is biologic injury to the endothelium that plays a major role [6].

The venous endothelium is normally antithrombotic. It produces prostaglandin i-2, TM, tPA, and glycosaminoglycan, which are antithrombogenic cofactors. The endothelium may become prothrombotic, producing TF, vWF, and fibronectin in favorable conditions. A procoagulant state that occurs because of endothelial hypoxia is caused by endothelial leukocyte adhesion during stasis. Thus, stasis can be a permissive factor for the events required for thrombosis.

An imbalance in the activation of the coagulation system is one of the most important factors underlying many episodes of acute DVT. There is continuity in the hemostatic system: it shows a precise balance between inhibitors and activators of fibrinolysis and coagulation, and confines thrombus formation to sites of local injury.

A prothrombotic state may result from activation exceeding antithrombotic capacity. This state is facilitated by the thrombin-T complex. Factors such as age, presence of malignancy, surgery, trauma, a primary hypercoagulable state, and oral contraceptive use can cause an imbalance in coagulation.

9.24 Treatment of DVT

Duplex ultrasound has been the most important development in characterizing the natural history of venous thrombi in humans. Valvular incompetence and persistent venous obstruction are the most important chronic manifestations of acute DVT [40].

Thrombosis in the venous bloodstream (systemic and pulmonary) is addressed by, firstly, prevention and, secondly, treatment of a thrombosis that has occurred.

Most of the drugs trialed and their clinical applications are in relation to the prophylaxis of VTE, and DVT is discussed in this context. However, a preventive/prophylactic approach and the treatment of an established DVT may be quite different.

Established acute DVT may be present in the most peripheral veins and may not have progressed to the main bloodstream. The aim is to evacuate the thrombus from the system, either by lysing it or by surgically removing it.

Very small thrombi will be treated by the body mechanism for natural lysis. When the thrombus load increases to a point whereupon the body mechanism finds it difficult to clear, other approaches come into play. Untreated DVT may progress to PE, or the thrombus may adhere to the vein wall in such a way that free fragmentation does not occur. Therefore, the natural outcome could be PE followed by chronic pulmonary hypertension or death due to PE [9] or PTS.

An adherent deep vein thrombus may resolve partially, resulting in valve destruction and chronic venous hypertension in the affected limb or organ. Or the thrombus may be completely lysed and leave behind a normal venous bloodstream. The outcome depends on the thrombus load in the system and the various factors described above.

The treatment centers on the prevention of PE, thereby preventing a life-threatening situation, while also preventing the development of chronic status, such as PTS, and preventing the imposition of a lifelong socioeconomic burden on the patient.

Three modalities are used to treat established acute DVT: heparin therapy, CDT, and surgical thrombectomy. All three modalities are followed by the long-term use of various anticoagulants.

9.25 Unfractionated Heparin

Heparin is available in unfractionated form and as fractionated low molecular weight heparin (LMWH).

Heparin, with a molecular weight of 10–16 kDa, is a pentasaccharide that inhibits thrombin and factor Xa by binding to antithrombin II (ATIII). Also, heparin catalyses the inactivation of thrombin by cofactor II. Other effects of heparin include the release of TF pathway inhibitors that bind to platelet proteins, endothelial cells, and leucocytes. Heparin increases vascular permeability. A therapeutic level of heparin achieved in the first 24 h after the diagnosis of venous thrombosis reduces the risk of recurrence; failure to reach this level entails a 23.3% risk of recurrence [41]. Heparin can cause bleeding (greater risk in those who are underweight and those aged above 65; independent risk factors), thrombocytopenia, and osteoporosis. Recent surgery, trauma, peptic ulcer, malignancy, liver disease, and hemostatic defects pose particular risks in the use of heparin.

9.25.1 LMWH

The molecular weight of LMWH is 4–5 kDa. Various LMWHs are prepared by different processes. A true comparison between the various varieties is still inconclusive and therefore the doses of different LMWHs are not comparable. LMWH, compared with heparin, is claimed to have better bioavailability, a prolonged half-life, and predictable clearance, resulting in twice-daily doses; also, it does not need laboratory monitoring. It has the capacity to inactivate platelet-bound Xa and to vascular permeability (leading to fewer hemorrhagic events). Repeated venographic studies have shown LMWH to be as effective as heparin in preventing thrombus extension and in increasing thrombus resolution.

9.25.2 Catheter-Directed Thrombolysis (CDT) (Fig. 9.4)

The best agent with which to lyse a thrombus is a tPA. With a tPA: plasminogen is activated to plasmin and plasmin degrades the fibrin in the clot. The maximum action of plasmin occurs when the tPA is directly sprayed on fibrin complexes. Therefore, systemic infusion and even use through a peripheral vein that drains into a thrombus do not have the maximum desired effect on clot lysis. To achieve the best result, the tPA should be delivered into the thrombus.

9.25.3 Rationale for Use of CDT

Extensive DVT, particularly in the ilio-femoro-popliteal segment of the vein, will have a massive thrombus load and will cause a painfully swollen extremity, and if not treated aggressively by thrombolysis will result in venous hypertension and loss of both valve function and deep vein refluxes. The outcome will be severe PTS [42].

Persistent obstruction increases the severity of PTS. Early lysis preserves valvular function. Two prospective studies have shown that patients who received thrombolytic therapy were free of PTS as compared with those who received anticoagulation alone [43, 44].

9.25.4 CDT Technique

Under ultrasound guidance, the posterior tibial vein and or popliteal vein is punctured with a needle and a 5fr or 8fr sheath is advanced over a wire. A catheter with multiple side holes is parked intra-thrombus and the preferred tPA is slowly infused, using a pump delivery system. Venograms for approximately 12-h checks are obtained, and the multihole catheter is advanced/repositioned as required. The most terminal portion is the common iliac vein and the help of a pigtail catheter may be needed. At the completion of thrombolysis if the check venogram shows any stenotic or occlusive lesion this is treated by balloon dilation or by the deployment of a stent—the choice depends on the patient's age and underlying disease. DVT of the upper limb and IVC can be treated similarly. Post-procedure, heparin cover is given for 48 h and a switch over to oral anticoagulant is then done. The newer anticoagulants—rivaroxaban and dabigatran—are now being used in place of drugs of the warfarin group. These newer oral anticoagulants

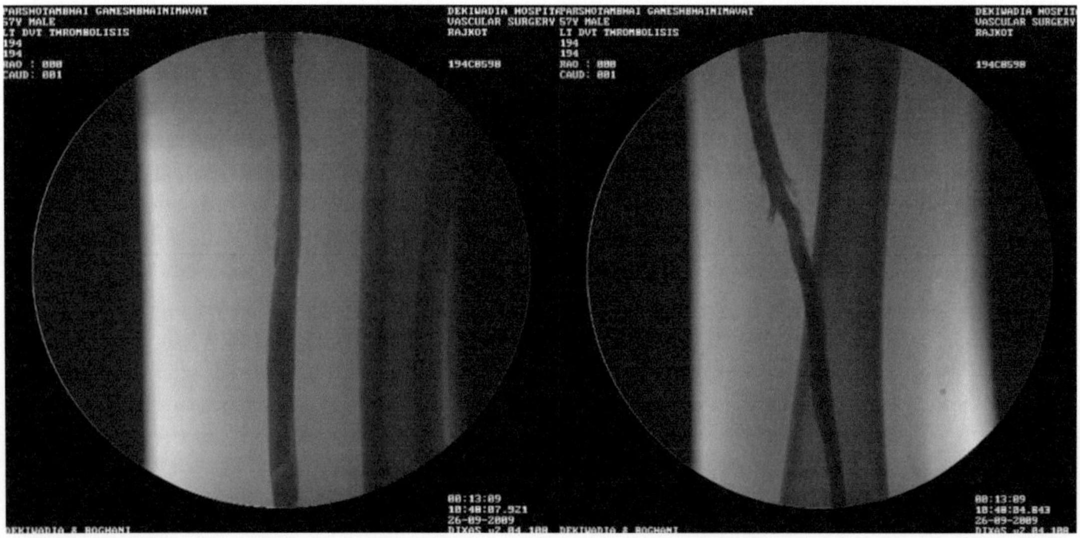

Fig. 9.4 Catheter-directed thrombolysis

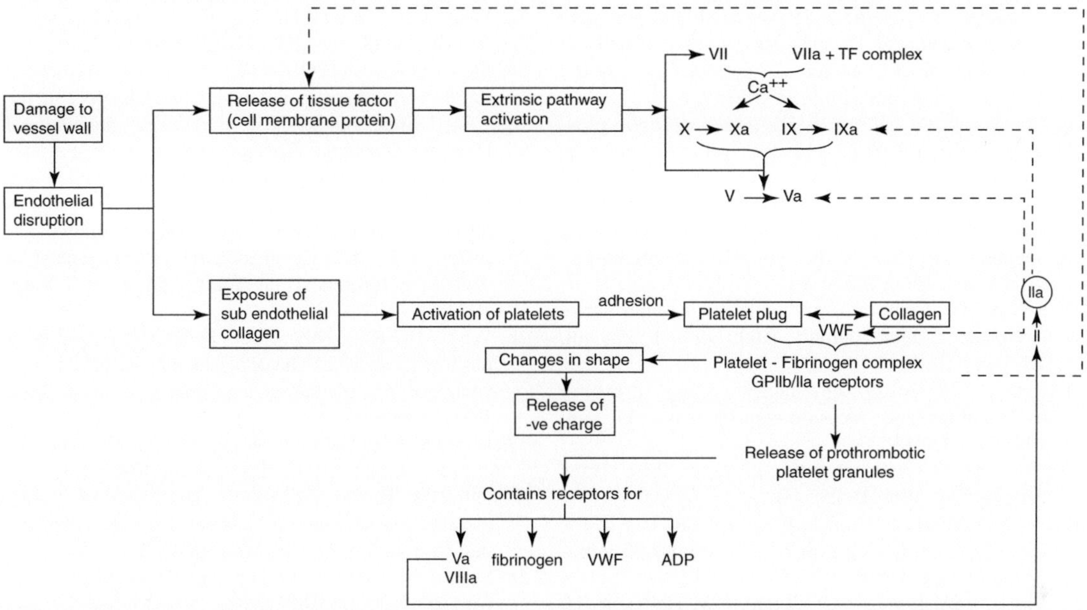

Fig. 9.5 Coagulation cascade

have obviated the need for repeated international normalized ratio (INR) checking.

The currently available literature and my personal experience support CDT as the preferred approach in patients with ilio-femoral DVT, axillo-subclavian DVT, SVC DVT, and IVC DVT. If there is any contraindication to this therapy, or if CDT fails, then venous thrombectomy may be considered.

9.25.5 Surgical Treatment of Acute Ilio-Femoral DVT

Prior to the endovascular era, massive DVT was treated surgically; the initial procedure in the treatment of this condition was ligation of the femoral vein or iliac vein. The aim was to prevent PE and to prevent reflux after re-canalization [45].

The newer surgical approach is in the form of exposure of the common femoral vein at the level of the inguinal ligament and its control. A venous Fogarty catheter technique is used to evacuate ilio-femoral thrombi after transverse venotomy. The thrombus load from the calf and lower thigh is evacuated by firm massage from calf to thigh, which will expel the thrombi from the venotomy. The sequence may have to be repeated several times before good evacuation occurs.

In patients with phlegmasia cerulea dolens a calf fasciotomy may be needed [46].

An IVC or a renal thrombus may need a retroperitoneal laparotomy or a subcostal retroperitoneal approach (Fig. 9.5).

Conclusion

DVT is a common phenomenon in hospital settings and may be a cause of sudden death because of PE. The aim should be to prevent the DVT, and if it occurs, to perform the required therapy, in terms of anticoagulation, thrombolysis, or thrombectomy.

References

1. Criado E, Passman MA. Physiological assessment of the venous system. In: Rutherford RB, editor. Vascular surgery. 3rd ed. Philadelphia: WB Saunders; 1989. p. 175–7.
2. Hjelmstedt A. The pressure in the veins of the dorsum of the foot in quiet standing and during exercise in limbs without signs of venous disorder. Acta Chir Scand. 1968;134:235–44.

3. Arnoldi CC, Linderholm H. Venous blood pressures in the lower limb at rest and during exercise in patients with idiopathic dysfunction of the venous pump of the calf. Act Chir Scand. 1969;135:601–9.
4. Hojensgard IC, Sturup H. Static and dynamic pressures in the superficial and deep veins of the lower extremity in man. Acta Physiol Scand. 1952;27:49–67.
5. Rothe CF. Physiology of venous return. Arch Intern Med. 1986;146:977–82.
6. Shepherd JT. Role of the veins in the circulation. Circulation. 1966;33:484–91.
7. Tyberg JV. How changes in venous capacitance modulate cardiac output. Arch Eur J Physiol. 2002;445:10–7.
8. Rothe CF. Mean circulatory filling pressure: its meaning and measurement. J Appl Physiol. 1993;74:499–509.
9. Attinger EO. Wall properties of veins. IEEE Trans Biomed Eng. 1969;16:253–61.
10. Persson AV, Jones C, Zide R, Jewell ER. Use of the triplex scanner in diagnosis of deep venous thrombosis. Arch Surg. 1989;124(5):593–6.
11. Mattos MA, Londrey GL, Leutz DW, Hodgson KJ, Ramsey DE, Barkmeier LD, Stauffer ES, Spadone DP, Sumner DS. Color-flow duplex scanning for the surveillance and diagnosis of acute deep venous thrombosis. J Vasc Surg. 1992;15(2):366–75.
12. Meissner MH, Moneta G, Burnand K, et al. The hemodynamics and diagnosis of venous disease. J Vasc Surg. 2007;46:4s–24s.
13. Nicolaides AN, Hussein MK, Szendro G, et al. The relationship of venous ulceration with ambulatory venous pressure measurements. J Vasc Surg. 1993;17:414–9.
14. Alimi YS, Barthelemy P, Juhan C. Venous pump of the calf: a study of venous and muscular pressures. J Vasc Surg. 1994;20:728–35.
15. Ludbrook J. The musculovenous pumps of the human lower limb. Am Heart J. 1966;71:635–41.
16. Pollack AA, Wood EH. Venous pressure in the saphenous vein at the ankle in man during exercise and changes in posture. J Appl Physiol. 1949;1:649–62.
17. Meissner MH, Eklof B, Coleridge-Smith P, et al. Secondary chronic venous disorders. J Vasc Surg. 2007;46:S68–83.
18. Barnes RW, Collicott PE, Mozersky DJ, et al. Noninvasive quantitation of maximum venous outflow in acute thrombophlebitis. Surgery. 1972;72:971–9.
19. Heit JA, Spencer FA, White RH. The epidemiology of venous thromboembolism. J Thromb Thrombolysis. 2016;41:3–14. https://doi.org/10.1007/s11239-015-1311-6.
20. Kreidy R. Influence of acquired and genetic risk factors on the prevention, management, and treatment of thromboembolic disease. Int J Vasc Med. 2014;2014:859726. https://doi.org/10.1155/2014/859726.
21. Leslie IJ, Dorgan JC, Bentley G, Galloway RW. A prospective study of deep vein thrombosis of the leg in children on halo-femoral traction. J Bone Joint Surg Br. 1981;63-B(2):168–70.
22. White RH. The epidemiology of venous thromboembolism. Circulation. 2003;107(23 Suppl 1):I4–8.
23. Stein PD, Kayali F, Olson RE, Milford CE. Pulmonary thromboembolism in Asians/Pacific Islanders in the United States: analysis of data from the National Hospital Discharge Survey and the United States Bureau of the Census. Am J Med. 2004;116(7):435–42.
24. Klatsky AL, Baer D. What protects Asians from venous thromboembolism? Am J Med. 2004;116(7):493–5.
25. Joffe SN. Racial incidence of postoperative deep vein thrombosis in South Africa. Br J Surg. 1974;61(12):982–3.
26. White JV, Katz ML, Cisek P, Kreithen J. Venous outflow of the leg: anatomy and physiologic mechanism of the plantar venous plexus. J Vasc Surg. 1996;24:819–24.
27. Burnand KG. The physiology and hemodynamics of chronic venous insufficiency of the lower limb. In: Gloviczki P, Yao JST, editors. Handbook of venous disorders. Guidelines of the American Venous Forum. 2nd ed. London: Arnold; 2001. p. 49–57.
28. Stegall HR. Muscle pumping in the dependent leg. Circ Res. 1966;19:180–90.
29. Caggiati A, Bergan JJ, Gloviczki P. Nomenclature of the veins of the lower limb: an international interdisciplinary consensus statement. J Vasc Surg. 2002;36:416–22.
30. Strandness DE Jr, Sumner DS. Hemodynamics for surgeons. New York: Grune & Stratton; 1975.
31. Sumner DS, Zierler RE. Vascular physiology: essential hemodynamic principles. In: Rutherford RB, editor. Vascular surgery. 6th ed. Philadelphia: WB Saunders; 2005. p. 75–123.
32. Mateo J, Oliver A, Borrell M, Sala N, Fontcuberta J. Laboratory evaluation and clinical characteristics of 2,132 consecutive unselected patients with venous thromboembolism – results of the Spanish Multicentric Study on Thrombophilia (EMET-Study). Thromb Haemost. 1997;77(3):444–51.
33. van Ommen H, Nowak-Göttl U. Inherited thrombophilia in pediatric venous thromboembolic disease: why and who to test C. Front Pediatr. 2017;5:50. https://doi.org/10.3389/fped.2017.00050.
34. Fardiazar Z, Hajizadeh K, Dinparvar S, Esmaili F. Thromboembolism and thrombosis during pregnancy and after delivery between 2009 and 2012 in Al-Zahra Educational Center. J Caring Sci. 2014;3(3):221–6. https://doi.org/10.5681/jcs.2014.024.
35. Lidegaard Ø, Løkkegaard E, Svendsen AL, Agger C. Hormonal contraception and risk of venous thromboembolism: national follow-up study. BMJ. 2009;339:b2890. https://doi.org/10.1136/bmj.b2890.
36. Nguyen GC, Sam J. Rising prevalence of venous thromboembolism and its impact on mortality among hospitalized inflammatory bowel disease patients. Am J Gastroenterol. 2008;103:2272–80.
37. Danese S, Papa A, Saibeni S, Repici A, Malesci A, et al. Inflammation and coagulation in inflammatory

bowel disease: the clot thickens. Am J Gastroenterol. 2007;102:174–86.
38. Gerkin TM, Beebe HG, Williams DM, Bloom JR, Wakefield TW. Popliteal vein entrapment presenting as deep venous thrombosis and chronic venous insufficiency. J Vasc Surg. 1993;18(5):760–6.
39. Álvarez SI, Ollero EB, Sanjuan FML, Martínez FL, Martín MTC. A deep vein thrombosis caused by 20209C>T mutation in homozygosis of the prothrombin gene in a Caucasian patient. Biochem Med (Zagreb). 2014;24(1):159–66. https://doi.org/10.11613/BM.2014.018.
40. van Ramshorst B, van Bemmelen PS, Hoeneveld H, et al. Thrombus regression in deep venous thrombosis: quantification of spontaneous thrombolysis with duplex scanning. Circulation. 1992;86:414–9.
41. Merli GJ. Treatment of venous thromboembolism. Am J Med. 2008;121:S2–9.
42. Raju S, Fredericks RK, Hudson CA, et al. Venous valve station changes in "primary" and post-thrombotic reflux: an analysis of 149 cases. Ann Vasc Surg. 2000;14:193–9.
43. Vedantham S, Piazza G, Sista AK, Goldenberg NA. Guidance for the use of thrombolytic therapy for the treatment of venous thromboembolism. J Thromb Thrombolysis. 2016;41:68–80. https://doi.org/10.1007/s11239-015-1318-z.
44. Enden T, Wik HS, Kvam AK, et al. Health-related quality of life after catheter-directed thrombolysis for deep vein thrombosis: secondary outcomes of the randomised, nonblinded, parallel-group CaVenT study. BMJ Open. 2013;3:e002984. https://doi.org/10.1136/bmjopen-2013-002984.
45. Labropoulos N, Leon M, Nicolaides AN, et al. Superficial venous insufficiency: correlation of anatomic extent of reflux with clinical symptoms and signs. J Vasc Surg. 1994;20:953–8.
46. Snyder MA, Adams JT, Schwartz SI. Hemodynamics of phlegmasia cerulea dolens. Surg Gynecol Obstet. 1967;125:342–6.

Post-Thrombotic Syndrome

10

Devendra Dekiwadia, Birju Patel,
and Dilip Vaghasia

10.1 Introduction

PTS may be considered as a postinflammatory stage of the venous system whereupon the venous tone and functioning of the valves of the veins are jeopardised. In the lower extremities, this results in deranged functions of the veins to perform antigravity venous drainage. Chronic venous congestion in the lower limbs ends into a large volume of deoxygenated blood stored in the veins. This results from poor performance of the venous pump capable of evacuating out the blood from the tissues. In superficial venous system derangements, varicose veins, the skin surface and the immediate deeper tissues mainly above the deep fascia are affected. When the entire system is affected, all the tissues of the limb are affected. Maybe the clinical manifestation could be of stasis ulcers, skin changes, varicose veins, etc., but at a depth all the tissues of the lower limb are affected. Age, infection, DVT, outflow obstruction and anomalous venous circulation are capable of chronic degenerative changes of the veins collectively called phlebosclerosis.

Phlebosclerosis disturbs haemodynamics. It can happen at various levels and with several aspects. This is described as 'post-thrombotic syndrome'—PTS. PTS is a chronic condition that develops in 20–50% of patients after untreated or poorly treated deep venous thrombosis (DVT) [1–3]. As such, it is the most common complication of DVT. However it is not always necessary that a clinically evident deep vein thrombosis has occurred. The level of venous segment affected decides the extent of the condition and local signs and symptoms.

Collectively the haemodynamics may result in central flow obstruction, valvular incompetence and reflux, incompetence of peripheral venous pump, venous hypertension and venous microangiopathy.

PTS reduces quality of life [4] and incurs significant direct and indirect societal costs [5]. To date, however, PTS has received little attention within the field of DVT and VTE research. For example, in the numerous clinical trials of therapies for VTE that have directly influenced our current-day clinical practices, PTS has almost never been included as a measure of outcome.

Possible reasons for the lack of attention to this common condition on the part of physicians and researchers include lack of knowledge of the high incidence of PTS, uncertainty as to how to diagnose PTS as no 'gold standard' test exists or the perception that PTS is untreatable, inevitable or takes years to develop after DVT (Table 10.1).

D. Dekiwadia (✉) · B. Patel · D. Vaghasia
Dekiwadia Hospital, Rajkot, Gujarat, India

A. K. Khanna, R. Jindal (eds.), *Venous Disorders*, https://doi.org/10.1007/978-981-13-1108-6_10

Table 10.1 Typical clinical features of the post-thrombotic syndrome

Leg symptoms	Signs
Heaviness	Oedema
Pain	Peri-malleolar telangiectasias
Swelling	Venous ectasia
Itching	Hyperpigmentation
Cramps	Redness
Paresthesia	Dependent cyanosis
Bursting pain	Lipodermatosclerosis
	Healed ulcer
	Open ulcer
Symptom pattern	
Worse with activity, standing, walking	
Better with rest, recumbency	

10.2 Clinical Presentation

Post-thrombotic syndrome is termed a 'syndrome' because it is associated with groupings of symptoms and clinical signs, which may vary from patient to patient. Common symptoms are pain, heaviness and swelling, cramps, itching or tingling in the affected limb. Symptoms may be present in various combinations and may be persistent or intermittent. Typically, symptoms are aggravated by standing or walking and improve with resting, leg elevation and lying down. On physical examination of the limb, usually one or many or all of the following may be present: oedema, telangiectasias, hyperpigmentation, eczema, varicose collateral veins and, in severe cases, lipodermatosclerosis and ulceration [6] (Fig. 10.1).

10.3 Pathophysiology of PTS

When DVT is diagnosed, standard anticoagulant treatment prevents thrombus extension and embolisation to the pulmonary arteries, but does not directly lyse the acute thrombus.

Follow-up studies of patients with DVT who were treated with anticoagulants have shown that in most cases, only partial clearance of thrombus occurs and return of normal physiological function of the vein is rare [7].

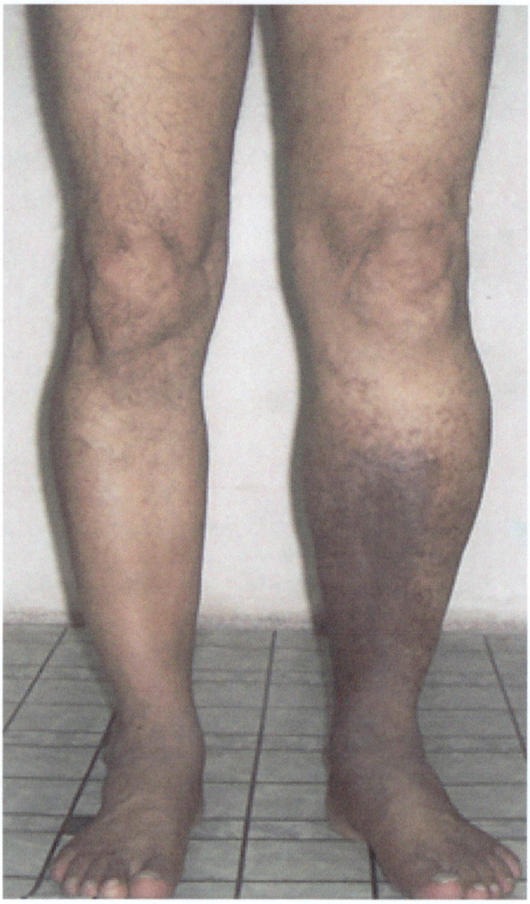

Fig. 10.1 PTS, chronic oedema of whole leg, dark pigmentation, varicose veins and ulcer scars

As such in treatment with anticoagulants, we are depending on the nature to perform physiologic thrombolysis, which, when the thrombus load is high, may be poor. Even in patients who do achieve clot lysis, permanent damage to venous valves occurs frequently, conceivably via thrombus-induced activation of inflammation [8] or scarring associated with acute and resolving thrombosis, leading to valve incompetence (reflux). The use of thrombolysis to treat DVT, while achieving high rates of clot lysis, has not been definitively shown to improve venous haemodynamics or reduce the risk of developing PTS.

Based on the above and on results of venous hemodynamic studies in patients with PTS, it is likely that the pathophysiology of this syndrome involves the interplay of two processes: (1) damage to delicate venous valves by the thrombus itself or by associated inflammatory mediators, which causes valvular reflux, and (2) residual venous obstruction because of incomplete thrombus clearance, which leads to impaired venous return. Both processes lead to increased centripetal or centrifugal venous pressure (venous hypertension), which results in reduced calf muscle postperfusion metabolite evacuation, increased tissue permeability and the associated clinical manifestations of PTS (e.g. pain, effort intolerance, swelling).

10.4 Diagnosis of PTS

By definition, there is no gold standard laboratory, imaging or functional test that establishes the diagnosis. In patients with a history of prior DVT who have typical symptoms and signs, PTS is usually the correct diagnosis. In some patients, it may take up to 3–6 months for the initial pain and swelling associated with acute DVT to resolve; hence a diagnosis of PTS should be deferred until after the acute phase has passed. Objective evidence of venous valvular incompetence by Doppler ultrasound or by plethysmography may help to confirm the diagnosis of PTS in symptomatic patients. PTS should not be diagnosed if clinical symptoms are absent. This is because, while many patients with symptomatic PTS have valvular incompetence, many DVT patients develop valvular incompetence but do not have symptomatic PTS [9, 10].

Three clinical scales for the diagnosis of PTS have been developed [11, 12] and are summarised in Table 10.2. These have been used to assess the presence and grade of the severity of PTS in a number of clinical studies, including trials of

Table 10.2 Clinical scales for the diagnosis of post-thrombotic syndrome (PTS)

PTS scale	Criteria used to diagnose PTS	Developed specifically for PTS	Rates severity of PTS
Villalta scale (Villalta et al. [11])	• Five symptoms (pain, cramps, heaviness, pruritus, paresthesia) • Six signs (oedema, skin induration, hyperpigmentation, venous ectasia, redness, pain during calf compression) • Each rated as 0 (absent), 1 (mild), 2 (moderate) or 3 (severe) • Points are summed to yield the total score: • 0–4: No PTS • 5–14: Mild/moderate PTS • 15 or more or presence of ulcer: Severe PTS	Yes	Yes
Ginsberg measure (Ginsberg et al. [14])	Pain and swelling of limb of ‡1 month duration, typical character (worse end of day or with prolonged sitting/standing, better after night's rest and leg elevation) that occurs ‡6 months after acute DVT	Yes	No
CEAP classification [12]	Patients with chronic venous disease classified into one of seven clinical classes (class 0–6) according to presence of clinical signs. Each class may include signs present in lower-order class. *Clinical* 0. Symptoms only; no visible or palpable signs of venous disease 1. Telangiectasias, reticular veins, malleolar flare 2. Varicose veins 3. Oedema, no skin changes 4. Skin changes (e.g. pigmentation, eczema, lipodermatosclerosis) 5. Skin changes with healed ulcer 6. Skin changes with active ulcer Each clinical class is then subclassified as to: *Aetiology* (congenital, primary, secondary) *Anatomy* (superficial, deep, perforator veins) *Pathophysiology* (reflux, obstruction, both)	No	No

therapies to prevent or treat PTS. However, none has undergone full evaluation of reliability, validity or responsiveness to change, and their use for the routine clinical monitoring of DVT patients has not been assessed. Moreover, differences in the test characteristics of these measures could help to explain the differing rates of PTS that have been reported in long-term follow-up studies of patients with DVT. For example, in a recent study of a population of patients evaluated 1 year after symptomatic DVT, the proportion of patients classified as having PTS was almost fivefold higher with the Villalta measure than with the Ginsberg measure, and the agreement between the two measures was poor [10]. Another recent study detected substantial differences in the ability of various PTS measures to discriminate between legs affected by DVT and those of controls [13]. Research aimed at validating and standardising diagnostic criteria for PTS to improve the uniformity of its diagnosis in clinical studies and to enhance the ability to compare results of different studies would be of value.

10.5 Which DVT Patients Are at Risk of Developing PTS?

Age Two studies found that increasing age was associated with a higher risk of developing PTS [15, 16]], but other studies did not [2, 4, 17].

Body Mass Index (BMI) Results of prospective studies suggest that higher BMI is associated with a greater risk of PTS. In a small cohort study of patients with symptomatic proximal DVT who were followed for 12 months, patients who developed PTS had significantly higher mean BMI than those who did not develop PTS. Long-term warfarin anticoagulation for unprovoked (idiopathic) proximal DVT also indicated that higher BMI was associated with increased severity of PTS [17]. Similarly, Van Dongen et al. [16] found that BMI >25 was a significant independent predictor of PTS after proximal DVT. As obesity is a potentially modifiable risk factor, the role of weight reduction in the prevention or management of PTS merits evaluation.

Thrombophilia Inherited and acquired thrombophilic disorders increase the risk of developing a first episode of VTE. In a longitudinal cohort study of predictors of PTS, there were no associations between the risk of developing PTS and deficiencies of antithrombin, protein C or protein S or the presence of lupus-like anticoagulants [1]. As this was an older study, testing for the common genetic thrombophilias was not yet available. In a recent cohort study, the presence of factor V Leiden, prothrombin gene mutation or elevated factor VIII levels was not predictive of the development of PTS [16]. From the limited data available, it does not appear that thrombophilia increases the risk of developing PTS.

Characteristics of the Initial DVT In recent prospective studies, the likelihood of developing PTS was not influenced according to whether DVT was idiopathic (unprovoked) or secondary (surgery, trauma or cancer) [2, 15, 16]. With regard to the relationship between the severity or location of the initial thrombus and the subsequent development of PTS, results have been inconsistent. In some studies, the risk of PTS was higher in patients with proximal rather than distal (calf) DVT [18, 19], while in other studies neither the site nor the extent of the initial thrombus predicted the development of PTS [20]. Indeed, some prospective studies reported higher rates of PTS after distal DVT [21, 22]. Hence, distal (calf vein) DVT appears to be associated with a higher risk of subsequent PTS.

Asymptomatic DVT Deep venous thrombosis is sometimes diagnosed in asymptomatic patients by performing screening imaging tests in high-risk situations, for example, postoperatively. Such imaging tests have included 125I-fibrinogen uptake testing, contrast venography or venous duplex ultrasound. A recent meta-analysis [23] pooled seven studies of patients with asymptomatic objectively confirmed postoperative DVT and reported that the overall relative risk of developing PTS was 1.6 [95% confidence interval (CI) 1.24–2.02] as compared with patients without asymptomatic DVT on imaging tests.

A study has been reported among total knee and hip arthroplasty patients. Those who were ultrasound-diagnosed, asymptomatic postoperative DVT and were treated, among these about 24% of patients had developed persistent oedema in the affected leg, compared with 1% of patients without postoperative DVT [24]. These findings indicate that asymptomatic DVT can lead to PTS, which could help to explain the lack of a clinical history of DVT in some patients who have post-thrombotic changes in their limbs.

Recurrent DVT The most important risk factor for PTS is recurrent ipsilateral DVT, which in a number of studies was found to increase the risk of PTS as much as tenfold [1, 15, 16], probably by causing further damage of compromised venous valves or by aggravating venous outflow obstruction. By extension, it is therefore important to prevent recurrent DVT by providing an adequate intensity and duration of anticoagulation for the initial DVT and by using thromboprophylaxis to prevent DVT in high-risk patients and settings as recommended in regularly updated evidence-based consensus guidelines [25].

Residual Thrombosis on Ultrasound The presence of residual thrombosis on ultrasound appears to be a risk factor for recurrent DVT after anticoagulant treatment of acute DVT [7] and could plausibly promote the development of PTS because of persistent venous obstruction or valve damage. However, in recent studies that have examined this issue, modest [odds ratio (OR) 1.69; 95% CI 1.23–2.32] [15] or no associations [17] between the presence of residual vein thrombosis and the development of PTS were found.

Persistent Elevation of D-Dimer Elevated D-dimer is a risk factor for first and recurrent DVT [26]. Elevated levels of D-dimer (defined as cutoff of >500 ng/ml on an enzyme-linked immunosorbent assay), measured 3 weeks after withdrawal of oral anticoagulant therapy, were found to be a modest risk factor (OR 1.9, 95% CI 1.0–3.9) for PTS [2]. These results require confirmation in large prospective studies.

10.6 How Often Does PTS Occur After DVT?

Over the last two decades, the annual incidence of VTE has remained stable and is estimated to be 1.0–1.6 per 1000 persons per year, with a per-person lifetime incidence of 0.5% [27]. Approximately 250,000 new cases of VTE occur in the United States each year. Hence, the prevalence of PTS is on the rise in the population. A recent population-based study showed that cumulative rates of venous stasis after DVT were 7% at 1 year, 14% at 5 years, 20% at 10 years and 27% at 20 years, and the cumulative risk of ulcer was 4% by 20 years [28].

More than a quarter of new cases of venous stasis per year are considered to represent cases of future PTS. Prospective studies have provided important information on the frequency of PTS after symptomatic DVT. In a longitudinal cohort study of patients with a first episode of symptomatic DVT, the cumulative incidence of PTS was 17% after 1 year (severe in 3%), 23% after 2 years, 28% after 5 years (severe in 9%) and 29% after 8 years [1]. In the control arm of a recent trial to evaluate the use of compression stockings to prevent PTS in patients with symptomatic proximal DVT, the cumulative rate of PTS at 2 years was 49%, and severe PTS occurred in 12% of patients by the end of 5-year follow-up [15]. In both studies, the majority of cases of PTS occurred within 2 years of the initial DVT. Prospectively followed DVT patients showed that the pooled incidence of any PTS was 46% and of severe PTS (including venous ulcers) was 15% and that in most cases, the condition developed within 1–2 years of the acute DVT [29].

10.7 Impact of PTS on Patients and Society

PTS is costly and burdensome to patients and society, both in terms of money spent and effect on quality of life and productivity. A US study estimated that the annual direct cost of PTS is at least $200 million dollars [30]. A Swedish study estimated that over a 15-year follow-up, the average cost of treating PTS was US$4700 or 75% of the cost of treating the primary DVT [5]. In a Brazilian study, the mean annual cost of treating PTS was the equivalent of US$426 for mild to moderate PTS and US$1188 for severe PTS [31]. In a recent Canadian study, the annual cost of venous ulcer care in Ottawa alone was >$1,000,000, and a large number of these cases are secondary to previous DVT [32]. The indirect costs of PTS are also significant as DVT and PTS affect persons of working age. For example, it is estimated that two million workdays are lost annually in the United States because of leg ulcers [33]. Patients with PTS have significantly poorer quality of life than DVT patients without PTS [4, 17], quality of life is lower than in patients with other forms of chronic venous disease [34], and impairment in quality of life is, on average, worse than in patients with osteoarthritis or chronic lung disease [4, 35].

10.8 Prevention of PTS (Table 10.3)

Thromboprophylaxis As PTS is a consequence of DVT and thromboprophylaxis is an effective means of preventing DVT, it is highly likely, by extrapolation, that use of thromboprophylaxis in high-risk patients and settings as recommended in evidence-based consensus guidelines [25] will prevent cases of PTS. However, practice audits continue to demonstrate that thromboprophylaxis is underutilised [36]. Further, while thromboprophylaxis is effective, its use does not eliminate the risk of VTE. Moreover, nearly 50% of VTE events occur unpredictably and are therefore not preventable with thromboprophylaxis. Strategies that focus on preventing the development of PTS after DVT are therefore more likely to be effective in reducing the frequency of PTS than are attempts to prevent the index DVT. As ipsilateral DVT recurrence is an important risk factor for PTS, preventing recurrent DVT by providing anticoagulation of appropriate intensity and duration for the initial DVT is an important goal [37].

Table 10.3 Strategies for the prevention and management of PTS

Prevention
• Prevent index DVT with the use of thromboprophylaxis in high-risk patients and settings as recommended in evidence-based consensus guidelines
• Prevent recurrent ipsilateral DVT by providing anticoagulation of appropriate intensity and duration for the initial DVT and by targeted used of appropriate thromboprophylaxis if long-term anticoagulation is discontinued
• Use of knee-length, 30–40 mmHg ECS elastic compression stockings for up to 2 years after DVT; optimal duration uncertain
• The role of thrombolysis for the prevention of PTS is not yet established. CDT requires further evaluation in properly designed trials before it is indorsed as being effective in reducing the risk of PTS
Management
• Elastic compression stockings reduce oedema and may improve PTS symptoms
• Intermittent pneumatic compression units are effective for severe symptomatic PTS
• Venoactive agents, such as micronised pulverised flavonoids, aescin (e.g. as found in horse chestnut) or rutosides, may offer short-term improvement of PTS symptoms; large controlled trials addressing long-term effectiveness and safety are needed
• Compression therapy, skin care and topical dressings are used to treat venous ulcer

Active and Passive Exercise Physical exercise is recommended by clinicians. Mobility reduces the acute symptoms of DVT and helps alleviate suffering. The chances of developing an ulcer also reduce.

Adequate Fluid Intake Maintaining fluid intake of minimum 2500 ml per day reduces the risk of occurrence of DVT and recurrence of DVT [38]. On diagnosis of PTS, multiple studies have shown that fluid intake should be maintained and monitored vigorously. An increase in BMI and fluid intake has been shown patient go in hyponatremia. Hypervolemic hyponatremia tends to create lower limb oedema.

Thrombolysis Thrombolytic therapy with tissue plasminogen activator used in conjunction with heparin for the treatment of acute DVT leads to higher rates of vein patency and better preservation of valve function than does the use of heparin alone [39]. However, the effectiveness and safety of thrombolysis for the prevention of PTS are as yet uncertain [40]. A few trials of systemic thrombolysis for the treatment of DVT have assessed PTS as a study endpoint. Among 51 patients with acute proximal DVT, symptoms and signs of PTS were less frequent at the 19-month follow-up in those who received streptokinase compared with those who received heparin alone (35% vs. 92%) [41]. Similarly, in a trial of 42 patients with acute proximal DVT, signs of PTS at 6-year follow-up were less frequent in streptokinase than in heparin recipients (24% vs. 67%) [42]. In a blinded trial of 83 proximal DVT patients, those treated with a 4-h systemic infusion of tissue plasminogen activator had higher rates of achieving >50% clot lysis than heparin-treated patients (58% vs. 0%, $P < 0.002$) and among trial patients who achieved >50% clot lysis, PTS occurred less frequently (25% vs. 56%, $P < 0.07$) [43]. While suggestive, these results are not considered to be definitive due to small numbers of patients studied, differing definitions of PTS and, for some trials, retrospective assessment for PTS.

Catheter-Directed Thrombolysis Catheter-directed thrombolysis, which involves direct delivery of a fibrinolytic drug into the clot via a catheter introduced within the thrombosed vein, may be safer and more effective than systemic thrombolytic therapy and could hold promise as a means of preventing PTS. Results of a nonrandomised study of 68 iliofemoral DVT patients enrolled in a registry who underwent successful catheter-directed thrombolysis suggested that such patients had fewer PTS symptoms, better physical functioning and less health distress at the 16-month follow-up than 30 similar patients who received anticoagulation alone [44]. In authors' own experience of a prospective, single-centre, nonrandomised study of 243 patients with acute iliofemoral DVT, those who chose to receive multimodality therapy that included catheter-directed thrombolysis with balloon angioplasty or stenting followed by anticoagulation had significantly better resolution of venous symptoms at 5 years than those who chose anticoagulation alone (78% vs. 30%, $P < 0.0015$) (personal experience Dekiwadia et al.) (Fig. 10.2).

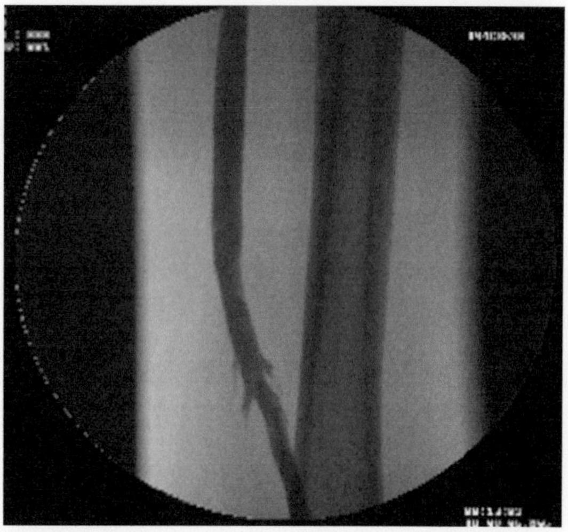

Fig. 10.2 Post thrombolysis preserved venous valves

While the above results are of interest, as yet, there is no clear, high-quality evidence to support the use of thrombolysis as a means to prevent PTS, and because of the lack of such evidence, consensus bodies are unable to recommend tissue plasminogen activators as a primary modality of treatment. In order to definitively address this important issue, large, rigorously conducted multicentre controlled trials of standard anticoagulation versus catheter-directed thrombolysis to prevent PTS are required.

Elastic Compression Stockings Graduated elastic compression stockings (ECS) decrease oedema and improve tissue microcirculation [45]. Knee-length and thigh-length ECS appear to have equal physiological effects, but the former are easier to apply and more comfortable. To date, three trials have evaluated the effectiveness of long-term use of ECS for the prevention of PTS after DVT. In the first, 194 patients with symptomatic proximal DVT were randomly allocated to daily use of a custom, made-to-measure 30–40 mmHg knee-length ECS for at least 2 years or no stocking [46]. PTS was diagnosed using a scoring system that incorporated symptoms and signs. The use of ECS resulted in a decrease from 47% to 20% of mild/moderate PTS and a decrease from 23% to 11% of severe PTS. A subsequent randomised trial conducted by Ginsberg et al. [14] compared the effect of active stockings to sham stockings (no haemodynamic effect; one or two sizes too large) to prevent PTS in proximal DVT patients who had venous valvular incompetence but no symptoms or signs of PTS 1 year after the initial event. PTS was diagnosed using the Ginsberg PTS measure. Finally, a recent trial by Prandoni et al. [15] evaluated the effectiveness of 'off the rack' 30–40 mmHg ECS versus no stockings in 180 patients with a first episode of symptomatic proximal DVT. The 2-year cumulative incidence of PTS, diagnosed using Villalta's scale, was 25% in the stocking group compared with 49% in the control group (hazard ratio 0.49; $P < 0.011$).

A number of important questions remain. Firstly, the lack of blinding in the two positive studies reduces confidence in the results because scales used to diagnose PTS and to assess its severity have subjective elements that are susceptible to bias reporting. Moreover, it is not yet known how long stockings need to be worn, which compression strength is optimal and whether they are of benefit to patients with distal DVT. Although elastic compression stocking are unlikely to cause harm, they are difficult to apply, uncomfortable, expensive and require replacement every few months. Pending results of ongoing multicentre, placebo-controlled studies, providing stockings to patients who have residual leg pain or swelling after DVT and continuing them for as long as the patient derives symptomatic benefit is a reasonable approach.

10.9 Treatment of PTS

There are few treatment options for PTS.

Diuretics To date, there is no evidence that long-term use of diuretics is effective for the treatment of PTS-related oedema. Clinicians often prescribe physical compression methods to counteract increased venous pressure.

Elastic Compression Stockings (ECS) On an as-needed basis, they may reduce swelling in some patients with PTS [47] and should be tried. However, their treatment benefit has not been definitively shown in the setting of PTS and is primarily extrapolated from studies of patients with chronic venous disease [6]. In the recent Cochrane review in 2017 [48], 10 RCTs with a total of 2361 participants evaluated compression therapy. Three studies compared elastic compression stockings (pressure of 30–40 mmHg at the ankle) versus no intervention. Two studies compared elastic compression stockings (pressure 20–40 mmHg) versus placebo stockings. Overall, use of elastic compression stockings led to a clinically significant reduction in the incidence of PTS (risk ratio (RR) 0.62, 95% confidence interval (CI) 0.38–1.01; $P = 0.05$; 1393 participants; 5 studies; low-quality evidence), no reduction in the incidence of severe PTS (RR 0.78, 95% CI 0.53–1.15; $P = 0.21$; 1224 participants; 4 studies; low-quality evidence) and no clear difference in DVT recurrence (RR 0.94, 95% CI 0.69–1.28; 1212 participants; 4 studies; $P = 0.69$; low-quality evidence). Two studies evaluated the effects of compression in the acute phase versus no compression treatment and found no differences in the incidence of PTS (RR 0.76, 95% CI 0.49–1.16; $P = 0.2$; 101 participants). One study reported that thigh-length stockings did not provide better protection against development of PTS than knee-length stockings (RR 0.92, 95% CI 0.66–1.28; $P = 0.6$; 267 participants). Another trial reported that wearing compression stockings for 2 years seemed to be superior to wearing them for 1 year in terms of PTS incidence. Two of the ten included studies described patient satisfaction and quality of life (moderate-quality evidence), using different measurement systems. The first study showed significant improvement in well-being and DVT-related quality of life with compression treatment ($P < 0.05$) compared with bed rest, and the second study showed no differences in quality of life scores between compression and placebo groups. Four studies poorly reported side effects (low-quality evidence) that included itching, erythema and other forms of allergic reaction and described no serious adverse events. Compliance with wearing of compression stockings was generally high but varied across studies. Low-quality evidence suggests that elastic compression stockings may reduce the occurrence of PTS after DVT. We downgraded the quality of evidence owing to considerable heterogeneity between studies and lack of or unclear risk of blinding due to clinical assessment scores. No serious adverse effects occurred in these studies. Large randomised controlled trials are needed to confirm these findings because of current lack of high-quality evidence and considerable heterogeneity.

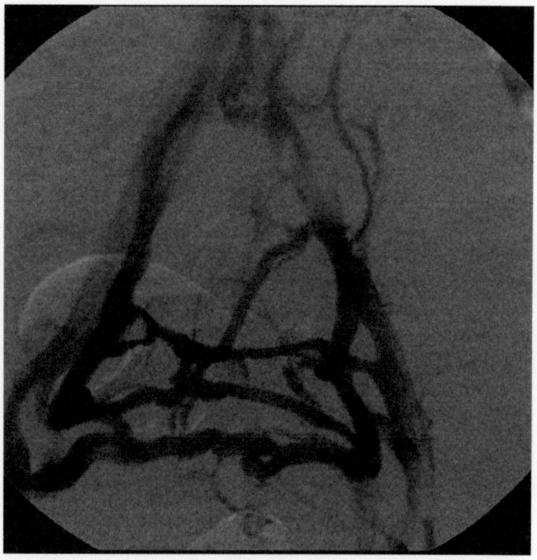

Fig. 10.3 If the large collaterals would fail, PTS will blow out (author's experience)

Intermittent Pneumatic Compression It may be of benefit for the management of severe, intractable PTS symptoms or severe oedema but lacks data on their long-term effects.

Oral Medications There is limited evidence that 'venoactive' may reduce symptoms of chronic venous insufficiency [49] and in one study improved PTS symptoms in the short term [50]. The long-term benefit and safety of these medications have not been evaluated in large controlled trials.

Post-Thrombotic Venous Ulcers They are generally treated with compression therapy, leg elevation and topical dressings but are often refractory to therapy and tend to recur [6]. Finally, surgical treatments for PTS, such as venous valve repair or venous bypass, have been evaluated primarily in small patient series at single, specialised centres, and its value is still case based [51].

10.10 Future Areas for Research

Post-thrombotic syndrome research has significantly lagged behind research in acute VTE. Studies are needed to better elucidate the pathophysiology and risk factors for PTS. Large-scale, ideally placebo-controlled, trials are needed to evaluate the effectiveness, optimal timing, strength and duration of use of ECS in preventing and treating PTS. Multicentre trials of catheter-directed thrombolysis to prevent PTS in patients with proximal DVT are also required. The potential value of venoactive agents, diuretics, anti-inflammatory medications and emerging novel therapies should be evaluated in well-designed trials that use a standardised approach to PTS diagnosis (Fig. 10.3).

10.11 Summary

Post-thrombotic syndrome is burdensome and costly to patients and society. At present, effective, evidence-based treatments for PTS are lacking, which is a source of difficulty and frustration for patients with PTS. Until effective treatments are found, prevention of PTS is the key to reducing its overall impact on patients and society. Preventing DVT recurrence is likely to reduce the risk of PTS. Daily use of graduated ECS after DVT may reduce the risk of PTS.

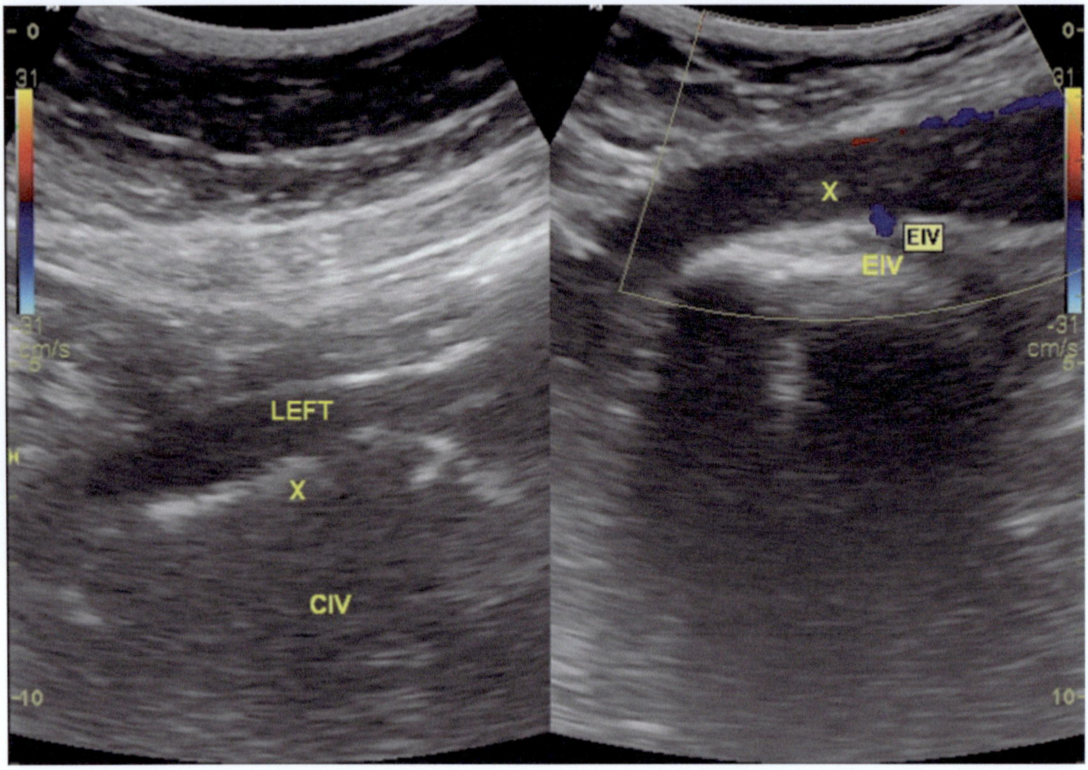

References

1. Prandoni P, Lensing A, Cogo A, Cuppini S, Villalta S, Carta M, Cattelan A, Polistena P, Bernardi E, Prins M. The longterm clinical course of acute deep venous thrombosis. Ann Intern Med. 1996;125:1–7.
2. Stain M, Schonauer V, Minar E, Bialonczyk C, Hirschl M, Weltermann A, Kyrle PA, Eichinger S. The post-thrombotic syndrome: risk factors and impact on the course of thrombotic disease. J Thromb Haemost. 2005;3:2671–6.
3. Schulman S, Lindmarker P, Holmstrom M, Larfars G, Carlsson A, Nicol P, Svensson E, Ljungberg B, Viering S, Nordlander S, Leijd B, Jahed K, Hjorth M, Linder O, Beckman M. Post-thrombotic syndrome, recurrence, and death 10 years after the first episode of venous thromboembolism treated with warfarin for 6 weeks or 6 months. J Thromb Haemost. 2006;4:734–42.
4. Kahn SR, Hirsch A, Shrier I. Effect of post-thrombotic syndrome on health-related quality of life after deep venous thrombosis. Arch Intern Med. 2002;162:1144–8.
5. Bergqvist D, Jendteg S, Johansen L, Persson U, Odegaard K. Cost of long-term complications of deep venous thrombosis of the lower extremities: an analysis of a defined patient population in Sweden. Ann Intern Med. 1997;126:454–7.
6. Kurz X, Kahn SR, Abenhaim L, Clement D, Norgren L, Bacaglini U, Berard A, Cooke JP, Cornu-Thenard A, Depairon M, Dormandy JA, Durand-Zaleski I, Fowkes GR, Lamping DL, Partsch H, Scurr JH, Zuccarelli F. Chronic venous disorders of the leg: epidemiology, outcomes, diagnosis and management - summary of an evidence-based report of the VEINES task force. Int Angiol. 1999;18:83–102.
7. Piovella F, Crippa L, Barone M, Vigano DS, Serafini S, Galli L, Beltrametti C, D'Angelo A. Normalization rates of compression ultrasonography in patients with a first episode of deep vein thrombosis of the lower limbs: association with recurrence and new thrombosis. Haematologica. 2002;87:515–22.
8. Roumen-Klappe E, der Heijer M, van Uum S, van der Ven-Jongekrijg J, van der Graaf F, Wollersheim H. Inflammatory response in the acute phase of deep vein thrombosis. J Vasc Surg. 2002;35:701–6.
9. Milne AA, Stonebridge PA, Bradbury AW, Ruckley CV. Venous function and clinical outcome following deep vein thrombosis. Br J Surg. 1994;81:847–9.
10. Kahn SR, Desmarais S, Ducruet T, Arsenault L, Ginsberg JS, VETO Study Investigators. Comparison of performance of two clinical scales to diagnose the post-thrombotic syndrome: correlation with patient-reported disease burden and valvular reflux. J Thromb Haemost. 2006;4:907–8.
11. Villalta S, Bagatella P, Piccioli A, Lensing A, Prins M, Prandoni P. Assessment of validity and reproduc-

ibility of a clinical scale for the post-thrombotic syndrome (abstract). Haemostasis. 1994;158a:24.
12. Porter JM, Moneta GL, An International Consensus Committee on Chronic Venous Disease. Reporting standards in venous disease: an update. J Vasc Surg. 1995;21:635–45.
13. Kolbach DN, Neumann HA, Prins MH. Definition of the post-thrombotic syndrome, differences between existing classifications. Eur J Vasc Endovasc Surg. 2005;30:404–14.
14. Ginsberg JS, Gent M, Turkstra F, Buller HR, MacKinnon B, Magier D, Hirsh J. Postthrombotic syndrome after hip or knee arthroplasty. Arch Intern Med. 2000;160:669–72.
15. Prandoni P, Lensing AWA, Prins MH, Frulla M, Marchiori A, Bernardi E, Tormene D, Mosena L, Pagnan A, Girolami A. Below-knee elastic compression stockings to prevent the post-thrombotic syndrome: a randomized, controlled trial. Ann Intern Med. 2004;141:249–56.
16. Van Dongen CJ, Prandoni P, Frulla M, Marchiori A, Prins MH, Hutten BA. Relation between quality of anticoagulant treatment and the development of the postthrombotic syndrome. J Thromb Haemost. 2005;3:939–42.
17. Kahn SR, Kearon C, Julian JA, MacKinnon B, Kovacs MJ, Wells P, Crowther MA, Anderson DR, Van Nguyen P, Demers C, Solymoss S, Kassis J, Geerts W, Rodger M, Hambleton J, Ginsberg JS. Predictors of the post-thrombotic syndrome during long-term treatment of proximal deep vein thrombosis. J Thromb Haemost. 2005;3:718–23.
18. Lindner DJ, Edwards JM, Phinney ES, Taylor LM, Porter JM. Long-term hemodynamic and clinical sequelae of lower extremity deep vein thrombosis. J Vasc Surg. 1986;4:436–42.
19. Monreal M, Martorell A, Callejas J, Valls R, Llamazares J, Lafoz E, Arias A. Venographic assessment of deep vein thrombosis and risk of developing post-thrombotic syndrome: a prospective study. J Intern Med. 1993;233:233–8.
20. Browse NL, Clemenson G, Thomas ML. Is the postphlebitic leg always postphlebitic? Relation between postphlebitic phlebographic appearances of deep-vein thrombosis and late sequelae. BMJ. 1980;281:1167–70.
21. Schulman S, Granqvist S, Juhlin-Dannfelt A, Lockner D. Long-term sequelae of calf vein thrombosis treated with heparin or low-dose streptokinase. Acta Med Scand. 1986;219:349–57.
22. McLafferty RB, Moneta GL, Passman MA, Brant BM, Taylor LM Jr, Porter JM. Late clinical and hemodynamic sequelae of isolated calf vein thrombosis. J Vasc Surg. 1998;27:50–6.
23. Wille-Jorgensen P, Jorgensen LN, Crawford M. Asymptomatic postoperative deep vein thrombosis and the development of postthrombotic syndrome. A systematic review and meta-analysis. Thromb Haemost. 2005;93:236–41.
24. Schindler OS, Dalziel R. Post-thrombotic syndrome after total hip or knee arthroplasty: incidence in patients with asymptomatic deep venous thrombosis. J Orthop Surg (Hong Kong). 2005;13:113–9.
25. Geerts WH, Pineo GF, Heit JA, Bergqvist D, Lassen MR, Colwell CW, Ray JG. Prevention of venous thromboembolism: the Seventh ACCP Conference on antithrombotic and thrombolytic therapy. Chest. 2004;126:338S–400S.
26. Cushman M, Folsom AR, Wang L, Aleksic N, Rosamond WD, Tracy RP, Heckbert SR. Fibrin fragment D-dimer and the risk of future venous thrombosis. Blood. 2003;101:1243–8.
27. Silverstein MD, Heit JA, Mohr DN, Petterson TM, O'Fallon WM, Melton LJ III. Trends in the incidence of deep vein thrombosis and pulmonary embolism: a 25-year population-based study. Arch Intern Med. 1998;158:585–93.
28. Mohr DN, Silverstein MD, Heit JA, Petterson TM, O'Fallon WM, Melton LJ III. The venous stasis syndrome after deep venous thrombosis or pulmonary embolism: a population based study. Mayo Clin Proc. 2000;75:1249–56.
29. Kahn SR, Ginsberg JS. Relationship between deep venous thrombosis and the postthrombotic syndrome. Arch Intern Med. 2004;164:17–26.
30. Heit JA, Rooke TW, Silverstein MD, Mohr DN, Lohse CM, Petterson TM, O'Fallon M, Melton LJ III. Trends in the incidence of venous stasis syndrome and venous ulcer: a 25-year population-based study. J Vasc Surg. 2001;33:1022–7.
31. Ramacciotti E, Gomes M, de Aguiar ET, Caiafa JS, de Moura LK, Araujo GR, Truzzi A, Dietrich-Neto F. A cost analysis of the treatment of patients with post-thrombotic syndrome in Brazil. Thromb Res. 2006;118:699.
32. Harrison M, Graham I, Friedberg E, Lorimer K, Vandevelde-Coke S. Assessing the population with leg and foot ulcers. Can Nurse. 2001;97:18–23.
33. Phillips T, Stanton B, Provan A, Lew R. A study of the impact of leg ulcers on quality of life: financial, social, and psychologic implications. J Am Acad Dermatol. 1994;31:49–53.
34. Kahn SR, M'Lan CE, Lamping DL, Kurz X, Be'rard A, Abenhaim L, VEINES Study Group. The influence of venous thromboembolism on quality of life and severity of chronic venous disease. J Thromb Haemost. 2004;2:2146–51.
35. Kahn SR, Ducruet T, Lamping DL, Arsenault L, Miron MJ, Roussin A, Desmarais S, Joyal F, Kassis J, Solymoss S, Desjardins L, Johri M, Shrier I. Prospective evaluation of health-related quality of life in patients with deep venous thrombosis. Arch Intern Med. 2005;165:1173–8.
36. Kahn SR, Panju A, Geerts W, Pineo GF, Desjardins L, Turpie AGG, Glezer S, Thabane L, Sebaldt RJ. Multicenter evaluation of the use of venous thromboembolism prophylaxis in acutely ill medical patients in Canada. Thromb Res. 2006;119:145.
37. Kearon C. Long-term management of patients after venous thromboembolism. Circulation. 2004;110:I10–8.

38. Davidson S. Davidson's principles and practise of medicine. 16th ed. Edinburgh: Churchill Livingstone; 1991.
39. Goldhaber S, Buring J, Lipnick R, Hennekens C. Pooled analyses of randomized trials of streptokinase and heparin in phlebographically documented acute deep venous thrombosis. Am J Med. 1984;76:393–7.
40. Wells P, Forster AJ. Thrombolysis in deep vein thrombosis: is there still an indication? Thromb Haemost. 2001;86:499–508.
41. Elliot MS, Immelman EJ, Jeffery P, Benatar SR, Funston MR, Smith JA, Shepstone BJ, Ferguson AD, Jacobs P, Walker W, Louw JH. A comparative randomized trial of heparin versus streptokinase in the treatment of acute proximal venous thrombosis: an interim report of a prospective trial. Br J Surg. 1979;66:838–43.
42. Arnesen H, Hoiseth A, Ly B. Streptokinase of heparin in the treatment of deep vein thrombosis. Follow-up results of a prospective study. Acta Med Scand. 1982;211:65–8.
43. Turpie AG, Levine MN, Hirsh J, Ginsberg JS, Cruickshank MK, Jay RM, Gent M. Tissue plasminogen activator (rt-PA) vs heparin in deep vein thrombosis. Chest. 1990;97:172S–5S.
44. Comerota AJ, Throm RC, Mathias SD, Haughton S, Mewissen M. Catheter-directed thrombolysis for iliofemoral deep venous thrombosis improves health-related quality of life. J Vasc Surg. 2000;32:130–7.
45. Pierson S, Pierson D, Swallow R, Johnson GJ. Efficacy of graded elastic compression in the lower leg. JAMA. 1983;249:242–3.
46. Brandjes DPM, Buller HR, Heijboer H, Hulsman MV, de Rijk M, Jagt H. Randomized trial of effect of compression stockings in patients with symptomatic proximal-vein thrombosis. Lancet. 1997;349:759–62.
47. Prandoni P. Elastic stockings, hydroxyethylrutosides or both for the treatment of post-thrombotic syndrome. Thromb Haemost. 2005;93:183–5.
48. Appelen D, van Loo E, Prins MH, Neumann MH, Kolbach DN. Compression therapy for prevention of post-thrombotic syndrome. Cochrane Database Syst Rev. 2017;9:CD004174. https://doi.org/10.1002/14651858.CD004174.pub3.
49. Diehm C. Comparison of leg compression stocking and oral horse-chestnut seed extract therapy in patients with chronic venous insufficiency. Lancet. 1996;347:292–4.
50. Prandoni P, Frulla M, Sartor D, Concolato A, Girolami A. Vein abnormalities and the post-thrombotic syndrome. J Thromb Haemost. 2005;3:401–2.
51. Eklof BG, Kistner RL, Masuda EM. Venous bypass and valve reconstruction: long term efficacy. Vasc Med. 1998;3:157–64.

Isolated Infrapopliteal Deep Venous Thrombosis

11

Madhuri Gore

11.1 Introduction

Though the gold standard of diagnostic modality and treatment of proximal deep vein thrombosis in leg veins is greatly established, the dilemma about approach to isolated distal deep vein thrombosis (IDDVT) still continues. The main reasons for the lack of clear guidelines are inadequate understanding of natural history of IDDVT, variable incidence reported in different studies, inferior sensitivity of diagnostic techniques and inconsistent outcomes of applied treatment.

This chapter is an effort to simplify different perspectives and to share some observations of the author too, with the hope that the readers would be able to reach some decision about this rather confusing situation.

11.2 Anatomy and Definition

The infrapopliteal deep veins include anterior and posterior tibial veins and peroneal veins. These are paired and accompany respective arteries. These veins coalesce with each other to form the trifurcation confluence that continues as popliteal vein. Also included are the muscular veins like medial and lateral soleal veins that empty into deep veins of calf and medial and lateral gastrocnemial veins that connect directly to the popliteal vein [1]. The author often wonders why the perforating veins that communicate directly with the deep veins are not included in this category. There is a possibility of extension of thrombosis from perforating veins to deep veins.

By definition, thrombosis of any of these veins below the trifurcation confluence without involvement of confluence or deep vein above the trifurcation falls in the category of isolated distal deep vein thrombosis. This is also referred to as isolated calf deep vein thrombosis. Some have further classified this entity into deep calf vein thrombosis (DCVT) encompassing tibial and peroneal veins and muscle calf vein thrombosis (MCVT) involving soleal and gastrocnemial veins [2].

To avoid confusion, this chapter would be using the term isolated distal deep vein thrombosis (IDDVT) for the condition under discussion unless specified.

11.3 Aetiology and Predisposing Factors

Idiopathic IDDVT is possible. But more often it is associated with recent surgery, immobilisation due to skeletal trauma, unconscious patients with

M. Gore
Consultant Surgeon, Former Professor and Chief of Surgery, LTMG Hospital, Mumbai, India

A. K. Khanna, R. Jindal (eds.), *Venous Disorders*, https://doi.org/10.1007/978-981-13-1108-6_11

minimal or no mobility and recent long duration travel [3]. Having worked in a busy trauma centre, this is author's observation too. In a study performed by the author in 100 patients in moderate-risk category undergoing general surgical procedure (no pharmaco-prophylaxis), the incidence of postoperative DVT was found to be 19%. Thirteen patients out of 19 (68.4%) were detected to have IDDVT—all unilateral, using compression Doppler ultrasound performed by the same trained investigator (unpublished data). The presence of leg varicosities has also been observed to be a predisposing factor for development of IDDVT by the author at the vein clinic at LTMGH since 1992 and then in her private setup as well.

IDDVT has been less commonly associated with presence of malignancy, pregnancy or postpartum period and in elderly population [3]. In patients with malignancy, IDDVT is more often bilateral. Existence of inherited thrombophilic state is more likely to be associated with proximal deep vein thrombosis rather than IDDVT, and if IDDVT occurs it is more often bilateral.

Palareti has opined that the risk factors for clot propagation and natural mechanisms for its lysis seem to be different in IDDVT and proximal DVT. So probably IDDVT should be considered as a different entity [3].

11.4 Incidence

The detection of IDDVT varies widely in different situations such as symptomatic or asymptomatic status of the patient, investigative modality used for confirmation, in-patient or outpatient location of the patient, patients receiving prophylactic anticoagulation and also the speciality involved in treatment of the patient. This explains the significant variation in reported incidence.

Symptomatic IDDVT rates ranging from 9 to 46% have been reported, while asymptomatic, nonobstructive IDDVTs were detected in 30% of patients subjected to surveillance during postoperative period or during prolonged hospitalisation [4]. The author has found asymptomatic unilateral IDDVT in 13 out of 19 patients detected to have postoperative DVT when total 100 were subjected to surveillance as mentioned above.

In 2011 Palareti reported detection of IDDVT to vary between 7 and 11% in outpatients suspected to have pulmonary embolism (PE), and it was 4–15% in patients suspected to have DVT. In patients diagnosed to have DVT, the occurrence of IDDVT was detected to vary between 23.4% and 59.7% [3].

A study involving 4035 lower limbs of 3146 patients, 716 scans revealed DVT. Out of these 304 (42.5%) were detected to have IDDVT, and PE was associated in 24 (7.9%) [5]. According to Galanaud et al., IDDVT accounts for 50% of patients with DVT [6], but this observation could be erroneous as many IDDVTs are asymptomatic and so may remain undetected and undiagnosed unless whole-leg compression ultrasound examination is performed.

The diagnostic modality alters the incidence of IDDVT as apparent by the observation that in patients undergoing total knee replacement without anticoagulation, IDDVT was detected in 58% on venography and 42% using ultrasonography [7].

So it appears that the incidence and prevalence of IDDVT vary variably and high level of suspicion and appropriate investigation in every suspected case of DVT is necessary to clinch the diagnosis.

11.5 Natural History

Due to significant personal variation in the treatment of IDDVT, the natural history of this condition is rather ill defined. Like proximal DVT, IDDVT may extend to involve proximal vein or gets lysed with recanalisation of the vein. IDDVT may lead to pulmonary embolism or have a possibility of recurrence. Development of incompetence leading to post-thrombotic syndrome is also a possibility. The course of natural history may depend on administration of treatment or the lack of it.

Proximal Extension of IDDVT In a review article published in 1995 [4], the incidence of proximal extension of IDDVT has been found to range from 5.6% to 30%. It was observed to be 10% in symptomatic patients and 20% in asymptomatic group. The author's study showed proximal extension occurring in 3 out of 13 patients (23%) with IDDVT on follow-up compression ultrasound on fifth and seventh postoperative day. All were asymptomatic and had not received any anticoagulation till extension was detected.

The incidence of extension was observed to be 0.6% in patients with IDDVT receiving anticoagulation, and it varied from 6% to 18% in those not receiving anticoagulation [4]. But some studies have reported extension in up to 20% even in patients receiving anticoagulation. In a retrospective study in which serial evaluation was performed in patients with IDDVT, the incidence of proximal extension was reported to be 15.5%. Association with malignancy was observed to be the major risk factor. Palareti quoted that in 2005 Righini et al. observed the incidence of extension to proximal veins as 10% in untreated and 4% in patients who received treatment [3]. Yet another review article published in 2017 mentions the extension was reported in 25–33% of individuals with IDDVT if untreated, while recent series shows it to occur in 8–15% of IDDVTs not receiving anticoagulation [1]. Cohen [7] mentions that proximal extension occurs in 8–23% of patients who are not treated for IDDVT. He also quotes that extension is rarely observed if the thrombus length is less than 5 cm. The only definite association found has been with smoking and malignancy. So it appears that the factors influencing the occurrence of extension are still unclear.

Lysis and Recanalisation The lysis of thrombus occurs due to natural fibrinolytic activity. It may take few hours to several months. Immediate lysis may prevent detection of thrombosis on investigative modality. In muscular calf vein thrombosis involving medial gastrocnemial vein and soleal vein, complete recanalisation was detected in 54.8% at 1 month, in 84.7% at 3 months and in 96% at 9 months [8]. The continuation of anticoagulation was decided based on findings at 1 month. In patients with aetiology restricted to short duration as postoperative status, spontaneous lysis of thrombus has been observed in 72–88% of patients within 3 months [7]. So generally, lysis seems to be the common fate of IDDVT while persistence and/or extension is more often associated with presence of malignancy.

Pulmonary Embolism The possibility of pulmonary embolism (PE) with proximal DVT is a well-documented complication. But the potential of IDDVT to cause PE is not clearly established yet. In 1995 Athanasios quoted incidence of PE to be 13–29% as reported in different series. Proximal extension of IDDVT to popliteal vein and above is considered necessary for occurrence of PE by many [4]. But review of literature has also revealed incidence of PE to the tune of 33% in pure IDDVT suggesting that this condition is not as innocuous as thought. This study also shows that this incidence increases to 66% when the thrombus extends to popliteal vein [4]. Change in V–Q ratio in serial examinations or positive pulmonary angiogram was used for diagnosis of PE. So it becomes imperative to identify the incidence of proximal extension of calf vein thrombosis to predict the incidence of PE. As mentioned above there is great variability in the incidence of proximal extension of IDDVT with a study mentioning the range as 0–40%! Another study by Gillet et al. observed that symptomatic PE occurred in 7% of patients with MCVT [8]. None of the PEs had clinical or haemodynamic alteration and were nonfatal. The risk factor identified for PE was thrombus diameter of more that 7–8 mm. Alhalbouni et al. reported incidence of PE to be 5.8% in patients with isolated calf muscle vein DVT, and there is no statistically significant difference in the incidence of PE between isolated proximal vein thrombosis and IDDVT [5].

In 2012 Palareti [3] reported detection of IDDVT in 7–11% patients with suspected PE. The author has observed PE in patients having IDDVT particularly with prolonged immobilisation due to skeletal trauma to leg, in patients using oral contraceptives and after long travel by bus or aeroplane. In 2017 after CALTHRO study, Palareti reported 1.6% incidence of PE in patients with IDDVT which was significantly less than association of PE with IDDVT at presentation as mentioned in Italian Master registry (26.5%) [1]. Palareti attributed this to overestimation due to missing of proximal extension prior to occurrence of PE. Worcester VTE study reports the incidence to be comparable with Palareti.

It can be concluded that IDDVT has a potential for development of PE and the clinician should be aware of this association.

Recurrence Just like all other aspects of IDDVT, the possibility of recurrence reported by different studies also varies significantly. In general the possibility of recurrence following the index event of DVT has been reported to be 67.5%. In the absence of anticoagulation, the incidence of recurrence has been observed to be 29%, and this could be reduced by 96% by anticoagulation administered for 3 months duration [4]. Gillet reported at least one episode of recurrence of thrombosis or PE in 18.8% patients during mean follow-up duration of 26.7 months. He could not detect any extension of thrombus or recurrence in patients with MCVT treated with anticoagulation [8].

Galanaud et al. [6] seem to have identified the factors influencing the incidence of recurrence more specifically. The possibility of recurrence reported was more than 3% per patient year when the index event of IDDVT was associated with affection of more than one vein in unilateral or bilateral lower extremities, age was more than 50 years and IDDVT was unprovoked. These factors tripled the occurrence of recurrence. No association with involvement of MCVT or DCVT or clot diameter was observed.

These studies indicate that the clinician should be aware of these influencing factors and not only administer anticoagulation for appropriate duration but also educate the patient about this possibility.

Post-Thrombotic Syndrome Occurrence of post-thrombotic syndrome following IDDVT is not rare. A review article published in 1995 [4] quoted a study by Browse et al. reporting incidence of post-thrombotic syndrome (PTS) as 20% after 5–10 years, and it was moderate to severe. This was followed by a study by Kakkar and Lawrence which detected PTS after IDDVT using foot volumetry 6 months after the index event. The incidence was 53% of which 38% were mild to moderate and 15% had severe haemodynamic affection. Continued pain and swelling were observed in more than 20% of patients even after 3–4 years. It appears that development of PTS is comparable after both IDDVT and proximal DVT as reported by Lindhagen et al. [4].

In 2008 Cohen [7] observed that PTS following IDDVT is underestimated and undervalued. He reported the incidence of PTS after IDDVT to be 30% and detected in all speciality clinics—medical, surgical, obstetrics and gynaecology. In a more recent study by Masuda published in 2012, the incidence of PTS has been reported as 10%, majority falling in CEAP Classes IV–VI, with very few having healed or active ulcer (CEAP C5/C6) [9].

Palareti in 2017 reported detection of PTS in 11% of patients 5 years after venographically confirmed, symptomatic IDDVT [1]. All of these patients with PTS belonged to CEAP Classes IV–VI. Generally the severity of PTS following IDDVT seems to be milder than PTS occurring after proximal DVT. Development of venous ulcer is not observed very often though pain and swelling is common.

11.6 Symptoms and Signs

A significant number of IDDVTs are asymptomatic. This applies particularly those associated with recent surgery, leg trauma, head injury and spine injury as these patients are often non-ambulatory. These may become symptomatic on extension to proximal veins or present as PE. This PE may be the first presentation and may be fatal or near fatal as these patients remain undiagnosed and untreated. So DVT prophylaxis has to be a routine practice in this category of patients.

Routine screening of high-risk patients to detect development of venous thrombosis is neither cost-effective nor practical. Sule et al. have observed that thrombi that are smaller and hence non-occlusive tend to be asymptomatic.

These tend to affect tibial veins, and their behaviour may be different from symptomatic thrombi [10].

IDDVT, when symptomatic, usually presents with swelling, leg pain and redness [10]. Galanaud also observed warm lower limb and localised pain in these patients [2]. The author has also observed similar symptoms in symptomatic IDDVTs along with tenderness on palpation of the limb. The severity of swelling is variable and is always much less than that associated with proximal DVT.

Some difference in presenting symptoms was observed by Galanaud depending on location of IDDVT [2]. MCVT presented less often with swelling as compared to DCVT. But localised pain was more commonly experienced with MCVT than DCVT. DCVT was rather more common with recent surgery, but other risk factors remained the same in both categories. The outcome was also comparable in both.

The possible differential diagnoses of IDDVT are calf muscle rupture, haematoma and popliteal cyst. The author has seen one case of tuberculous tenosynovitis, and the patient was being treated with anticoagulants with suspicion of IDDVT till confirmation.

11.7 Diagnosis and Investigations

The diagnosis can be confirmed by the following methods:

1. Clinical suspicion
2. Wells score
3. D-dimer estimation
4. Imaging techniques—venography

I^{125}-labelled fibrinogen uptake studies
Compression ultrasound
Magnetic resonance imaging—venography

1. *Clinical suspicion*: Symptomatic IDDVT is not very common, and signs are neither common nor specific. So high level of clinical suspicion in high-risk group is the only way that can lead to further investigations for confirmation of diagnosis. Appropriate administration of DVT prophylaxis is very essential in this group of patients and will be discussed later in this chapter.
2. *Wells score*: Wells described this scoring system for DVT risk stratification and has been evaluated by many by this time [11, 12]. It is very practical and easy to apply. It is based on history and clinical evaluation, and the patients are categorised into high probability of DVT with score of 3–8 points, moderate probability with 1–2 points and low probability with −2–0 points. It is author's practice to attach a chart of Wells score to the record of high-risk patient group and those with clinical suspicion and mark the score on it to make a decision about further course of action. The low probability score certainly helps in avoiding further testing. If Wells score reveals high or moderate probability, depending on protocol followed, the next investigation is either D-dimer assay or imaging technique. The author prefers D-dimer assay particularly in asymptomatic patients without recent surgery or trauma. It is cheaper than imaging investigations.
3. *D-dimer assay*: It is a fibrin degradation product detected in plasma and so is expected to rise in patients with DVT. But raised values are also observed following trauma, surgery and in presence of malignancy and pregnancy. So its specificity for making a definitive diagnosis of DVT is low. But it has very high negative predictive value. So low values (normal >500 ng/ml) of D-dimer rule out the need for further imaging, particularly when combined with clinical probability score.

The most commonly used test for quantitative evaluation of D-dimer is enzyme-linked immunosorbent assay (ELISA). For bedside qualitative testing, two tests are available whole-blood agglutination test—SimpliRED and Simplify—an immunochromatography D-dimer test. Simplify has been introduced recently, and evaluation studies are not yet available. The bedside tests provide positive or negative result in 10 min. Some studies also suggest D-dimer estimation after completion of anticoagulation treatment. This may help in evaluating the possibility of recurrence [13].

Ebadi et al. have quoted a study reporting 35% of patients having normal D-dimer levels even in the presence of IDDVT [14]. This suggests that normal D-dimer levels may have lesser sensitivity in patients with IDDVT. But the same review article also quotes other studies showing much higher sensitivity, thus continuing to support use of D-dimer estimation for ruling out IDDVT. As the confusion continues, the author continues to decide the further course of investigations based on D-dimer values.

Imaging Techniques In the 1960s contrast venography was the main diagnostic modality for DVT. But possibility of complications, allergic reactions, radiation exposure, and interobserver variation in interpretation and emergence of ultrasonography—all changed the scene.

In 1970, I^{125}-labelled fibrinogen uptake study was extensively studied by Kakkar et al. and was accepted as the gold standard for diagnosis of DVT, particularly asymptomatic calf vein thrombosis. Impedance plethysmography was another technique that was enthusiastically accepted. But both had their limitations and complications and were replaced by ultrasonography [4].

Today compression ultrasonography (CUS) is accepted as the new gold standard for diagnosis of proximal DVT and also for IDDVT in majority of situations. The technique to be mastered for evaluation of calf veins is described in details later in this chapter. But in certain situations, it may still be difficult, e.g. limb trauma with immobilisation or plaster, postoperative limb status. In these conditions ascending venography may still have a place. But this is also may be rapidly replaced by venography using spiral computerised tomography or magnetic resonance imaging (MRI) technology [4, 13].

Compression Ultrasound (CUS) The vein lumen can be completely compressed by gentle pressure of probe if there is no thrombus occupying the vein. This is the main principle of compression ultrasound. One may or may not combine ultrasound with colour coding or Doppler. This method of CUS is now established as the new gold standard for diagnosis of DVT. Majority of the studies have been done by comparing its specificity and sensitivity with ascending venography (the previous gold standard). Though the sensitivity and specificity of CUS for proximal DVT have been reported as 97%, it is observed to be 75% for symptomatic IDDVT [13]. A review article in 1995 quoted colour-flow Doppler imaging to have sensitivity of 86% and specificity of 91% for IDDVT. Another study reported this to be 100% in symptomatic IDDVT. But in asymptomatic patients, the sensitivity has been reported to be just 42% [4]. In 2007, Gillet has reported CUS sensitivity and specificity to be 87% in MCVT [8].[1] So CUS is now accepted as the new gold standard for confirming the diagnosis of symptomatic IDDVT.

Though CUS is highly specific (98%) and sensitive (97%) for proximal DVT, it reduces to 50–75% sensitivity and 90–95% specificity for IDDVT [14].

Protocol for Leg CUS The outcome of distal leg CUS obviously depends on the type of equipment, the skill and experience of the operator. It also depends on the type of patient as evaluation is very difficult in bedridden intensive care unit patient or patient with recent orthopaedic surgery. Hence it is necessary that the operator knows the appropriate technique for evaluation of lower leg veins. The position of the patient during the evaluation should be sitting on examination table with leg hanging down or standing on a stool of suitable height. This position allows filling and distension of the leg veins with blood due to gravity. The leg veins are examined from popliteal fossa downwards to ankle in cross section following the venous anatomy. Gentle probe pressure is applied to judge the vein compressibility on identification of veins. This examination protocol has been quoted to show the failure rate of CUS to be less than 0.5% at 3 months [1]. CUS of leg also helps to identify popliteal cyst, muscle rupture or haematoma in patients suspected to have IDDVT.

Protocol for Investigations Different guidelines have been recommended by different groups and individuals for approaching the final diagnosis of IDDVT.

ACCP guidelines [15] suggest that if Wells score and normal value of D-dimer are present, no further investigation should be done for confirmation of DVT and alternative diagnosis should be looked for. With Wells score and higher than normal D-dimer value both suggesting DVT, CUS of proximal veins should be performed immediately. If this is negative, the patient should be evaluated with whole-leg CUS within 48–72 h, or the patient should be called back after 1 week for proximal vein CUS to detect proximal extension of probable calf vein thrombosis. Prospective controlled studies with application of these guidelines are yet awaited [16].

NICE guidelines [17] from UK also suggest evaluating Wells score for estimating the probability of DVT to begin with. NICE guidelines categorise Wells score in only two groups—high and low. The low-risk group undergoes D-dimer estimation. If it is normal, no further investigation is performed.

In high-risk group, CUS of proximal veins is performed, and if found positive, anticoagulant therapy is started. But if CUS is negative, now D-dimer is estimated. If it is normal, no further investigation for DVT is done. If D-dimer is high, CUS is repeated after 1 week again for proximal veins. If this is also negative, no further work-up for DVT is done. But, NICE guidelines don't seem to consider existence of IDDVT in any limb of the guidelines.

Neither ACCP nor NICE guidelines recommend use of bridging anticoagulation during the waiting period for high-risk patients. If whole-leg CUS is performed, the incidence of thromboembolic event is 0.5–0.3%. Righini also reported that distal DVT was detected in 50% patient with DVT in such studies, thus increasing the number of patients receiving anticoagulation [18]. But getting CUS done twice is very expensive and difficult.

Considering common Indian patient population and their reluctance to travel for investigations repeatedly along with their compromised financial status, both of these guidelines are not suitable for them. Limited availability of operators who are appropriately trained for performing CUS is another limiting factor. So in author's opinion, the visits to medical facility before reaching the treatment decision need to be as few as possible. Or the patient with IDDVT may be lost for follow-up and then may suddenly present with extension of thrombus or PE. So the author prefers to proceed for whole-leg CUS in patients with high or moderate risk for DVT based on Wells score and D-dimer levels. The patients with unlikely probability and low D-dimer levels are not subjected to any further investigation for DVT, and alternative diagnosis is considered.

Above approach may lead to over use of anticoagulant therapy, but I think it is worth it as the possibility of life-threatening PE and development of troublesome PTS is certainly not desirable particularly in the absence of any long-term studies related to Indian population.

11.8 Management and Outcome

Management of IDDVT is the most debated aspect of this condition. There are two main groups—one that doubts the need for anticoagulation in patients with IDDVT, mainly out of concern regarding haemorrhagic complications of the therapy. This group recommends anticoagulation only if proximal extension is detected or the patient belongs to high-risk category. This needs repeated CUS of whole leg. The second group believes in proceeding with anticoagulation once the diagnosis of IDDVT is confirmed without waiting for proximal extension.

If we consider the guidelines, NICE guidelines don't seem to consider IDDVT as an entity, and the investigation protocol does not address this at all. So the question of treating IDDVT does not arise as it is not diagnosed unless it leads to proximal extension [17]. ACCP guidelines recommend anticoagulation of all diagnosed IDDVT patients with initial parenteral agent like unfractionated or low molecular weight heparin or fondaparinux (Grade IA) followed by oral anticoagulation for 3 months [15].

It is not surprising that with completely divergent guidelines and confusing, unclear natural history, different workers in this field are following and recommending different management protocols based on presence of symptoms, location and length or diameter of thrombus and presence or absence of risk factors. This has further added to unclear outcomes and natural history of IDDVT.

Singh et al. report that asymptomatic ICVT should not be anticoagulated but observed. But the study also observed higher possibility of proximal extension in association with malignancy, orthopaedic surgeries and immobility [19]. As these are the situations that are more likely to be associated with asymptomatic IDDVT due to immobility, withholding anticoagulation is difficult to accept.

In 1992, Solis et al. had reported that anticoagulation did not change the incidence of proximal extension of IDDVT after arthroplasty. So they suggested that postoperative IDDVT need not be treated. Repeated CUS was recommended to detect proximal extension, and then anticoagulation was suggested. This appears inconvenient from many angles [20] including cost and availability.

A review article by Giannoukas et al. quoted significant increase in incidence of proximal extension and recurrence of asymptomatic and hence untreated IDDVT as compared to symptomatic and treated IDDVT [4]. This article quoted incidence of proximal extension to be 32% and that of PE as 5% as suggested by ventilation perfusion scan. With risk of bleeding being 4–10% with anticoagulation, it was recommended that all patients detected to have IDDVT should be anticoagulated for 3 months. Only the patients with high risk of haemorrhagic complications were followed with repeat CUS. In the end this article states that in the absence of properly controlled prospective randomised trials, no conclusion about treatment recommendation could be reached [4].

In 2012 Singh et al. report that asymptomatic ICVT should not be anticoagulated but observed. But the study also observed higher possibility of proximal extension in association with malignancy, orthopaedic surgeries and immobility [19] as these are the situations that are more likely to be associated with asymptomatic IDDVT due to immobility, withholding anticoagulation is difficult to accept.

MCVT tends to be more often symptomatic compared to ICVT, but the outcome on follow-up as regard to death, recurrence and bleeding is the same as reported by Galanaud et al. So the author sees no reason to apply different treatment protocol to each of these entities [2].

Cohen and his group base the treatment decision on length and location of IDDVT. Hence patients with IDDVT which is close to the venous confluence, thrombus longer than 10 cm in those with no symptoms and asymptomatic thrombus with length between 5 and 10 cm, but associated with higher risk for propagation (immobility, malignancy) are all anticoagulated [7]. This group does not recommend anticoagulation for MCVT or small ICVT, instead suggest close observation of these patients and repeated CUS. These patients also receive thromboprophylaxis for variable time period. This protocol obviously involves much more effort and expertise on the part of clinician and more expenses for the patients. All patients whether symptomatic or asymptomatic receive graduated compression stockings and are ambulated as early as possible. This is very acceptable and applicable for all patients.

In 2007 Righini detected the incidence of IDDVT to be 50% of all DVTs when whole-leg CUS of both legs was performed. But he commented that though the advantages of performing calf CUS are very valid, diagnosing these IDDVTs would increase the number of patients receiving anticoagulation and hence the possibility of overtreatment. So we need randomised controlled trials [18]. After 10 years in 2017, Righini and Ebadi reviewed some randomised trials and observed increased risk of haemorrhagic complications in symptomatic IDDVT patients who received anticoagulation. This approach did not prove to be superior in decreasing the incidence of venous thromboembolism (VTE) when compared to group treated with placebo [14]. So the recommendation of this study was to conduct more randomised controlled trials to identify the optimal therapy particularly for high-risk patients.

Actually this means that treatment concepts about IDDVT are in the same confused state today as they were in 1995!

In 2012, Masuda et al. recommended an ambiguous approach [9]. They suggested acceptance of all reported methods of management of IDDVT as there is no study providing strong evidence to recommend either repeated CUS or anticoagulation.

While deciding the agent for anticoagulation, ACCP guidelines support use of unfractionated (UFH) or low molecular weight heparin (LMWH) or fondaparinux either throughout the treatment period or followed by oral anticoagulants (vit K antagonist, VKA). A study using nadroparin did not reveal superiority over placebo in symptomatic low-risk patients. It did not decrease the incidence of proximal extension or VTE. But it increased the risk of haemorrhage. So the study concluded that avoiding systemic anticoagulation would have important effect on patient and would also reduce the cost of treatment benefitting the public health expenditure [21].

One aspect of management of IDDVT that is uniformly agreed upon is use of graduated pressure elastic compression stockings (Class II below knee). This helps in relieving the edema and pain particularly during initial period. Available evidence does not support continued long-term use of compression stockings after IDDVT [1, 14].

Addressing the duration of anticoagulant therapy, Sule et al. have quoted an open labelled, randomised trial that concluded that anticoagulation for 6 weeks is adequate in patients with IDDVT [10]. The outcome would certainly guide the management protocol. Sule et al. have quoted that 5% of patients presenting with PE were associated with IDDVT. So though the possibility of PE is more with proximal DVT, it is not negligible with IDDVT. This study also mentions the incidence of major bleeding following anticoagulation to be 1–7%. The independent factors responsible for higher likelihood of bleeding were past history of stroke or gastrointestinal bleeding, age more than 65 years and presence of one or more comorbid conditions. The incidence of major bleeding at 48 months varied from 3% to 53% depending on number of risk factors detected in the patient. After evaluating the low incidence of proximal extension of IDDVT and the significant risk of bleeding after anticoagulation, Sule et al. recommended observation and follow-up CUS in patients with IDDVT. The CUS should be done at 2 weeks, 1 month and 3 months. Any evidence of extension of thrombus or augmentation of symptoms should prompt anticoagulation [10].

After study of all available data about management of IDDVT, conclusion drawn by Ebadi and Righini seems logical. They suggest that symptomatic, low-risk patients with IDDVT should receive compression stockings and follow-up CUS to detect proximal extension and no anticoagulation. Though the available evidence is inadequate, symptomatic, high-risk patients with previous VTE, malignancy and unprovoked DVT as well as patients with low risk of haemorrhage should receive anticoagulation in therapeutic dose [14].

So the pendulum swings from no anticoagulation even after diagnosis of IDDVT to anticoagulation of all patients confirmed to have IDDVT! Palareti accepts the fact that optimal management of IDDVT is still a debated topic and probably same protocol cannot be applied to all patients. Though CALTHRO study has shown that use of Class II compression stockings alone has shown very low incidence of VTE, the therapeutic and prophylactic utility of this modality has not been studied yet [3]. The need to diagnose and treat each patient with IDDVT and the agent and duration of anticoagulation has not yet been established. So we have two options—one is to detect and treat only proximal DVT or the second being to perform whole-leg CUS in all suspected cases and treat all IDDVTs that are detected. If first CUS is negative, second CUS after 1 week would be needed in 80–90% of patients, and it's difficult to obtain this compliance. But if only the patients with high D-dimer are called back then, the number reduces to 30% [3], and better compliance may be achieved with appropriate counselling.

The management protocol used by Palareti seems practical and more suitable for Indian scenario [1]. He opposes the ACCP guidelines that recommend serial CUS after diagnosis of IDDVT to detect proximal extension (Grade 2C). His patients as well as mine would want treatment of their diagnosed, symptomatic IDDVT, and it has to be in appropriate dose using appropriate medication. Palareti also reports low diagnostic accuracy of Wells score for IDDVT and good negative predictive value of D-dimer assay. He recommends that all patients confirmed to have IDDVT should be evaluated for any contraindications for anticoagulation, and if none are detected, the patient should be anticoagulated initially with UFH or LMWH or fondaparinux followed by VKA in titrated dose for period of 1–3 months. In selected high-risk cases like presence of malignancy and pregnancy, the parenteral therapy is continued throughout the treatment period and even later in prophylactic dose [1]. He recommends reduction in the dose of parenteral anticoagulant to 50% after 2 months in high-risk patients and after 10 days in transient-risk patients. The author does not perceive the need to do this dose modification. All patients are instructed to use Class II below knee compression stockings. CUS is performed on completion of anticoagulation period to evaluate the effect of therapy and status of thrombosed veins.

11.9 The Author's Approach

Prophylaxis All methods of mechanical and pharmacological prophylaxis are strictly followed according to risk stratification. Adequate hydration, early ambulation, calf and ankle exercises in bed and appropriate use of calf pump if needed are strictly observed. Pharmacoprophylaxis using LMWH is administered in appropriate dose to all moderate-, high- and very high-risk patients unless contraindicated. The time of administration and withdrawal of neuraxial blockade access is adjusted suitably.

Diagnosis of IDDVT In-hospital or outpatients with suspicion of IDDVT undergo calculation of Wells score and evaluation of D-dimer levels. D-dimer levels may not be dependable particularly in postoperative or trauma patients. Whole-leg CUS is performed in all the suspected patients based on Wells score and D-dimer. Main problem is experienced in patients who can't sit and those with cast on leg due to orthopaedic surgery or trauma. Radiologists or technicians well versed with correct method of performing whole leg CUS are very few even in metropolis like Mumbai. It is necessary to encourage them to learn the methodology, and a document describing the method is provided to them. Even then it is difficult and repeated serial evaluation is almost impossible. It is also expensive, and outpatients particularly from out of Mumbai find it very difficult to comply with follow-up. Occasionally the author is forced to ask for MR venography (though it's expensive) as application of CUS technology is difficult due to patient's condition. Such a situation may force dependence on proximal CUS and repeat CUS at 1 week interval if the first evaluation is negative for DVT.

Our Treatment Protocol All ambulatory patients are provided with Class II below knee compression stockings with complete explanation about its use and care.

In all patients with diagnosed IDDVT, anticoagulation is initiated (unless contraindicated) using LMWH and rarely UFH with dose calculation according to the molecule and weight of patient. Patients with malignancy and pregnancy are continued on LMWH. Others start receiving VKA from day 1, and the overlap continues for at least 5–6 days till the INR reaches 2 on three consecutive evaluations done daily. The INR is maintained in the therapeutic range between 2.5 and 3 by dose titration if needed. INR is evaluated every 15 days after therapeutic range is achieved and stabilised. This is continued for 3 months, and CUS is obtained to confirm satisfactory response before withdrawal of anticoagulation.

Patient and family are educated about the anticoagulant medication, its effects and possible haemorrhagic complications, need for regular monitoring and precautions to be taken. A contact phone number is provided for emergency contact. Instructions about follow-up schedule are explained. All these instructions are also provided on a sheet written or printed in the language that the patient or the family can read and understand. I have observed that patient education is the most important aspect of improving patient compliance.

Newer oral anticoagulants available in India are rivaroxaban, apixaban and dabigatran. The availability is rather restricted, and cost is high. But fixed dose, no requirement for repeated dose titration and no need to monitor the therapeutic effect make these agents easy to use if patients can afford the cost and ensure availability. The author uses these agents particularly factor Xa inhibitors (as direct thrombin inhibitors have really limited availability) whenever the patient can afford it. Patient education is certainly desirable.

Conclusion

Due to wide variation in the treatment protocol, the outcomes reported vary over a wide range. The fear of haemorrhagic complications seems to have overwhelming effect on the treatment and actually overlooks the possibility of proximal extension of thrombus, possibility of PE, development of PTS and recurrent VTE. All these outcomes, though less than proximal DVT, are not nonexistent.

It appears that over the last several years, very little progress has been made regarding our understanding of natural history, appropriate treatment and optimal dosage of anticoagulants as well as the outcome of IDDVT. So each one still is forced to follow his or her own protocol.

The protocol has to depend on accrued experience, availability and affordability of investigative modalities and pharmacological agents, financial and educational status of patient population and availability of trained and interested medical personnel.

But we do need standard guidelines that can be easily applied and are acceptable. For this purpose appropriately designed, randomised, controlled trials enrolling large patient population are desperately needed. These should preferably be conducted in different countries with application of same trial design and protocol. This would make it possible to pool the results and may be prepare guidelines specific for each participating country. These guidelines based on the conditions specific to that country could then be recommended as the standard of care for that country. That would be the ideal solution to this condition which is in dilemma for years!

References

1. Palareti G. How I treat isolated distal deep vein thrombosis (IDDVT). www.bloodjournal.org by guest on 3 Sep 2017.
2. Galanaud J-P, Sevestre M-A, Genty C, Laroche J-P, Zizka V, Quéré I, Bosson J-L, OPTIMEV SFMV Investigators. Comparison of the clinical history of symptomatic isolated muscular calf vein thrombosis versus deep calf vein thrombosis. J Vasc Surg. 2010;52(4):932–8, 938.e1-2. https://doi.org/10.1016/j.jvs.2010.05.019. Epub 2010 Jul 13.
3. Palareti G, Schellong S. Isolated distal deep vein thrombosis: what we know and what we are doing. J Thromb Haemost. 2012;10:11–9. https://doi.org/10.1111/j.1538-7836.2011.04564.x.
4. Giannoukas AD, Labropoulos N, Burke P, Katsamouris A, Nicolaides AN. Calf deep venous thrombosis : a review of the literature. Eur J Vasc Endovasc Surg. 1995;10:398–404.
5. Alhalbouni S, Hingorani A, Shiferson A, Marks N, Ascher E. Infra-popliteal deep venous thrombi and the risk of symptomatic pulmonary embolism in hospitalized patients. Vascular. 2011;19:29.
6. Galanaud JP, Sevestre MA, Genty C, Kahn SR, Pernod G, Rolland C, Diard A, Dupas S, Jurus C, Diamand JM, Quere I, Bosson JL, OPTIMEV-SFMV Investigators. Incidence and predictors of venous thromboembolism recurrence after a first isolated distal deep vein thrombosis. J Thromb Haemost. 2014;12:436–43. https://doi.org/10.1111/jth.12512.
7. Cohen AT, Balaratnam S, Fassiadis N. Are isolated distal deep-vein thromboses clinically significant? Therapy. 2008;5(2):151–7. https://doi.org/10.2217/14750708.5.2.151.
8. Gillet J-L, Perrin MR, Allaert FA. Short-term and mid-term outcome of isolated symptomatic muscular calf vein thrombosis. J Vasc Surg. 2007;46:513–9.
9. Masuda EM, Kistner RL, Musikasinthorn C, Liquido F, Geling O, He Q. The controversy of managing calf vein thrombosis. J Vasc Surg. 2012;55:550–61.

10. Sule AA, Chin TJ, Handa P, Earnest A. Should symptomatic, isolated distal deep vein thrombosis be treated with anticoagulation? Int J Angiol. 2009;18(2):83–7.
11. Wells PS, Anderson DR, Bormanis J, et al. Value of assessment of pretest probability of deep-vein thrombosis in clinical management. Lancet. 1997;350(9094):1795–8.
12. Wells PS, Owen C, Doucette S, Fergusson D, Tran H. Does this patient have deep vein thrombosis? JAMA. 2006;295(2):199–207.
13. Tovey C, Wyatt S. BMJ. 2003;326(7400):1180–4. https://doi.org/10.1136/bmj.326.7400.1180.
14. Robert-Ebadi H, Righini M. Management of distal deep vein thrombosis. Thromb Res. 2017;149:48–55. https://doi.org/10.1016/j.thromres.2016.11.009.
15. Bates SM, Jaeschke R, Stevens SM, et al. Diagnosis of DVT: antithrombotic therapy and prevention of thrombosis, 9th ed. American College of Chest Physicians Evidence-Based Clinical Practice Guidelines. Chest. 2012;141:e351S–418S.
16. Kitchen L, Lawrence M, Speicher M, Frumkin K. Emergency department management of suspected calf-vein deep venous thrombosis: a diagnostic algorithm. West J Emerg Med. 2016;17(4):384–90. https://doi.org/10.5811/westjem.2016.5.29951.
17. In Clinical Questions by David Wonnacott, March 21, 2017, 3 Comments. Isolated distal DVT – diagnosis and management. https://canadiem.org/isolated-distal-dvt-diagnostic-and-management.
18. Righini M. Is it worth diagnosing and treating distal deep vein thrombosis? No. J Thromb Haemost. 2007;5(s1):55–9. https://doi.org/10.1111/j.1538-7836.2007.02468.x.
19. Singh K, Yakoub D, Giangola P, DeCicca M, Patel CA, Marzouk F, Giangola G. Early follow-up and treatment recommendations for isolated calf deep venous thrombosis. J Vasc Surg. 2012;55:136–40.
20. Solis MM, Ranval TJ, Nix ML, Eidt JF, Nelson CL, Ferris EJ, Lavender RC, Barnes RW. Is anticoagulation indicated for asymptomatic postoperative calf vein thrombosis? J Vasc Surg. 1992;16(3):414–8; discussion 418-9.
21. Righini M, Galanaud JP, Guenneguez H, Brisot D, Diard A, Faisse P, Barrellier MT, Hamel-Desnos C, Jurus C, Pichot O, Martin M, Mazzolai L, Choquenet C, Accassat S, Robert-Ebadi H, Carrier M, Le Gal G, Mermilllod B, Laroche JP, Bounameaux H, Perrier A, Kahn SR, Quere I. Anticoagulant therapy for symptomatic calf deep vein thrombosis (CACTUS): a randomised, double-blind, placebo-controlled trial. Lancet Haematol. 2016;3:e556.

Novel Biomarkers in Deep Vein Thrombosis

12

Ajay K. Khanna, Manbendra Vaidya, and Soumya Khanna

Venous thromboembolic disease (VTE) remains a significant source of morbidity and mortality. As non-specific subjective complaints and a paucity of objective clinical examination findings complicate the diagnosis of both deep venous thrombosis (DVT) and pulmonary embolism (PE), diagnostic modalities remain essential. Symptoms suggestive of deep vein thrombosis are extremely common in practice but unfortunately non-specific. The modified Wells score remains the most supported clinical decision rule for risk stratifying these concerns. Compression ultrasound remains the gold standard for diagnosis of DVT. Reliable imaging is not always available, so making a serologic diagnosis, or biomarker, is highly desirable. While D-dimer, a highly sensitive biomarker, is useful for excluding acute VTE, it lacks the specificity necessary for diagnostic confirmation. As such, ongoing research efforts target and support the utility of alternative plasma biomarkers to aid in the diagnosis of VTE including selectins, microparticles, IL-10, and other inflammatory markers. These molecular markers may also predict recurrence risk, guide length and modality of treatment, and predict which thrombi will resolve spontaneously or recanalize, thus potentially identifying patients who would benefit from more aggressive therapies than standard anticoagulation [1].

Currently, the only biomarker used in the diagnosis of deep vein thrombosis (DVT) is plasma D-dimer. D-dimer, a product of fibrin degradation, is a sensitive biomarker that, when low or absent, can be used to exclude or "rule out" the diagnosis of DVT in patients with a low Wells score. However, this biomarker is not specific for DVT as it is frequently elevated in the setting of non-specific inflammation such as cancer, pregnancy, surgery, trauma, etc. Because of the low specificity of D-dimer, elevated levels alone cannot be used to confirm the diagnosis of DVT, and in such instances, an imaging study is needed for definitive diagnosis. The current gold standard for diagnosis of DVT is compression duplex ultrasound. However, the availability of this diagnostic modality is limited at smaller medical centers, outpatient settings, and on nights and weekends and also person-to-person expertise. In these circumstances, a chemical or laboratory diagnosis to "rule in" the diagnosis of DVT without having to rely on duplex ultrasound would be helpful. Using the biology of platelet and leukocyte activation, inflammation, and thrombosis, it has been identified that soluble P-selectin (sPsel) and microparticles (MP) are potential novel biomarkers to make the diagnosis of DVT. Of these, sPsel has shown the greatest promise. D-dimer, a fibrin degradation product, has been thoroughly investi-

A. K. Khanna (✉)
Department of General Surgery, Institute of Medical Sciences, Banaras Hindu University, Varanasi, India

M. Vaidya · S. Khanna
Institute of Medical Sciences, Banaras Hindu University, Varanasi, India

A. K. Khanna, R. Jindal (eds.), *Venous Disorders*, https://doi.org/10.1007/978-981-13-1108-6_12

gated and performs well in select populations, although it is best as a rule-out test because of its generally low specificity. Soluble P-selectin, a marker of endothelial activation, has shown good diagnostic performance in several studies but has not yet been adopted widely. Others, including cellular adhesion molecules, tissue factor, circulating microparticles, and C-reactive protein, are under investigation, with varying results in a few studies [2].

12.1 D-Dimer

D-dimer is the most common and widely accepted biomarker to rule out deep vein thrombosis. When assayed by a quantitative ELISA or by some automated turbidimetric assays, D-dimer is highly sensitive (more than 95%) in excluding acute deep vein thrombosis or pulmonary embolism, usually below a threshold of 500 μg/L. Hence, a concentration lower than this value rules out acute venous thromboembolism (VTE), at least in patients with low or intermediate clinical probability [3]. ELISA-based tests can be of two types, whole-blood or plasma latex agglutination tests. Sensitivity of these tests ranges from 84 to 97%, but again, specificity is low [4]. Recently D-dimer values are being used as an indicator to determine the duration for anticoagulation therapy in patients with DVT or VTE. It has been still a matter of debate because while extending oral anticoagulation therapy reduces the risk of recurrence by 90%, it is associated with an increased clinically important risk of major bleeding. In 2005, Cosmi et al. [5] investigated D-dimer levels in combination with residual venous obstruction and the risk of recurrence after anticoagulation withdrawal for a first idiopathic DVT. Authors concluded that abnormal D-dimer levels at 1 month after therapy withdrawal are an independent risk factor for recurrent VTE. They also noted that residual venous obstruction on duplex ultrasound at the time of oral anticoagulation withdrawal, despite a normal or abnormal D-dimer after 1 month, does not influence the rate of recurrence.

12.2 Soluble P-Selectin

Soluble P-selectin (sPsel), a member of the selectin family of cell adhesion receptors, has been proposed as a key molecule in hemostasis and thrombosis mediating platelet rolling, generating procoagulant microparticles, and enhancing fibrin deposition. Recently soluble P-selectin (sPsel) has emerged to be a very promising biomarker in diagnosing DVT. P-selectin is an adhesion glycoprotein present in platelet α-granules and endothelial cell Weibel-Palade bodies that is responsible for the initiation of leukocyte rolling. The sPsel has been proposed not only as a marker of inflammation or platelet activation but also as a direct inducer of procoagulant activity associated with vascular and thrombotic diseases [6]. P-selectin is the major receptor supporting constitutive leukocyte rolling and promotes platelet adhesion to stimulated vessel wall. It also enhances fibrin formation thereby leading to formation of venous thrombosis. The sPsel, when combined with the Wells score, may represent the best combination for the diagnosis of VTE. With a suspicion of DVT, a high Wells score (≥2) and sPsel above 90 ng/mL) may establish the diagnosis of DVT for the first time, with a positive predictive value (PPV) of 100%. Furthermore, sPsel has evidenced even a very high sensitivity (99%) in some cases [7]. However, high sPsel concentrations have been observed in other diseases including ischemic heart disease, atherosclerosis, and acute ischemic stroke [8]. Furthermore, high levels of sPsel were recently associated with an increased risk for recurrence of DVT.

George et al. [9] studied 11 studies, comprising of 586 VTE patients, and 1843 controls were deemed eligible. The sPsel was significantly increased after VTE (OR = 2.89, 95%CI = 2.31–3.61, $p < 0.001$) or DVT only (OR = 2.64, 95%CI = 1.95–3.56, $p < 0.001$). Subgroup analysis evidenced that sPsel was also increased after VTE when evaluating only studies with patients that had no prior medical history (OR = 2.88, 95%CI = 1.98–4.19, $p < 0.001$). Exclusion of studies including patients with solid organ tumor and HIV or lupus anticoagulant-positive patients did not alter the findings. Pooled sensitivity and specificity of sPsel were 0.57 (95%CI = 0.30–082, $p < 0.001$) and 0.73 (95%CI = 0.51–0.90, $p < 0.001$), respectively, and DOR was 4.31 (95%CI = 2.22–8.37, $p < 0.01$). SROC curve yielded in significant accuracy of sPsel performance (AUC = 0.74, $p = 0.05$). The sPsel was significantly elevated in patients with DVT, both uncomplicated and complicated with PE, and presented with high levels of diagnostic performance.

Knut et al. [10] investigated the plasma levels of the endothelium-specific biomarkers soluble E-selectin and endocan in a consecutive and unselected group of 120 patients admitted to the hospital for suspected deep vein thrombosis. DVT patients showed evidence for an acute phase reaction with increased serum C-reactive protein levels, but this was similar to many other patients admitted with suspected but not verified thrombosis. Plasma endocan and E-selectin levels did not differ between patients with thrombosis, healthy controls, and the patients without verified thrombosis (i.e., patients with other causes of their symptoms, including various inflammatory and non-inflammatory conditions). However, the combined use of endothelial biomarkers, C-reactive protein, and D-dimer could be used to identify patient subsets with different frequencies of venous thrombosis. Thus, analysis of plasma biomarker profiles including endothelial cell markers may be helpful in the initial evaluation of patients with deep vein thrombosis.

12.3 Homocysteine

Another biomarker which has shown its close relation with DVT is homocysteine. More than 40 years ago, it has been reported that some patients suffering from mental retardation had homocystinuria and hyperhomocysteinemia. This group of people also shared other specific phenotypic characteristics, including skeletal and ophthalmic abnormalities, as well as an increased predisposition to thrombosis [11].

Homocysteine is a nonessential sulfated amino acid that is not directly involved in protein synthesis. It is ubiquitously produced by all cells and has been preserved throughout the evolution. Mild to moderate hyperhomocysteinemia may be a result of acute occlusive events such as myocardial infarction and thromboembolic stroke [11]. Homocysteine leaks from damaged tissue, and it also tends to accumulate during the repair process. The latter is possibly due to the essential methylation reactions required to form new DNA, RNA, and proteins. High homocysteine levels are also present in malignancies, including breast cancer, gliomas, and acute lymphoblastic leukemia. Total homocysteine concentration in plasma falls during uncomplicated pregnancy. The physiology of this is unclear, but it may be hormonally driven since a similar effect is observed with combined oral contraceptive pill use and hormone replacement therapy. A contributory factor could be the use of folate supplements to prevent neural tube defects.

Den et al. [12] studied 24 retrospective studies, which included a total of 3289 subjects with hyperhomocysteinemia. There was significant heterogeneity between the reports, but overall these studies have shown that each 5 μmol/L increase in measured homocysteine is associated with a 60% increased risk of venous thrombosis.

12.4 CRP (C-Reactive Protein)

In 1930 after the publication of the seminal article by Tillett et al. [13] which clearly suggested that CRP was not really a pathogenic secretion of bacteria but rather a non-specific physiochemical reaction to bacterial infection, there have been a lot of studies which have shown CRP as a predictor in arterial thrombotic events [14]. Clinical data on the association between increased plasma CRP concentrations and venous thrombosis are conflicting.

Vormittag et al. [15] studied two case-control studies and reported a positive univariate association between CRP and VTE, but not after multivariable adjustment. Similarly, Tsai et al. [16] studied two other cohort studies, with limited numbers of VTE events, and reported no association between CRP and VTE. However, a subsequent analysis of the prospective population-based

ARIC study which included a larger number of VTE cases and longer follow-up found that increased CRP concentrations were independently associated with an increased risk of VTE [17]. In a recently published case-control study, Luxembourg et al. [18] showed that markers of inflammation, including fibrinogen, factor VIII, and CRP, were at higher concentrations in patients with idiopathic compared to secondary VTE, supporting the hypothesis that idiopathic VTE and arterial thromboembolism share common risk factors. Finally, the prospective Copenhagen City Heart Study (CCHS) and the cross-sectional Copenhagen General Population Study (CGPS) by Zacho et al. [19] observed that nongenetically increased CRP concentrations were robustly associated with increased risk of VTE.

Although still a matter of debate, the potential role of CRP in the pathogenesis of cardiovascular disorders is currently considered plausible, because inflammation represents one of the underlying mechanisms leading to the formation of human atheroma, favoring both the destabilization of vulnerable plaques and formation of occlusive thrombi. Although it has been hypothesized that VTE and arterial thromboembolism share common risk factors, there is scarce and mostly conjectural evidence supporting the contribution of increased CRP to the development of venous thrombosis. Therefore, for cardiovascular disorders, the crucial and unresolved question is whether CRP represents an independent risk factor for VTE and may therefore play a causal role or rather does it reflect mutual associations with established VTE risk factors.

12.5 Factor VIII

Modern thrombophilia testing fails to identify any underlying prothrombotic tendency in a significant number of patients presenting with objectively confirmed VTE. This observation has led to a search for other novel inherited or acquired human thrombophilia markers. An increasing body of work supports the hypothesis that increased plasma factor VIII (FVIII) levels may be important in relation to DVT. An association between elevated plasma FVIII levels and VTE was first described in the Leiden Thrombophilia Study (LETS). Cumulatively, studies have clearly demonstrated that high FVIII levels constitute a prevalent, dose-dependent risk factor for VTE. Furthermore, more recent studies have shown that the risk of recurrent venous thrombosis is also significantly increased in patients with high FVIII levels.

In a retrospective study, Kraaijenhagen et al. [20] studied 60 patients with recurrent VTE, 65 patients with a single episode of thrombosis, and 60 age- and sex-matched controls. The authors calculated that for each 10 iu/dL increment in plasma FVIII level, the risk for a single and recurrent episode of VTE increased by 10% and 24%, respectively. Furthermore, for patients with FVIII levels above 200 iu/dL, the odds ratio for a recurrent thrombotic episode was markedly elevated at 45. Kyrle et al. [21] studied 360 patients with a first episode of objectively confirmed VTE. Plasma FVIII levels were significantly increased in the cohort of patients who developed recurrent VTE. However the relationship between increased FVIII levels and risk of recurrent thrombosis was nonlinear. Consequently, patients with plasma FVIII levels above the 90th percentile (>234 iu/dL) were at particular high risk for developing recurrent VTE. Cristina et al. [22] in his prospective cohort study also observed that the risk of recurrent venous thrombosis was significantly increased in patients with elevated FVIII.

12.6 Microparticles (MPs)

Microparticles (MPs) are small (0.1–1.0 μm) membrane vesicles constitutively released from the surface of cells after activation and apoptosis. The clinical research on MPs is hampered by the limitations of the currently available detection methods. A correlation between MPs and venous thromboembolism (VTE) has been observed. The effects of MPs on thrombogenesis involve the exposure of phosphatidylserine, the vehiculation of tissue factor, and MP-induced intercellular cross talk between inflammation and coagulation [23].

12.7 MicroRNAs (miRNAs)

MicroRNAs (miRNAs) are endogenous small (about 22 nucleotides in length) noncoding RNAs that play important regulatory roles by targeting mRNAs for cleavage or translational repression. Recent studies have found that miRNAs play crucial roles in many cellular processes, such as development, proliferation, differentiation, and apoptosis. Due to its high stability in plasma or serum and potential for highly sensitive measurement, circulating miRNAs have been intensively investigated as noninvasive biomarker for diseases, such as cancers, neurodegenerative diseases, and cardiovascular diseases. Recent studies have also explored the biomarker value of miRNAs in the diagnosis of pulmonary embolism. Few studies explored the diagnostic value of elevated plasma miR-134 in PE, indicating that plasma miR-134 could be an important biomarker for the diagnosis of PE. However, all those studies were limited to a small sample size. Therefore, the actual diagnostic power of miRNAs in PE is still unclear [24].

Serum microRNA-1233 is a specific biomarker for diagnosing acute pulmonary embolism [25]. Rapidly and accurately diagnosing acute PE would be an extremely helpful tool, especially at emergency departments. Ideally, miRNA-1233 could identify acute PE patients early as a bedside test so that correct treatment could be initiated timely, consequently reducing mortality and morbidity. As of now, most laboratories use RT-qPCR-based methods for detecting serum miRNAs. RT-qPCR is very sensitive on one hand but also difficult to standardize on the other. To date, a housekeeping miRNA to normalize miRNA content to is lacking. The current practice of supplementing external controls (for instance, spiking of miRNAs for normalization in PCR-based measurements) might not be sufficient enough to provide an accurate bedside measurement of circulating miRNAs. For the clinical routine, well-defined cutoff values and reliable measurements are most crucial and would be needed.

12.8 Combination of Parameters

Ramacciotti et al. [7] studied the various combinations of the parameter to get the best results (Table 12.1).

In 2005, Rectenwald et al. [26] hypothesized that plasma microparticles, P-selectin, and D-dimer levels, alone or in combination with patient risk stratification, would accurately predict the presence or absence of DVT when compared to the current gold standard of duplex ultrasound examination. Rectenwald et al. [26] enrolled 73 patients in his pilot study, of which 30 were healthy controls, 22 had acute DVT present on duplex ultrasound, and 21 had clinical symptoms supporting DVT but with a negative ultrasound. The authors established threshold values for all the biomarkers investigated (including D-dimer) that provided the highest sensitivity while maintaining the highest specificity: soluble P-selectin values of 0.68 ng/mg per mg total protein, total microparticles levels 125% of control, and D-dimer levels of 3 mg/L. The preliminary data presented suggested that the sensitivity (73%) and specificity (81%) of sPsel, total microparticles, and d-dimer used in combination as dichotomous values for diagnosing DVT, although less sensitive and specific than duplex ultrasound, were an improvement over D-dimer alone (64% sensitivity, 76% specificity).

We studied various parameters in 43 proved patients of DVT. We saw that D-dimer test alone has a detection sensitivity of 88.3% in patients with DVT. But when this test is combined with soluble P-selectin test, the detection sensitivity increases to 95.35%. When three tests were combined (D-dimer + sPsel + WBC), detection sensitivity increased to 100%. Similarly D-dimer + sPsel + factor VIII had a detection sensitivity of 100%. So we concluded that combination of these biomarkers can increase the detection sensitivity of cases with deep vein thrombosis (Table 12.2).

So there have been a few biomarkers which show their role in diagnosis of deep vein thrombosis. All these biomarkers have stood to their respective tests when used alone, and there have been quite a few studies which support their role

Table 12.1 Statistical significance of individual parameter and combination of parameters

Variable	*p*-value (regression)	Sensitivity (%)	Specificity (%)	NPV (%)	PPV (%)
sPsel (‡90 ng/mL)	<0.0001	28	96	72	72
sPsel + Wells score (‡90 ng/mL + ‡ 2)	<0.0001	33	95	70	100
sPsel + Wells score (<60 ng/mL + <2)	<0.0001	99	33	96	47
D-dimer (£ 0.5 mg/L	<0.0001	98	29	80	40
D-dimer + Wells score (£ 0.5 mg/L + <2)	<0.0001	93	45	81	44
Wells score (‡2)	<0.0001	41	93	79	33
sPsel + D-dimer (‡90 ng/mL + £ 0.5 mg/L)	<0.0001	43	81	81	58

DVT deep venous thrombosis, *NPV* negative predictive value, *PPV* positive predictive value, *sPsel* soluble P-selectin

Table 12.2 Detection sensitivity of combinations of various biomolecular markers in deep vein thrombosis

Combination of markers	No of positive cases	Sensitivity (%)
D-dimer	38	88.37
D-dimer + sPsel	41	95.35
D-dimer + factor VIII	41	95.35
D-dimer + WBC	40	93.02
D-dimer + sPsel + WBC	43	100
D-dimer + sPsel + factor VIII	43	100

in diagnosing DVT. Moreover there exist positive correlations among all these markers which again indicate the importance of these biomarkers in the pathophysiology of DVT. But still their involvement and accepting them to be a specific biomarker in ruling in DVT are under evaluation. Each of the biomarker has their limitation and has limited sensitivity and specificity in diagnosing DVT. On the contrary when these biomarkers are being used in combination, they have shown to be much more promising in diagnosing DVT.

12.9 Biomarkers in Cancer

While cancer patients suffer from a high burden of VTE, the D-dimer and Wells score are less helpful in this group. This is due to non-specific D-dimer elevations in these patients and cancer being part of the Wells risk stratification scheme. D-dimer > 500 with Wells score ≥ 2 was less specific for the diagnosis of DVT among cancer patients compared to non-cancer patients ($p = 0.003$). However, D-dimer ≥ 500 with sPsel ≥ 90 showed not only high specificity, but that specificity was not different between the cancer and non-cancer populations ($p = 0.88$). sPsel ≥ 90 and Wells ≥2 had similar performance characteristics in both groups as well ($p = 0.54$ for specificity, $p = 0.14$ for positive predictive value (PPV)). Results concur with the finding that the D-dimer, combined with a clinical prediction rule, is not as helpful for DVT in cancer patients. Moreover, this study further supports sPsel as a specific test for DVT that can be combined with clinical information (Wells score) or other laboratory data (D-dimer) to reflect the presence of DVT and potentially rule in clot; the test seems equally useful for both cancer and non-cancer populations [27].

12.10 Summary

D-dimer is the only clinically applied biomarker for DVT diagnosis, with soluble P-selectin a promising novel biomarker. Recent studies have identified several other potential biomarkers. Ultrasound remains the imaging modality of choice, but CT, MRI, or nuclear medicine tests can be considered in select scenarios [28].

References

1. Coleman DM, Thomas W. Biomarkers for the diagnosis of deep vein thrombosis. Expert Opin Med Diagn. 2012;6(4):253–7.
2. Jacobs B, Obi A, Wakefield T. Diagnostic biomarkers in venous thromboembolic disease. J Vasc Surg Venous Lymphat Disord. 2016;4(4):508–17.

3. Righini M, Le Gal G, Aujesky D, et al. Diagnosis of pulmonary embolism by multidetector CT alone or combined with venous ultrasonography of the leg: a randomized non-inferiority trial. Lancet. 2008;371:1343–52.
4. Bockenstedt P. D-dimer in venous thromboembolism. N Engl J Med. 2003;349:1203–4.
5. Cosmi B, Legnani C, Cini M, et al. D-dimer levels in combination with residual venous obstruction and the risk of recurrence after anticoagulation withdrawal for a first idiopathic deep vein thrombosis. Thromb Haemost. 2005;94(5):969–74.
6. Andre P, Hartwell D, Hrachovinova I, Saffaripour S, Wagner DD. Procoagulant state resulting from high levels of soluble P-selectin in blood. Proc Natl Acad Sci U S A. 2000;97:13835–40.
7. Ramacciotti E, Blackburn S, Hawley AE, Vandy F, Ballard-Lipka N, Stabler C, et al. Evaluation of soluble P selectin as a marker for the diagnosis of deep venous thrombosis. Clin Appl Thromb Hemost. 2011;17:425–31.
8. Nadar SK, Lip GY, Blann AD. Platelet morphology, soluble P selectin and platelet P selectin in acute ischaemic stroke. The West Brimingham Stroke Project. Thromb Haemost. 2004;92:1342–8.
9. Sfyroeras GS, Kakisis JD, Moulakakis KG, Liapis CD. The role of soluble P selectin in the diagnosis of venous thromboembolism. Thromb Res. 2014;133(1):17–24.
10. Mosevoll KA, Lindås R, Wendelbo Ø, Bruserud Ø, Reikvam H. Systemic levels of the endothelium-derived soluble adhesion molecules endocan and E-selectin in patients with suspected deep vein thrombosis. Springerplus. 2014;3:571. http://www.springerplus.com/content/3/1/571
11. Dudman NP. An alternative view of homocystiene. Lancet. 1999;354:2072–4.
12. Den Heijer M, Lewington S, Clarke R. Homocystiene, MTHFR and risk of venous thrombosis: a meta-analysis of published epidemiological studies. J Thromb Haemost. 2005;3:292–9.
13. Tillett WS, Goebel WF, Avery OT. Chemical and immunological properties of a species-specific carbohydrate of pneumococci. J Exp Med. 1930;52(6):895–900.
14. Casa JP, Shah T, Hingorani AD, Danesh J, Pepys MB. Creative protein and coronary heart disease: a critical review. J Intern Med. 2008;264:295–314.
15. Vormittag R, Vukovich T, Schonauer V, Lehr S, Minar E, Bialonczyk C, et al. Basal high sensitivity C- reactive protein levels in patient with spontaneous venous thromboembolism. Thromb Haemost. 2005;93:488–93.
16. Tsai AW, Cushman M, Rosamond WD, Heckbert SR, Polak JF, Folsom AR. Cardiovascular risk factors and venous thromboembolism incidence: the longitudinal investigation of thromboembolism etiology. Arch Intern Med. 2002;162:1182–9.
17. Folsom AR, Lutsey PL, Astor BC, Cushman M. C-reactive protein and venous thromboembolism. A prospective investigation in the ARIC cohort. Thromb Haemost. 2009;102(4):615–9.
18. Luxembourg B, Schmitt J, Humpich M, Glowatzki M, et al. Cardiovascular risk factors in idiopathic compared to risk-associated venous thromboembolism: a focus on fibrinogen, factor VIII, and high-sensitivity C-reactive protein (hs-CRP). Thromb Haemost. 2009;102(4):668–75.
19. Zacho J, Tybjaerg-Hansen A, Nordestgaard BG. C-reactive protein and risk of venous thromboembolism in the general population. Arterioscler Thromb Vasc Biol. 2010;30(8):1672–8.
20. Kraaijenhagen RA, Anker PS, Koopman MM, Reitsma PH, Prins MH, van den Ende A, Buller HR. High plasma concentration of factor VIII:C is a major risk factor for venous thromboembolism. Thromb Haemost. 2000;83:5–9.
21. Kyrle PA, Minar E, Hirschl M, Bialonczyk C, Stain M, Schneider B, Weltermann A, Speiser W, Lechner K, Eichinger S. High plasma levels of factor VIII and the risk of recurrent venous thromboembolism. N Engl J Med. 2000;343:457–62.
22. Cristina L, Benilde C, Michela C, Mirella F, Giuliana G, Gualtiero P. High plasma levels of factor VIII and risk of recurrence of venous thromboembolism. Br J Haematol. 2004;124:504–10.
23. Campello E, Spiezia L, Radu CM, Simioni P. Microparticles as biomarkers of venous thromboembolic events. Biomark Med. 2016;10(7):743–55. https://doi.org/10.2217/bmm-2015-0063
24. Deng H-Y, Li G, Luo J, Wang Z-Q, Yang X-Y, Lin Y-D, Liu L-X. MicroRNAs are novel non-invasive diagnostic biomarkers for pulmonary embolism: a meta-analysis. J Thorac Dis. 2016;8(12):3580–7.
25. Kessler T, Erdmann J, Vilne B, Bruse P, Kurowski V, Diemert P, Schunkert H, Sager HB. Serum microRNA-1233 is a specific biomarker for diagnosing acute pulmonary embolism. J Transl Med. 2016;14:120.
26. Rectenwald JE, Myers DD, Hawley AE, et al. D-dimer, P-selectin and microparticles: novel markers to predict deep venous thrombosis. Thromb Haemost. 2005;94:1312–7.
27. Schaefer JK, Angelini DE, Hawley A, Blackburn SA, Lusk E, Braun TM, Wakefield TW, Sood SL. Biomarkers and clinical prediction rules in the diagnosis of suspected deep vein thrombosis: a comparison of cancer and non-cancer patients. Blood. 2016;128:3804.
28. Schaefer JK, Jacobs B, Wakefield TW, Sood SL. New biomarkers and imaging approaches for the diagnosis of deep venous thrombosis. Curr Opin Hematol. 2017;*24*(3):274–81.

13 Newer Oral Anticoagulants

Ravul Jindal and Piyush Chaudhary

13.1 Introduction

Anticoagulants are widely used for the prevention and treatment of venous and arterial thrombosis. Vitamin K antagonists such as warfarin and Acitrom though effective are associated with numerous drawbacks including narrow therapeutic window. Therefore, frequent International normalized ratio (INR) monitoring is required which is a huge financial burden. There are multiple food-drug and drug-drug interactions with VKAs which also complicate the treatment with these drugs. Also TTR (time in therapeutic range) value maintained should be more than 60% to have an effective anticoagulation. In most of the studies, required percentage of >60% TTR (time in therapeutic range) value is not maintained [1].

This was overcome with discovery of NOACs which work with inhibition of thrombin and factor Xa. They have rapid onset of action within 30 min to 2 h. Another good thing is that it has least drug-drug interaction and patient does not have to change its dietary plan due to less food-drug interactions.

Another important point is that they don't require INR monitoring and are given to a patient in a fixed dose. Therefore therapy is much simpler for both patient and medical staff. There are some drawbacks with this also which we will explain later in the chapter.

R. Jindal (✉) · P. Chaudhary
Vascular and Endovascular Surgery, Fortis Hospital, Mohali, India

13.1.1 Why Anticoagulation

Anticoagulant is used for prophylaxis of thrombosis in patients who are undergoing surgery or are immobilized. It is also used as a treatment in patients with thrombosis to prevent further propagation. This can be used in both arterial and venous thromboses which can affect coronary, cerebrovascular, visceral and limb circulation.

13.1.2 Discovery and Development of Anticoagulants

Heparin

In 1916 McLean discovered that liver extracts contained a powerful anticoagulant which was later named as heparin (from the Greek word *Liver) by* Howell and Holt in 1918 [2, 14].

This heparin was impure and was associated with severe toxic reactions. Jorpes in Stockholm (1935) and Best in Toronto (1959) prepared pure heparin resulting in fewer side effects. Initially heparin was prepared from lungs of beef but later on was derived from pig intestine [3].

A. K. Khanna, R. Jindal (eds.), *Venous Disorders*, https://doi.org/10.1007/978-981-13-1108-6_13

Warfarin-VKA

Schofield in 1924 found that spoiled sweet clover hay was the cause of bleeding in cattle in the USA. This bleeding was stopped by fresh transfusions and by removing clover hay from feed of cattle [2]. It was found that bleeding occurred due to plasma prothrombin defect.

In 1941 Campbell and Link identified that bacterial contamination of hay converted natural coumarin to hydroxyl coumarin which resulted in formation of an anticoagulant (dicoumarol). Dicoumarol resulted in bleeding in cattle [2].

This led to research by Link's group to find a compound which can have the effect of dicoumarol-warfarin (Wisconsin Alumni Research Foundation initials) that was found to be very effective and at that point was used as a rat poison [2].

LMWH (Low-Molecular-Weight Heparin): Subcutaneous Anticoagulant

LMWH is produced by chemical splitting of heparin into one third of its size. It is more effective than heparin with fewer side effects since it is injected subcutaneously in fixed doses and do not need monitoring, so it can be used at home as well [4].

Rivaroxaban (NOAC)

The new anticoagulants target the activated serine proteases factor Xa. Rivaroxaban was approved for clinical use in 2008 as first direct factor Xa inhibitors. It is now used in preventions of VTE in adult patients undergoing hip or knee replacement surgery [4–6] as well as for treatment of VTE.

Dabigatran Etexilate (NOAC)

Dabigatran provides long anticoagulation duration but was not active orally due to its polarity. The compound, dabigatran etexilate, is its orally active prodrug. It has shown promising results both in prophylaxis and treatment of VTE [7].

Apixaban (NOAC)

This compound was discovered by Bristol-Myers Squibb and is a factor Xa selective inhibitor. This is being produced now in alliance with Pfizer and is a very effective antithrombotic agent [8, 16].

13.2 Comparison Between NOACS and VKAs

From the last many years, VKAs were the only oral anticoagulants which were used. They include coumarin derivatives (warfarin and acenocoumarol). New generation of oral anticoagulants like NOACs have been shown to be effective in prevention of stroke and systemic embolization in patients with non-valvular atrial fibrillation (NVAF) and treatment of venous thromboembolism [15]. They have more predictable anticoagulant response. NOACs are termed as direct oral anticoagulants (DOACs) due to direct inhibition of factor IIa (F IIa)/thrombin and factor X (F Xa).

VKA dose is not fixed, whereas NOACs are administered in fixed doses. NOACs with various advantages are still not considered ideal because of the presence of certain disadvantages compared to VKA (Table 13.1).

Table 13.1 Table showing advantages and disadvantages of warfarin and NOACs

	Advantage	Disadvantage
Warfarin	• High bioavailability • Anticoagulation can be monitored (INR) • Reversal agent available (vitamin K) • Can use in all group ages • Long clinical experience with VKAs • Price is less	• Great drug-drug interactions and food-drug interaction • Frequent monitoring of INR is required • Narrow therapeutic window • Slow onset and offset • Long half-life
NOACs	• Predictable pharmacokinetics • Low drug-drug and food-drug interactions • Rapid onset and offset • Short half-life • Wide therapeutic window • No lab monitoring required	• Difficult monitoring • Antidote not commonly available • High cost • Not enough experience

13.3 Newer Oral Anticoagulants

NOACs are a revolution in the world of oral anticoagulant therapy, whereas their rate of expansion is slow due to lack of effective antidote, their cost, and reservations in renal patients. Their use depends on experience and good knowledge of their indications.

13.3.1 Classification of Newer Oral Anticoagulants

NOACs are divided into two classes – the oral direct thrombin inhibitors (DTIs, e.g., dabigatran) and oral direct factor Xa inhibitors (e.g., rivaroxaban and apixaban). These drugs block the activity of one single step in coagulation cascade compared to multiple steps in VKA. Indications with doses, safety profile and pharmacological properties are given in Tables 13.2, 13.3, and 13.4 respectively [13].

Dabigatran Etexilate

Dabigatran was the first NOAC studied and FDA approved. It is a highly specific and competitive direct thrombin inhibitor. It is orally inactive but is converted to its active form – dabigatran etexilate – in the body.

It has rapid onset of action (1–2 h), reaches peak plasma levels in 2–3 h, has a short half-life (12–13 h), and has 80% renal excretion.

Rivaroxaban

Rivaroxaban is the second NOAC approved by the FDA. It is a competitive and dose-dependent direct inhibitor of factor Xa. It is rapidly absorbed with 30% renal clearance. It is contraindicated in severe renal impairment. It is administered as single 20 mg dose, which is adjusted in mild renal impairment patients.

Apixaban

Apixaban is a direct, selective inhibitor of factor Xa. It is well absorbed and reaches peak plasma concentration in 1–4 h. It is prescribed in a dose of 5 mg twice a day, and dose is modified if age >80 years, weight is <60 kg, and serum creatinine >1.5 mg/dL. It is mainly metabolized in the liver, and therefore drugs capable of inhibiting CYP 3A4 should be carefully administered with apixaban.

Edoxaban

Edoxaban is a factor Xa inhibitor with its effect reaching peak in 1–2 h. It is excreted mainly by the kidney and has got drug interaction with quinidine, amiodarone, and verapamil which can result in significant higher levels of edoxaban.

13.3.2 Antidotes for NOAC [17]

Idarucizumab (Reversal of Factor II Inhibitor)

Idarucizumab (Praxbind®), approved by the FDA in October 2015, is a monoclonal antibody fragment that binds to dabigatran with high affinity. It is used for reversal of factor II inhibitor. Dose of 5 mg of it completely reverses the anticoagulant effect within minutes of drug administration and restores normal homeostasis [9, 10].

Table 13.2 Approved indications for and doses of the Newer oral anticoagulants

Indication	Dabigatran	Rivaroxaban	Apixaban
Atrial fibrillation	150 mg BD 75 mg BD If creatinine clearance is 15–30 mL/min	20 mg once a day 15 mg once a day If creatinine clearance Is 15–50 mL/min	5 mg BD
Prevention of venous thromboembolism	Not indicated	10 mg once a day	2.5 mg BD
Treatment of venous thromboembolism	150 mg BD after LMWH for 7 days	15 mg BD for 21 days and then 20 mg once a day	10 mg BD for 7 days and then 5 mg BD
Preventing recurrence of venous thromboembolism	150 mg BD	20 mg once a day	2.5 mg BD

Table 13.3 Safety outcomes of NOACs

	Dabigatran 150 mg BD	Dabigatran 110 mg BD	Rivaroxaban 20 mg OD	Apixaban 5 mg BD
Major bleeds	Low	Very low	Low	Very low
Major GI bleeds	Slightly high	Low	Slightly high	Low
Life-threatening bleeds	Very low	Very low	NA	Very low
ICH	Very low	Very low	Very low	Very low
Total bleeds	Very low	Very low	Low	Very low

Table 13.4 Absorption and Metabolism of NOACs

	Dabigatran	Apixaban	Rivaroxaban
Bioavailability	3–7%	50%	66% without food Almost 100% with food
Absorption with food	No effect	No effect	+39% more
Intake with food recommended?	No	No	Mandatory
Prodrug	Yes	No	No
Clearance nonrenal/renal of absorbed dose	20/80%	73/27%	65/35%
Liver metabolism: CYP3A4 involved	No	Yes (elimination, moderate contribution)	Yes (elimination, moderate contribution)
Elimination half-life	12–13 h	12 h	5–9 h (young) 11–13 h (elderly)
Absorption with H2B/PPI	−12 to 30%	No effect	No effect
Asian ethnicity	+25%	No effect	No effect
GI tolerability	Dyspepsia 5–10%	No problem	No problem

Table 13.5 Reversible agent: Pharmacological properties

	Idarucizumab	Andexanet Alfa	Ciraparantag (PER 977)
Target	Dabigatran	FXa inhibitors	FXa inhibitors, dabigatran, and heparins
Administration	IV bolus or short infusion	IV, bolus, and/or continuous infusion	IV
Mechanism of action	Specific humanized fab: binds dabigatran	Nonspecific recombinant activated FX: competitive affinity for direct FXa inhibitors	Nonspecific synthetic small molecule; hydrogen bonds (NOACs): charge-charge interactions (heparin)
Reinitiate anticoagulation	Possible	No data available	No data available
Inclusion criteria in patient trial	Uncontrolled bleeding or requiring emergency surgery	Uncontrolled bleeding only	No patient trial yet

Andexanet Alfa (Reversal Factor Xa Inhibitor)

Modified recombinant factor Xa acts as decoy protein when it binds to factor Xa inhibitors due to lack of procoagulant activity. Because of its short half-life, it is given as bolus plus a 1–2-h infusion.

This drug reduces anti-factor XA activity (of anticoagulant) by >90% in patients taking either apixaban or rivaroxaban and restores normal hemostatic function. It is still not FDA approved.

Activated Charcoal

Activated charcoal when administered within few hours of drug ingestion reduces drug absorption. Pharmacological properties of these reversible agents are given in Table 13.5.

Perioperative management of NOACS is a very important aspect of the treatment. One has to consider type of surgery and the comorbidities of the individual patient. In some patients one must see renal or hepatic function of the patient (Table 13.6).

Shifting from one anticoagulant to another is called switching. Usually it is done when some surgery is required on patient taking anticoagulants. After surgery patient is reverted back on previous anticoagulant which is called bridging therapy. Bridging of NOACS is commonly done with LMWH which is best for perioperative period. Table 13.7 shows the recommendations.

For the safety of the patient one must have knowledge about reaction of NOACs with various drugs. These reactions can either enhance or diminish the effects of NOACs. Drugs having interactions with NOACs are shown in Table 13.8.

Usually NOACs don't require monitoring of coagulation. On basis of these parameters dose and dosage interval should not be changed. Sometimes its important to measure anticoagulant effect in specific situations like hepatic or renal insufficiancy and suspected overdosing. Samples taken 3 hrs after the intake of NOAC (peak levels) will show much larger impact on the coagulation test. Various assays which can be used are shown in Table 13.9. We are

Table 13.6 Perioperative management with NOACs

	Minor surgery		Major surgery	
NOAC	Preoperative	Postoperative	Preoperative	Postoperative
Dabigatran	Stop 2 days before surgery Stop 3 days before surgery	Restart 24 h after surgery	Stop 3 days before surgery Stop 4–5 days before surgery	Restart 48 h after surgery
Apixaban (CrCl>30 mL/min)	Stop 2 days before surgery	Restart 24 h after surgery	Stop 3 days before surgery	Restart 48 h after surgery
Rivaroxaban	Stop 2 days before surgery	Restart 24 h after surgery	Stop 3 days before surgery	Restart 48 h after surgery

Table 13.7 Recommendation on how to switch between different anticoagulant regimens

Switching	How?
Low-molecular-weight heparin (LMWH) to newer anticoagulants	At the due time of next LMWH dose
Warf/Acitrom to newer anticoagulants	When INR is <2
Unfractionated heparin (UFH) to newer anticoagulants	2 h after last dose of UFH except in renal disease
Newer anticoagulants to parenteral anticoagulant (UFH, LMWH)	At the predicted time of next dose of newer anticoagulants
One newer anticoagulant to another	At the next due dose of newer anticoagulants except in renal disease
Newer anticoagulants to warf/Acitrom	Treatment with both until INR is between 2 and 3

Table 13.8 Drug interactions of different NOACs

	No dose adjustment	Contraindicated	Age of adjustment (%)
Rivaroxaban	Amiodarone, antacids, atorvastatin, carbamazepine, digoxin, diltiazem, phenytoin, phenobarbitone, rifampin, verapamil	Clarithromycin/erythromycin, cyclosporine/tacrolimus, HIV protease inhibitors, ketoconazole, itraconazole, voriconazole, posaconazole	Quinidine (+50%)
Apixaban	Amiodarone, antacids, atorvastatin	Carbamazepine, HIV protease inhibitors, ketoconazole, itraconazole, voriconazole, posaconazole, phenytoin, phenobarbitone, rifampin	Diltiazem (+40%)
Dabigatran	Antacids, atorvastatin, clarithromycin/erythromycin, digoxin, diltiazem	Carbamazepine, dronedarone, ketoconazole, itraconazole, voriconazole, posaconazole, phenytoin, phenobarbitone, rifampin	Amiodarone (+12–60%), quinidine (+53–56%), verapamil (+12–180%)

Table 13.9 Monitoring assays for NOAC

	Yes	No
Dabigatran	aPTT, ECT, TT, dTT	INR, anti-FXA ASSAYS, PT
Rivaroxaban	Anti-FXA ASSAYS, PT	aPTT, ECT, INR, TT, dTT
Apixaban	Anti-FXA ASSAYS	aPTT, ECT, INR, TT, dTT, PT

aPTT activated partial thromboplastin time, *dTT* diluted thrombin time, *ECT* ecarin clotting time, *FXa* factor Xa, *INR* international normalized ratio, *PT* prothrombin time, *TT* thrombin time

Table 13.10 Important clinical trials with NOACs [18]

	Name of trial	Enrolled patients	Dosage
Dabigatran	RE-COVER I and II	5128	Dabigatran 150 mg twice daily for 6 months
Apixaban	AMPLIFY	5400	Apixaban 10 mg twice daily for first 7 days, followed by 5 mg twice daily for 6 months
Rivaroxaban	EINSTEIN-DVT, EINSTEIN-PE	8282	Rivaroxaban: 15 mg twice daily for 3 weeks, followed by 20 mg once daily for 12 months

also showing the various clinical trials which has been done with Dabigatran, Apixaban and Rivaroxaban which have been shown in Table 13.10.

13.4 NOACs in Specific Conditions

13.4.1 NOACs for Children

Children have various physiologic protective mechanisms involved which prevent thromboembolic disorders in them. Pharmacokinetic parameters such as distribution, binding, half-life, and clearance are age dependent. Also compliance is difficult in children [11].

Safety and effectiveness of dabigatran and rivaroxaban in children have not been established. Apixaban has the least renal clearance around 25% among all. Due to lack of pharmacological studies in children, the clinical decision regarding the best anticoagulant is taken after consulting specialist anticoagulation services. Dosing of LMWH in children is depicted in Table 13.11.

Table 13.11 Dosing of low-molecular-weight heparins

LMWH	Prophylaxis dose	Treatment dose
Dalteparin (U/kg/dose every 24 h)	92 ± 52	129 ± 43
Enoxaparin (mg/kg/dose every 12 h)	<2 months: 0.75 >2 months: 0.5	<2 months: 1.5 >2 months: 1

13.4.2 Pregnancy

Pregnant women should avoid NOACs and VKAs. Instead they should be switched to LMWH or UFH. When pregnant, NOACs should be used only if the potential benefit outweighs the potential risk to the mother and fetus. Anticoagulant therapy should be discontinued at the onset of spontaneous labor.

NOACs should not be used in breastfeeding women and other alternative anticoagulants LMWH/UFH/warfarin/acenocoumarol should be considered [4].

13.4.3 Cancer

There is very limited data present to support the use of NOACs in cancer patients on chemotherapy. There are some randomized trials which showed similar benefits with dabigatran as warfarin in acute VTE. Also no significant difference in efficacy was seen between the drugs during the study [4, 6, 10].

13.4.4 Renal Failure

NOACs are not appropriate in some patients, such as who have liver or kidney disease.

Table 13.12 Approved dosing in CKD

	CrCl>50 mL/Min	CrCl 30–49 mL/min	CrCl 15–30 mL/min	CrCl <15 mL/min
Dabigatran	150 mg BD	110 mg BD	75 mg BD	Not recommended
Apixaban	5 mg BD	5 mg BD	2.5 mg BD	Not recommended
Rivaroxaban	No adjustment	15 mg OD	15 mg OD	Not recommended

Approximately 80% of dabigatran, 33% of rivaroxaban, and 25% of apixaban are eliminated through the kidneys as an active drug.

Renal function must be assessed before applying any of the NOAC drugs with the help of creatinine clearance (the Cockroft-Gault formula). Therefore, the application of NOACs in renal disease should be performed with caution, especially in elderly patients [12] (Table 13.12).

13.4.5 Liver Failure

NOACs can be used in patients with mild and moderate liver insufficiency but requires dose adjustment. Apixaban and rivaroxaban are contraindicated in hepatic disease as associated with coagulopathy and high bleeding risk.

Rivaroxaban is contraindicated in severe hepatic impairment (e.g., Child-Pugh Class C) and cirrhotic patients with Child-Pugh Class B or C.

13.4.6 Elderly

Elderly patients of age ≥75 treated with NOACs did not have an increased recurrence compared to younger patients. Meta-analysis of all patients ≥75 showed that NOACs were found to be more effective compared to warfarin [5, 6, 8, 9].

13.4.7 Patients on Antiplatelet Therapy

Low-dose concomitant aspirin can be used according to the NOAC VTE treatment trials, and dual antiplatelet therapy was allowed in the dabigatran and rivaroxaban trials. Concomitant usage of antiplatelets should be done only if it is necessary.

13.5 How to Choose Between Different NOACs

There is no head-to-head comparing data on these agents, picking one agent over another. There isn't any data to support. All anyone can do is compare its efficacy to warfarin. All four NOACs are approved for treatment of venous thromboembolism (VTE), but only rivaroxaban and apixaban are approved for VTE prevention.

Cost, renal function, and bleeding risk are the factors which we consider while making our choice.

13.5.1 Choice

- Is patient a candidate for a NOAC?
- Does the patient have comorbid illnesses (that would preclude NOAC use)?
- Is patient compliant and able to afford the medication?

Choice will be among apixaban, dabigatran, and rivaroxaban (edoxaban hasn't been on the market long enough for clinicians to get comfortable using it). Clinicians will narrow their options based on familiarity of the drug they use. Rivaroxaban's once-a-day dosing also is a factor compared with twice-daily apixaban and dabigatran.

13.5.2 The Cost Equation

Whereas VKAs are by far the cheapest option for patients, the three NOACs haven't differed much in price. They are comparatively costlier than VKAs, but as now generic drugs are available, there is good market competition making these drugs cheaper.

13.5.3 Bleeding Risk

Bleeding risk with NOACs increases if patient is already on some antiplatelet therapy due to coronary artery disease or peripheral vascular disease. In our practice, when there are patients on dual antiplatelet therapy, for example, after drug-eluting stent placement specifically aspirin and a P2Y12 antagonist, we do not elect to use a novel anticoagulant. We think warfarin is probably the safest choice, but ease of administration and other advantages are pushing the physicians to prescribe these drugs more and more.

There is minimal data with NOACs in these settings, and triple anticoagulant therapy significantly increases risk for major bleeds.

While still highly controversial, we switch patients to clopidogrel (Plavix) and warfarin after stenting if they come in on a NOAC. After 6 or 12 months, we will switch to aspirin and a NOAC. Studies are in progress to get a better sense of what the best regimen should be in these complicated settings. As clinicians, we should not let marketing dictate which drugs we choose for our patients. This should be a joint decision between the doctor and his/her patient.

Conclusion

Each of the NOACs is slightly different, enabling us to further individualize and optimize therapy for each patient. Dabigatran has a higher chance of dyspepsia (11.3%) along with GI bleed compared to warfarin, so patients with a history of GERD, gastritis, or GI bleed may do better with warfarin or apixaban and/or consider starting a proton-pump inhibitor.

Rivaroxaban needs to be taken with food for better bioavailability, so patients who do not eat a full meal, such as those with a history of gastric bypass, might not have full bioavailability. Daily dosing of rivaroxaban may be a better option for those patients in whom twice-daily dosing might lead to compliance issues. Rivaroxaban has a higher rate of GI bleed than warfarin, so once again consider avoiding in those with a history of GI bleed.

The amount of GI bleeds was not statistically significant between apixaban and warfarin, so it might be a better consideration than the other NOACs for those with a history of GI bleeds. So as a physician, you can decide which NOAC to use depending on your knowledge about the drug and clinical experience.

References

1. Jeffrey I, Weitz F. Expanding use of new oral anticoagulants. 1000 Prime Rep. 2014;6:93. https://doi.org/10.12703/P6-93.
2. Wardrop D, Keeling D. The story of the discovery of heparin and warfarin. Blackwell Publishing Ltd. Br J Hematol. 2008;141:757–63.
3. Mannucci PM, Poller L. Venous thrombosis and anticoagulant therapy. Br J Haematol. 2001;114(2):258–70. https://doi.org/10.1046/j.1365-2141.2001.02961.
4. Bates SM, Greer IA, Middeldorp S, Veenstra DL, Prabulos A-M, Vandvik PO. VTE, thrombophilia, antithrombotic therapy, and pregnancy. Chest. 2012;141(2):e691S–736S.
5. Perzborn E, Roehrig S, Straub A, Kubitza D, Misselwitz F. The discovery and development of rivaroxaban, an oral, direct factor Xa inhibitor. Nat Rev Drug Discov. 2011;10(1):61–75.
6. Ageno W, Gallus AS, Wittkowsky A, Crowther M, Hylek EM, Palareti G. Oral anticoagulant therapy. Chest. 2012;141(2):e44S–88S.
7. van Ryn J, Goss A, Hauel N, Wienen W, Priepke H, Nar H, Clemens A. The discovery of dabigatran etexilate. Front Pharmacol. 2013;4:12.
8. Hanna MS, Mohan P, Knabb R, Gupta E, Frost C, Lawrence JH. Development of apixaban: a novel anticoagulant for prevention of stroke in patients with atrial fibrillation. Ann N Y Acad Sci. 2014;1329(1):93–106.
9. Roca B, Roca M. The new oral anticoagulants: reasonable alternatives to warfarin. Cleve Clin J Med. 2015;82(12):847–54.
10. Heidbuchel H, Verhamme P, Alings M, Antz M, Diener H-C, Hacke W, Oldgren J, Peter S, John Camm A, Kirchhof P. Updated European Heart Rhythm Association practical guide on the use of non-vitamin K antagonist anticoagulants in patients with non-valvular atrial fibrillation. Europace. 2015;17(10):1467–507.
11. Dabbous MK, Malaeb DN, Sakr FR. Anticoagulant therapy in pediatrics. J Basic Clin Pharm. 2014;5(2):27.
12. Mekaj A, Mekaj Y, Duci S, Miftari E. New oral anticoagulants: their advantages and disadvantages compared with vitamin K antagonists in the prevention and treatment of patients with thromboembolic events. Ther Clin Risk Manag. 2015;11:967.

13. Masotti L, Pampanini M. Pharmacology of new oral anticoagulants: mechanism of action, pharmacokinetics, pharmacodynamics. Ital J Med. 2013;7(8S):1–7. https://doi.org/10.4081/itjm.s8.1.
14. Hirsh J, Warkentin TE, Shaughnessy SG, Anand SS, Halperin JL, Raschke R, Christopher G, Magnus Ohman E, Dalen JE. Heparin and low-molecular-weight heparin mechanisms of action, pharmacokinetics, dosing, monitoring, efficacy, and safety. Chest. 2001;119(1):64S–94S.
15. Connolly SJ, Ezekowitz MD, Yusuf S, Eikelboom J, Oldgren J, Parekh A, Pogue J, Reilly PA, Themeles E, Varrone J, Wang S, Alings M, Xavier D, Zhu J, Diaz R, Lewis BS, Darius H, Diener H-C, Joyner CD, Wallentin L. Dabigatran versus warfarin in patients with atrial fibrillation. N Engl J Med. 2009;361(12):1139–51.
16. Wong PC, Pinto DJP, Zhang D. Preclinical discovery of apixaban, a direct and orally bioavailable factor Xa inhibitor. J Thromb Thrombolysis. 2011;31(4):478–92.
17. Dolgin E. Antidotes edge closer to reversing effects of new blood thinners. Nat Med. 2013;19(3):251.
18. Hinojar R, Jiménez-Natcher JJ, Fernández-Golfín C, Zamorano JL. New oral anticoagulants: a practical guide for physicians. Eur Heart J Cardiovasc Pharmacother. 2015;1(2):134–45.

14 Therapeutic Alternatives for Venous Ulcer

Fernando Vega Rasgado

14.1 Introduction

The usual definition of venous ulcer is "an open skin lesion of the leg or foot that occurs in an area affected by venous hypertension" sic [1]. In epidemiological reports the prevalence of leg ulceration in the population C5–C6, shown by the CEAP score (Clinic estadification method for venous insufficiency, C5 Healed ulcer and C6 Open ulcer), is about 1–2%. The etiologic factors that can produce leg ulcers are diverse, but the majority of the patients have venous disease in different stages of evolution. Chronic venous insufficiency is ten times more frequent than arterial ulcers [2]. Venous ulcers affect approximately 10–35% of the total United States population, and 4% of the population who are older than 65 years show active ulcers [3]. The economic cost of this disease in the United States is one billion dollars per year. Recent epidemiological studies on chronic venous disease have been conducted in England, Sweden, and Australia; the studies included between 12,000 and 434,699 individuals. The average point prevalence for venous ulceration was 0.29%, and some interesting aspects of venous ulcer were reported: there was a strong relationship between the prevalence of arterial hypertension ulcers (63.2%) and the prevalence of venous ulcers (arterial-venous), which approached 80%. Healing was less frequent for the mixed-etiology ulcers, at 26%, than for venous ulcers alone, at 41% [4]. In regard to etiology, Koerber and Schadendorf [5] found 75.25% venous leg ulcers, 3.66% arterial leg ulcers, 14.66% ulcers of mixed origin, and 13.5% vasculitic ulcers in their study population. Diabetic leg ulcers and ulcers with an inflammatory border and skin necrosis are often associated with chronic inflammatory diseases such as ulcerous colitis or rheumatoid arthritis. Leg ulcers may also occur in patients with Klinefelter's syndrome; in these patients with hypogonadism and testosterone deficit, slow-healing ulcers may occur with or without chronic venous disease. There is some evidence that abnormal platelet aggregability or fibrinolysis with elevated plasminogen activator inhibitor-1 activity may play an important role in these cases. The most important differential diagnosis of leg ulcers is that of ulcerations caused by malignant or semi-malignant diseases, in which ulcerating tumors such as basal cell carcinoma or melanoma may mimic venous ulcerations [5]. For the correct treatment of venous ulcers we need to have the most accurate possible diagnosis, and in some cases the diagnosis is not 100% accurate. The single most helpful confirmatory test is the duplex Doppler examination; the diagnosis should not only evaluate the great saphenous vein (GSF) but all the superficial, deep, and perforating venous systems. In the Skövde study only 25% of patients with venous ulcers had

F. Vega Rasgado
Instituto Mexicano de Flebología, Academia Mexicana de Flebología y Linfología, Clínica de Várices y Ulceras de México, Mexico City, Mexico

A. K. Khanna, R. Jindal (eds.), *Venous Disorders*, https://doi.org/10.1007/978-981-13-1108-6_14

detectable deep venous incompetence (DVI) [6], in contrast to the Skaraborg study, in which 60% of such patients had DVI [7]. In (a previous report about) young people with venous ulcers, 50 to 75% had only superficial and/or perforator venous incompetence (SVI/PVI) [8]. Clinical association with deep venous thrombosis occurred in 5 to 22% of the patients [9]. All these are sufficient reasons to complicate the ethiologic diagnostic in venous ulcers; in the cases where only exist venous problems, we need to locate the sources of reflux (unique o mixed). The most difficult aspect of diagnosis is that the failure of a system affects others; for example, in saphenofemoral reflux with an reentry insufficient perforating vein, can be corrected totally the perforant insufficiency by eliminating reflux in the saphenofemoral junction, while in other cases does not occur and the perforator vein remain insufficient. Similarly, in the deep venous system, there may be insufficiency in the thigh and the venous hypertension may be deflected to the superficial system in the leg or vice versa. In other cases, deep vein insufficiency of the tibialis posterior veins may be associated with post-thrombotic sequelae and perforator veins may develop a superficial circuit to compensate the changes in the venous circulation and pressure, wich them become insufficient later.

This difficulty in diagnosis can lead to insufficient treatment of the venous system, with subsequent recurrence. Not only is the venous diagnosis important, but also important is the evaluation of other factors, such as the arterial circulation, the ankle-brachial index, gait biomechanics, and other disorders such as chronic illness or any other factors that may prevent complete healing or cause recurrence. In this section we outline different methods for the treatment of venous ulcers. However, I recommend that we not lose sight of the main goal: "Decrease the distal venous hypertension and correct the source of reflux" [10].

14.2 Compression

In almost all reviews of venous ulcer treatment, compression therapy is considered to be the basis of phlebology therapy, especially in the conservative treatment of venous ulcers and the prevention of recurrences, even after other treatments. However, the effectiveness of compression therapy requires patient education and the patient's complete acceptance, as many patients do not agree to maintain adequate compression for the required time and discontinue the compression as soon as they feel better; in some cases the compression systems prevent the patient from working and interfere with their daily activities. Leg ulcers are not only a health problem but they also entail economic, psychological, and social problems.

In any case, classic compression bandages remain the most useful and economical—although not the fastest—way to treat a venous ulcer. However, when compression is combined with other techniques such as surgery, laser, sclerotherapy, and radiofrequency, the results are much better. In a broad review, O'Meara et al. [11] conclude: … "Compression improves the healing of ulcers when compared with no compression: Multicomponent compression systems are more effective than single-component compression systems; high compression is more effective than lower compression and medical compression stockings (MCS) are more effective than compression with short stretch bandages…."

Thus, it is very important to decide what kind of compression will be used in each case; for example, whether the compression treatment is used alone, whether it is combined with other procedures, or whether it is applied before or after another treatment. Commonly compression bandages are only used during the intensive phase of decongestive therapy within a period of 2–4 weeks and then treatment is changed to MCS, although some patients need a multilayer system for longer periods; personally, I use MCS when the wound is almost healed. Inelastic bandages such as the Unna boot lose the initial pressure of 60 mmHg by the next day (dropping to less than 20 mmHg) and although this pressure is still high, the standing and walking pressure may still be up 50 mmHg. This system could represent another important action mechanism, known as the "massaging effect", that produces high pressure peaks, like an intermittent pneumatic pressure pump, during gait [12]. Compression has many effects on the tissues in the ulcer: it promoted an increase in the number of nutritive capillaries, while the diameters of the capillaries and the dermal papillae were reduced [13]. With compression, there is a release of growth factors and neuropeptides, which are essential for tissue repair and for significant improvement in the transcutaneous partial pressure of oxygen and in electrical cutaneous perception thresholds. Compression improves the microcirculation by preventing the Capillary filtration on intact capillaries and compression also leads to better venular flow volume. It has been seen that high levels of compression can activate the unmyelinated sensory nerves (C fibers) and produce neurogenic inflammation and the release of growth factors and neuropeptides, which, as stated above, are fundamental for tissue repair. The C-fiber stimulation might explain the beneficial effect of the compression therapy; against this background, we share the opinion that the effect of compression on neuronal function contributes significantly to the healing of venous leg ulcers [14].

Applying inelastic bandages with a pressure of 40 mmHg is significantly more effective for increasing the ejection fraction (EF) than applying elastic bandages; the EF improved by 33% with elastic material and by up to 90% with inelastic material. The pressure exerted by inelastic materials in a person in the standing position is significantly higher than that in the supine position, even when pressures of less than 40 mmHg are employed so as not to damage the arterial circulation [15]. The Coban 2 bandage induced ulcer healing within a 3-month observation period, and this effect was not different from that of the Unna boot, which is considered the "gold standard bandage" in compression therapy for venous ulcers [16].

In Mexico, we have introduced the Unna boot modified with coumarin and other oily components that allow greater mobility of the foot. Changes are made every week, and patients show a healing rate of 75% in 8 weeks of treatment, with total healing reached in 16 weeks, showing that the use of a bandage impregnated with coumarin and zinc oxide is a good choice as treatment for veno-lymphatic ulcers. First we apply a coumarin and zinc oxide bandage from the toes to the anterior tibial tuberosity, then immediately put on a low compression bandage with sufficient pressure, extending the bandage over the previous one; finally, we put on a third low compression bandage over the above unstretched bandage, and we leave this system in place for a week; we do changes and cleaning and protection of the skin with a nutritive dermal preparation DIABEM® cream (By Integral Health Services Co. México City) [17].

The use of sequential gradient intermittent pneumatic compression for a few hours daily can complement elastic compression and heal venous ulcers to the same extent as the Unna boot, without its drawbacks; the problem is that carrying the equipment to the patient's home or the patient's attendance for daily sessions at the medical office is burdensome, and the machine is not cheap [18].

When surgical treatment was compared with compression only (conservative treatment) in patients with venous ulceration, the ulcer recurrence rates were substantially lower in the surgical group, and this effect could last for 10 years. The recurrence rates were 48.9% for the surgical group and 94.3% for the conservative group [19].

14.3 Surgical Procedures

Most guidelines recommend endovenous laser treatment and radiofrequency ablation as the first option in the treatment of varicose veins and truncal reflux, while foam sclerotherapy is reserved for patients in whom the previous methods are not accessible. In the guidelines of the Society for Vascular Surgery and the American Venous Forum, also endorsed by the American College of Phlebology and the International Union of Phlebology, it is recommended that, for the treatment of active leg ulcers and axial reflux that produces incompetent superficial veins, ablation of these veins should be performed, adding compression therapy to improve the ulcer healing [20]. Endovenous (EV) ablation has several advantages over surgical saphenectomy, particularly in obese patients, elderly patients, and patients with other diseases that make open surgery risky. EV ablation is done under local anesthesia, is less invasive than surgery, and the patient is discharged quickly and with minimal postoperative pain. The procedure also has few complications and the patient returns early to daily activity, with high satisfaction; with EV ablation of incompetent superficial veins, chronic venous ulcers show healing 6 to 12 months after the procedure, and the recurrence rates decrease significantly during this time frame. Recurrent ulcers can be managed with EV laser ablation (EVLA) as an alternative option after surgery. Of 25 leg ulcers with reflux identified by duplex Doppler ultrasound and treated with EV ablation, only 1 leg ulcer did not heal—a success rate of 96%. Sufian et al. [3] also had one leg ulcer recurrence, which by insufficient perforator which healed with the ablation with a success rate of 4%; on the other hand, in a 7-year study in 173 patients with chronic venous ulcers, classic open surgery for interruption of the refluxing veins showed an 87% ulcer healing rate and 4.6% recurrence in 5 years. EV ablation is useful to treat incompetent superficial veins with venous ulcers [3]. The use of EVLA for the management of refractory ulcers after venous surgery appears to be a good option that needs more evidence. Eighty-five percent of 52 legs had healed during follow up; moreover, 27 (52%) of all the limbs did not require subsequent continuous compression, and there was clinical improvement in 98% of the patients. Ambulatory venous pressure (AVP) has excellent predictive value for the recurrence of venous ulcers; for postoperative AVP above or below 60 mmHg, the sensitivity in assessing the likelihood for recurrent ulceration, after initial healing was 0.80, and the specificity was 0.50. The ulcer-free period for the whole group was 76% (3 years). There was a significant relationship between decreased AVP with ulcer-free periods (89%) and recurrences when the AVP was greater than 60 mmHg. When AVP does not normalize with the treatments used, this suggests persistent venous hypertension and an increased risk of venous ulcer recurrence [21].

14.4 Sclerotherapy

Sullivan et al. [22] used mechanico-chemical endovenous ablation to treat recurrent and persistent venous ulcers in patients who had previous ablation closure of the great saphenous vein (GSV); they explain that this method used for below-knee insufficiency can selectively treat these pathologic veins or their branches to accelerate wound healing. They used a catheter to apply a sclerosing agent close to the ulcer and the insufficient veins [22]. In a more recent publication, Grover et al. [20] report results for patients with long-term venous ulcers who received treatment with foam sclerotherapy and compression bandaging. Their method of foam sclerotherapy is interesting, and we quote:

The foam was prepared by mixing air or physiological gas (carbon dioxide and oxygen) and 3% or 1% sodium tetradecyl sulphate (STS; Fibrovein, STD Pharmaceuticals Ltd, Hereford, UK), in a ratio of 3:1. GSV treatment was primarily a combination of 3% and 1% STS with a greater ratio volume of 3% as compared to short saphenous vein (SSV) alone. Gas and STS were oscillated manually between two 5 ml syringes connected by a 5 mm filter, a minimum of 20 times. With the patient then in the Trendelenburg position, foam was injected in 3 ml aliquots with intervals and plantar and dorsi- flexion exercises between injections, under ultrasound supervision. Post treatment, patients were asked to plantar and dorsiflex their ankle to clear any foam from the deep system. All patients were placed into a multilayer compression bandaging, or a thigh length Class II compression stocking with appropriate non-adherent ulcer dressing.

In another study of 57 legs treated for venous ulcer, with a median follow up of 2.7 months, at first follow-up, 90% had achieved complete closure of the truncal veins with one treatment session. Following the first ultrasound-guided foam sclerotherapy (UGFS) treatment, recurrence was seen in only 4 of the 50 legs (8%) at 12 months (with a median follow-up of 15.2 months). These results highlight the important role of foam sclerotherapy in the treatment of chronic venous ulcer and give some evidence that foam sclerotherapy in experienced hands can be useful, with minimal risk, in these patients [20]. In this sense other authors have reported similar results; Owens comments that in patients with severe venous insufficiency the venous ulcers responded quickly to UGFS, and their preliminary observations have shown that large ulcers with many years of evolution respond quickly to this method [23]. Catheter-directed sclerotherapy is an alternative treatment for superficial venous reflux in refractory venous leg ulcers, according to the results of Williamsson et al., who report that the treatment is safe and leads to fast healing [24]. In Perú Dr. Juan Chunga Chunga does not use ultrasound; however, he applies sclerotherapy under direct vision or palpation to localize the varicose veins around the ulcer, with excellent results. In our experience direct sclerotherapy or UGFS is a good option for the first treatment of leg ulcers and for the treatment of recurrent leg ulcers, and polidocanol, at 1–3%, is the main sclerosing agent used in Latin America [25]. Another technique used to identify the veins around the ulcers is transillumination, which is very useful to identify the small veins around the injury in recurrent ulcers. When ultrasound and transiluminator equipment is not available, the most commonly used procedure is to apply small punctures with foam sclerotherapy around the ulcer to try sclerosing some veins; however, this is a blind procedure and may produce sclerosing necrosis.

14.5 Dressings

Dressings are items specially designed to promote the healing of scars; there are many different kinds of dressings for many purposes—for dry or wet wounds, for the promotion of tissue growth, and for the evacuation of wound secretions. Many studies and technologies have been employed to develop different dressings; however, in the management of venous ulcers the usefulness of dressings is still questionable. The first consideration is that venous or lymphatic ulcers are exudative and therefore wet. The second consideration is that the ulcers result from venous hypertension and not from infection, nutritional deficiencies, or biochemical disturbances as the primary etiologic source. Thus, the ideal dressing for venous wounds must remove excess exudate, protect against external contamination, and maintain an appropriate environment for tissue growth, and removal of the dressing must be accomplished without damaging the new growing cells. Usually a venous ulcer is not an infected wound; it can be a colonized wound but not infected. This kind of wound heals by "second intention"; this means that the growing tissues fill the wound and it just needs to be kept clean so it can heal without the necessity for antibiotics. Despite these theoretically positive effects on ulcer healing, wound dressings have failed to show any clinical benefit on the ulcer healing rate, as stated by a Cochrane review [26]. However, today the publication has withdrawn these findings, although in another Cochrane publication, O'Meara et al. conclude: "The current evidence does not suggest that foam dressings are more effective than other wound dressing treatments in the healing of venous leg ulcers." [27], and in another review the same author concludes about alginate dressings: "There is no evidence to suggest that alginate dressings are more or less effective in healing leg venous ulcers than simple hydrocolloid or non-adherent dressings, nor is there any difference between different patented alginate dressings." [28]. In another Cochrane review about negative pressure therapy the authors conclude: "There is not enough evidence regarding the use of negative pressure wound therapy (NPWT) for the treatment of leg ulcers, only one small trial that compared the use of NPWT with standard care was found. Given the current uncertainties, practitioners may elect to consider various characteristics such as costs and symptom management properties when choosing between alternative treatment options for leg ulcers." [29]. Mosti reviewed different dressings without reaching specific conclusions, but he states that the Cochrane review did not find significant advantages for dressings when non-adherent dressings and compression were compared [30]. Biofilm (a hydrocolloid dressing by Clinimed) was not found to be significantly different from Jelonet (Paraffin gauze dressing by Smith and Nephew) and Betadine (antiseptic of iodopovidone) in terms of the time taken for complete ulcer healing, and the total cost of treatment over the 4-month duration of the trial was similar for both treatments for small ulcers, but for large ulcers Biofilm cost about three times as much as Jelonet and Betadine [31].

As simple dressings, we use small portions of zinc-oxide-coumarin bandage or gauze bandage impregnated with Lassar's paste to cover the wound and then put on a two-layer bandage with an inelastic system. This dressing system allows the wound to be isolated; the excess secretion emerges and is contained in the outer band and does not adhere to the delicate tissue growth. This method is easy and inexpensive.

14.6 Circannual Fluctuations in Venous Ulcers

In a very interesting study, Simka [32] describes circannual variations in the healing rates of venous ulcers. He found, in Poland, a significant increase in healing rates in spring (April–May) and in autumn (September–October), although the rates exhibited a higher frequency during the warmer part of the year. Moreover, he reported the following interesting findings:

"Non-statistically significant peaks in spring and autumn observed for ulcers were similar to the pattern observed for peptic ulcer disease and autoimmune disorders (e.g. lupus erythematosus or multiple sclerosis). These data may imply that although venous ulcers are related to abnormal venous circulation, the triggering factor might be of another kind and not be associated with the vascular system" [32].

This annual variation can explain the different healing rates of venous ulcers and could change the method of treating these ulcers according to the time of year in which they are presented.

14.7 Ankle Motility

It is well known that the venous circulation requires the participation of the foot plant pump and of the calf; in their initial study Barwell et al. [33] considered ankle function to be important for the proper function of the plant pump, and they studied the relationship between ankle motility, calf muscle pump function, and calf muscle bulk.

The mean (range) values for ankle motility, the calf-ankle circumference ratio, and calf pump power were 35° (5–60°), 1.47 (1.06-1.77) and 3.5% (0.3-11.0%) respectively. Ankle motility was correlated with the calf-ankle circumference ratio. The 24-week healing rate was significantly reduced in patients with limited ankle motility, at 13% in legs with an ankle motility under 35°; ankle motility was an independent risk factor for chronic venous ulcer healing rate when adjusted for age, ulcer chronicity, and popliteal vein reflux. Restricted ankle motility has previously been a recognized phenomenon in patients with chronic venous ulceration, and its deleterious effect on venous hemodynamics is relatively well understood. This study by Barwell et al. confirms that good ankle mobility is an important factor for leg ulcer healing [33]. Gait biomechanics is an important factor that affects the function of the plantar and calf pumps; the gait characteristics have important effects on the intramuscular venous system, the walking in "varus" or "valgus" not only affects osteoarticular function in the pelvis or spine but affects the function of the leg muscles, mainly the gastrocnemius. A large number of patients with venous ulcers have limited function of the ankle and this is a restrictive factor in the healing of these ulcers.

14.8 Electrotherapy

Electrical muscle stimulation (EMS) has been used successfully to promote venous return in the legs. Electrical muscle stimulation demonstrated high efficacy and good tolerance and significantly reduced pain severity, the venous clinical severity score (VCSS), and ankle edema, as well as showing a threefold increase in the number of healed venous ulcers compared with control group. In Russia, Bogachev and Lobanov [34] applied electrostimulation to post-thrombotic syndrome ulcers, in addition to compression therapy and the oral intake of micronized purified flavonoid fraction (1000 mg daily). They had two groups in the study: the study group, which received EMS with Veinoplus® V.I. for at least 3 times a day; and the control group that did not receive electro-stimulation. Pain decreased significantly in the electrostimulation patient group (study group), as did ankle circumference, which decreased from 270.9 ± 4.6 mm to 257.1 ± 4.2 mm in the study group and from 269.7 ± 5.3 mm to 263.4 ± 5.2 in the control group; the healing rates were significantly higher in the study group. At 3 months, the number of open venous ulcers in the electrostimulation group was one-third that in the control group (4 vs. 12). Electrical muscle stimulation is well tolerated, reduces pain, and is effective in the treatment of venous ulceration, as well as improving the VCSS and decreasing ankle edema. In our experience this is an especially useful method for obese or elderly patients with limited mobility, to be used before the application of a three-layer compression system or to prevent recurrence; the ankle edema decrease by 0.5–1.0 cm after 30 min of electrostimulation [34].

14.9 Platelet-Rich Gel

The use of platelet-rich gel (PRG) is a novel procedure for the treatment of several types of wounds; the platelets are obtained from the patient's own blood by centrifugation and separation from the dense plasma layer on the bottom, at this point plasma calcium gluconate is added and the resultant gel is applied to the wound. Villa and Froio [35] used a PRG for arterial and post-thrombotic or vasculitic ulcers in 16 patients with non-healed wounds not responsive to conventional treatment. In their study, platelet gel, obtained from platelet concentrates from whole blood or from plateletpheresis concentrates, was applied to the wound and then a soft dressing was applied. Three patients required amputation, five patients had healed ulcers, and in eight ulcer size was decreased, and almost all patients had reduced pain. The authors concluded that this treatment was effective in many patients and was without side effects. The ease of its application, and the almost total absence of side effects, as well as its low cost, make the platelet gel approach very convenient for the treatment of chronic non-healing ulcers [35].

14.10 Fasciotomy

A study by Christenson [36] showed that patients with severe chronic venous insufficiency and lipodermatosclerosis who were resistant to therapies such as compression, had chronic or recurrent venous ulcers when they showed a significant increase of intramuscular or subcutaneous pressure. When compartment pressure exceeds deep vein pressure, the tibial veins may be impaired, and the increase in compartment pressure leads to progressive local venous hypertension, a decreased arteriovenous pressure gradient, and disrupted capillary flow, which can cause ischemia and necrosis of the skin [36]. In another study by Christenson [37], in Switzerland, in patients with post-thrombotic syndrome and deep reflux, all the limbs had an intramuscular tissue pressure of 15 mmHg or higher. Subcutaneous fasciotomy was performed via a small paratibial incision, then the fascias of the anterior and posterior tibial compartments were opened with a long Metzenbaum scissor all the way down to the ankle level under the ulcer. Intramuscular tissue pressure in ten healthy limbs was 9.2 mmHg (+4.9) and the corresponding subcutaneous tissue pressure was 0.2 mmHg (+1.2). The tissue pressures were significantly decreased following surgery, from 23.5 (+6.1) to 5.5 (+3.1) for intramuscular tissue pressure and from 9.8 (+3.2) to 0.6 (+1.1) mmHg for subcutaneous tissue pressure, and the values remained low at 3 months after surgery [37]. A high intramuscular pressure is a possible condition in hypodermitis and non-healing ulcers; we use this subcutaneous fasciotomy procedure in other cases of venous congestion of the foot. The release of the pressure allows better muscle work and better pump calf function.

14.11 Venoactive Drugs: Pentoxifylline and Sulodexide

Venoactive drugs are used as complementary treatment in the management of chronic venous insufficiency; however, flavonoids and other coumarin derivatives have not been shown to be useful in the treatment of venous ulcers. The use of pentoxifylline in venous ulcer healing is controversial; a Cochrane review of 864 trials found that pentoxifylline was more effective for complete ulcer healing or improvement than placebo (response rate [RR] 1.70; 95% confidence interval [CI] 1.30–2.24). Pentoxifylline with compression was more effective than placebo with compression (RR 1.56; 95% CI 1.14–2.13). Pentoxifylline without compression seemed to be more effective than placebo or no treatment (RR 2.25; 95% CI 1.49–3.39) [38]. Another study, in Spain, concluded something similar: at 8 weeks ulcers were healed in 33.33% of patients with combination therapy of pentoxifylline and compression and in 22.22% of patients with compression-only therapy,and at 24 weeks ulcers were healed 63.31% of the patients with combination therapy versus a healing rate of 45.39% in the patients with compression-only therapy [39]. This may be a justification for the systematic use of pentoxifylline, although its gastrointestinal side effects are considerable. The likely reason that the combination therapy works is that 30% of ulcers that are classified as venous are actually of mixed type (arterial and venous) and this treatment can be very useful in hemorheological disorders.

More recently, a new agent, known as sulodexide, has been introduced. Sulodexide (a naturally occurring molecule) is a highly purified glycosaminoglycan that has antithrombotic and profibrinolytic properties (it reduces the formation of blood clots), as well as anti-inflammatory effects. In an Italian study, after 2 months of treatment, venous ulcers were healed in 15 patients (36%) in the control group and in 30 patients (58%) in the sulodexide group ($p = 0.03$). Life table analysis showed that the healing times in the sulodexide group were shorter in the first 2 months of treatment. Total healing times were 110 days in the control group and 72 days in the sulodexide group ($p = 0.08$) and the results were proportional to the initial severity of the lesion [40]. The Cochrane review concluded that sulodexide may increase the healing of venous ulcers as long it is used together with local wound care, although these observations are not yet reliable and may change with new research. It is not known if sulodexide has adverse effects [41]. In our experience, sulodexide is useful for decreasing edema and for the prophylaxis or treatment of post-thrombotic syndrome; however, an increase in the healing rate was not clear with either oral, intramuscular, or even in situ use, and some patients reported mild gastrointestinal discomfort or rash, although in some patients clinical improvement was observed with the use of oral sulodexide.

14.12 Short Gastrocnemius Syndrome: A New Consideration

We recently started a study in patients whose venous ulcers did not close after conventional treatment with intravenous chemical ablation (sclerotherapy) and compression. We observed that in these patients the ankle mobility index was diminished and for these patients flexion of the foot (mainly in a standing position) was almost impossible. We designed a test to verify the limit of dorsiflexion; this test consisted of placing the patient in the standing posture and, without them swinging back or folding the trunk, ask them to lift the tips of the feet; if the patient cannot do this or if the lift is less than 10° the maneuver is positive for short gastrocnemius syndrome; between 10 and 20° the maneuver is moderately positive, and if they can lift the toes without difficulty (+20°) the maneuver is negative. We observed gait alterations in these patients, either excluding the foot or for the entire walking mechanism. These alterations correspond to a series of conditions caused by shortness of the gastrocnemius muscle or dysfunction of the soleus muscle. A report by the podiatrists Carrizosa and Antonio from Mexico [42] described that in some patients an operation to elongate the gastrocnemius medially alleviated the pain of venous ulcers.

We designed a study to corroborate these observations and to look for their causes and other variables. For this study, we selected patients with venous ulcers and a positive test for short gastrocnemius, as previously described, and a positive result on the Silfverskiold test [43, 44]; the patients underwent Doppler ultrasound and measurements were made of the diameters and venous blood velocity in the great saphenous, popliteal, and femoral veins before and after gastrocnemius ultrasound morphology was determined. Short gastrocnemius syndrome was confirmed in all the patients and they were prepared for surgery, in which release of the medial tendon of the gastrocnemius was performed under local anesthesia, and a short cut was made in the popliteal fossa skin. This surgery releases the tendon of the gastrocnemius muscle, elongating it and recovering adequate function, with which we are able to get the calf muscle pump to work normally again, improving gait biomechanics. With this procedure the musculoskeletal defect was corrected and subsequently the muscular pump worked again in better conditions [45]. We obtained the approval of the Ethics Committee and the patients' informed consent for the procedure. The initial results are very encouraging; the venous ulcers closed within 1–4 weeks after the procedure, and gait improved considerably, as did the dorsiflexion angles of the foot, making the test for short gastrocnemius negative. The diameter of the great saphenous vein decreased and the diameter of the gastrocnemius veins also decreased. The study has not yet been completed. Some aspects of the study that deserve attention are that the patients need to re-learn to walk; we have seen that they are afraid to walk "normally" and they lean forward to move the foot. The gastrocnemius veins are usually tortuous or enlarged, and determination of this aspect could be a way of diagnosing pump failure; however, more details about the normal and pathologic features of gastrocnemius veins will be required [46]. The elongation of the internal tendon gives the gastrocnemius muscle better capacity to contract and consequently better capacity to pump the venous blood, and the venous hypertension is rapidly decreased simply by walking. In the light of this study, we can ask ourselves some questions about venous ulcers: Is venous hypertension and valvular damage secondary to malfunction of the leg muscles? And do all the venous problems have their origin in alterations of the biomechanics of walking? (Figs. 14.1, 14.2, and 14.3).

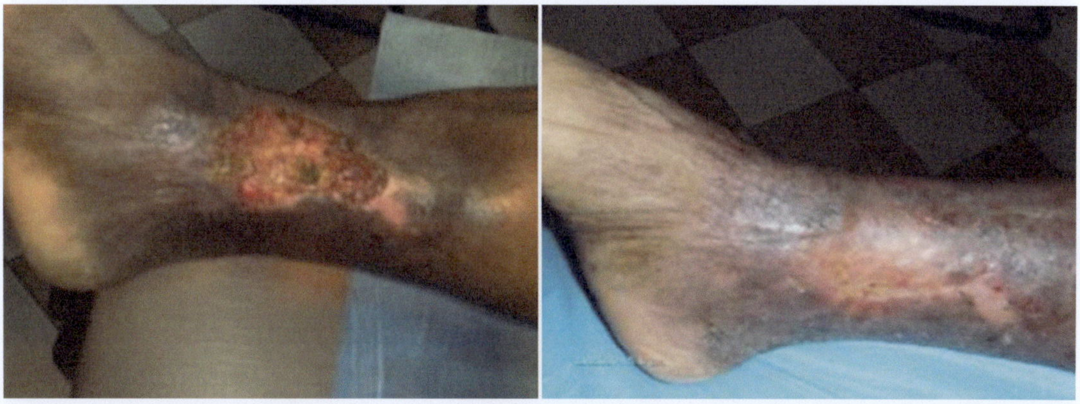

Fig. 14.1 Before and after release of the medial gastrocnemius tendon in a patient with venous ulcer

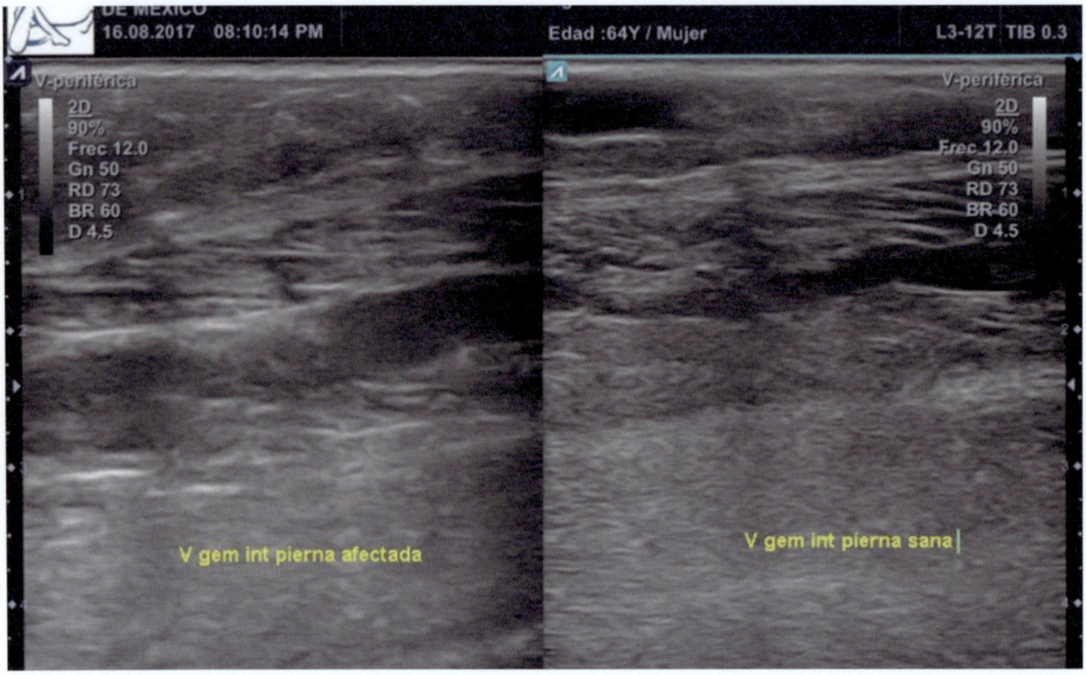

Fig. 14.2 Left, abnormal gastrocnemius vein in Venous Chronic Insufficiency (VCI); right contralateral gastrocnemius vein is normal (same patient)

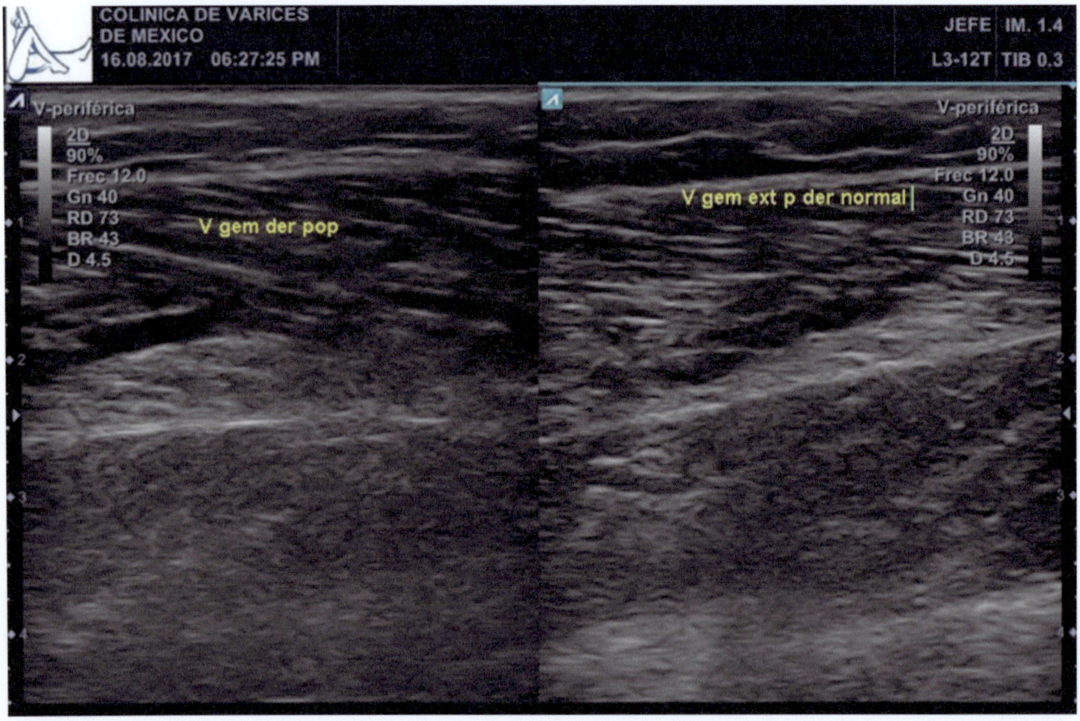

Fig. 14.3 Left gastrocnemius vein postoperatively; right normal gastrocnemius vein in contralateral leg

Conclusions

The treatments for venous ulcer are many and varied; the main point in regard to treatment is to obtain the correct diagnosis, as many ulcers that are classified as venous do not meet the criteria for this classification. In 354 leg ulcers, Koerber found the prevalence of venous leg ulcers to be 75.25%, of which 3.66% were arterial leg ulcers, 14.66% were mixed ulcers (venous and arterial), and 13.5% were vasculitic ulcers [5]. There is a close relation of high rate of arterial hypertension's comorbidity (63.2%) and leg ulcers and this with the prevalence of ulcers with venous or mixed (arterial-venous) etiology (about 80%). The cure rate varies from 41% for venous ulcers and decreases to 26% in ulcers of mixed etiology [47]. For this reason, drugs may be useful as general treatments in ulcers of indeterminate etiology, but if only treat ulcers from venous ethiology the treatment needs to take into account other causes of venous hypertension. With this in mind, the disconnection of reflux points on the venous system would be the most important treatment, but as a venous ulcer is a delayed consequence of chronic venous insufficiency, compression also plays an essential role in the treatment of disease, not only alone but as an adjunct with other therapies. The three-layer system of bandaging remains as the best method, while other therapies such as drugs and exercise can be helpful. The integral management of venous ulcers is not a "magic procedure," it is a logical matter that requires common sense, a little science, and a lot of patient care. To provide better treatment for our patients, we also need to consider additional factors, such as gait biomechanics, mobility of the leg joints, muscle function, concomitant diseases, and many other causes or complications of venous ulcers.

References

1. O'Donnell TF Jr. Management of venous leg ulcers: clinical practice guidelines of the Society for Vascular Surgery and the American Venous Forum. J Vasc Surg. 2014:60 3S–59S.
2. Zimmet SE. Venous leg ulcers: modern evaluation. Dermatol Surg. 1999;25:236–41.
3. Sufian SL, Lakhanpal S, Marquez J. Superficial vein ablation for the treatment of primary chronic venous ulcers. Phlebology. 2011;26:311–6.
4. Apollonio A, Antignani PL. Epidemiology and healing of vascular ulcers in Italy. Preview of the SUV study results (AIUC September 2012): short report. Acta Phlebologica. 2012;13(2):101–3.
5. Koerber A, Schadendorf D. Genese des ulcus cruris. Hautarzt. 2009;60:488.
6. Nelzén O, Bergqvist D, Fransson I, Lindhagen A. Prevalence and aetiology of leg ulcers in a defi ned population of industrial workers. Phlebology. 1996; 11:50–4.
7. Nelzén O, Bergqvist D, Lindhagen A. Leg ulcer etiology—a cross-sectional population study. J Vasc Surg. 1991;14:557–64.
8. Nelzén O, Bergqvist D, Lindhagen A. The prevalence of chronic lower-limb ulceration has been underestimated: results of a validated population questionnaire. Br J Surg. 1996;83:255–8.
9. Nelzenn O. Epidemiology of venous ulcers. In: En CK, Bergan JJ, editors. Venous ulcer. London: Elsevier; 2007. p. 34–6.
10. Vega F. Fundamentos de Flebología. México: Instituto Mexicano de Flebología; 2013.
11. O'Meara S,CN. Compression for venous leg ulcer. Cochrane Database Syst Rev. 2012;11:CD000265.
12. Partsch H. Compression for the management of venous leg ulcers: which material do we have? Phlebology. 2014;29(1S):140–5.
13. Jünger M, Steins A, Hahn M, Häfner HM. Microcirculatory dysfunction in chronic venous insufficiency (CVI). Microcirculation. 2000;7(S1): S3–S12.
14. Ogrin R, Darzins P, Khalil Z. Neurovascular changes after four-layer compression bandaging in people with chronic venous leg ulcers. Phlebology. 2007;22(2):49–55.
15. Mosti G. Compression in mixed ulcers: venous side. Phlebology. 2014;29(1S):13–7.
16. Mosti G, Cavezzi A. A prospective multicenter randomized controlled trial comparing the new 2-component bandage system Coban 2 with a zinc oxide bandage. Acta Vucanologica. 2010;8(3):119–27.
17. Vega Rasgado F, Rendón F-R. Treatment of venolymphatic ulcer with compression system of coumarin-zinc-oxide. Spanish J Surg Res. 2007;X(3):161–5.
18. Schuler JJ, et al. Treatment of chronic venous ulcers using sequential gradient intermittent pneumatic compression. Phlebology. 1996;11:111–6.
19. van Gent WB, Catarinella FS, Nieman FHM, Toonder IM, van der Ham AC, Wittens CHA. Conservative versus surgical treatment of venous leg ulcers: 10-year follow up of a randomized, multicenter trial. Phlebology. 2015;30(1S):35–41.
20. Grover G, et al. Chronic venous leg ulcers: effects of foam sclerotherapy on healing and recurrence. Phlebology. 2016;31(1):34–41.

21. Akesson H. Long-term clinical results following correction of incompetent superficial and perforating veins in patients with deep venous incompetence and ulcers. Phlebology. 1993;8:128–31.
22. Sullivan PL, et al. Retrograde mechanico-chemical endovenous ablation of infrageniculate great saphenous vein for persistent venous stasis ulcers. Phlebology. 2014;29(10):654–7.
23. Owens PA. Ultrasound-guided foam sclerotherapy. Phlebology. 2007;22(1):24–9.
24. Williamsson C, et al. Catheter-directed foam sclerotherapy. Phlebology. 2014;29(10):688–93.
25. Vega RF, Ramirez C, et al. First Mexican sclerotherapy consensus. Primer Consenso Mexicano de Escleroterapia. Phlebologie. 2014;1:1–12.
26. Palfreyman SJ, Nelson EA. Dressings for healing venous leg ulcers. Cochrane Database Syst Rev. 2006;19(3):CD001103.
27. O'Meara S. Foam dressings for venous leg ulcers. Cochrane Database Syst Rev. 2013;31(5):009907.
28. O'Meara S, Martyn-St James M. Alginate dressings for venous leg ulcers. Cochrane Database Syst Rev. 2015;30(8):CD010182.
29. Dumville JC, Land L, Evans D, Peinemann F. Negative pressure wound therapy for treating leg ulcers. Cochrane Database Syst Rev. 2015;14(7):CD011354.
30. Mosti G. Wound care in venous ulcers. Phlebology. 2013;28(Suppl 1):79–85.
31. Smith M, et al. Biofilm dressing for venous leg ulcers. Phlebology. 1992;7:108–13.
32. Simka M. Chronobiology of venous ulcers. Phlebology. 2010;25:29–34.
33. Barwell R, et al. Ankle motility is a risk factor for healing of chronic venous leg ulcers. Phlebology. 2001;16:38–40.
34. Bogachev VY, Lobanov VN. Electrical muscle stimulation with Veinoplus® device in the treatment of venous ulcers. Int Angiol. 2015;34(3):257–62.
35. Villa V, Froio A. Application of autologous platelet-rich gel to non healing vascular ulcers. Ital J Vasc Endovasc Surg. 2011;18(1):31–8.
36. Christenson JT. Postthrombotic or non-postthrombotic severe venous insufficiency. J Vasc Surg. 2007;46(2):316–21.
37. Christenson JT. Subcutaneous fasciotomy and eradication of superficial venous reflux. Phlebology. 2011;26:197–202.
38. Jull AB. Pentoxifylline for treating venous leg ulcers. Cochrane Database Syst Rev. 2012;1(12):CD001733.
39. Marinel-lo-Roura J, et al. Pharmacoeconomic analysis of pentoxifylline in venous leg ulcers treatment. Angiologia. 2007;59(1):45–54.
40. Scondotto G. Treatment of venous leg ulcers with sulodexide. Angiology. 1999;50(11):883–9.
41. Wu B, et al. Sulodexide for treating venous leg ulcers. Cochrane Database Syst Rev. 2016;6:CD10694.
42. Carrizosa Q, Antonio H. Relación del Sistema Aquíleo-Calcáneo-Plantar en las Úlceras venosas, valoración y tratamiento. Tesina de Diplomado. México: Instituto Mexicano de Flebología, Escuela Superior de Medicina I.P.N. Ciudad de México; 2015.
43. Barouk LS, Barouk P. Gastrocnemios cortos. Revista del pie y tobillo. 2012;XXVI(2):7–13.
44. Barouk LS, Barouk P. Gastrocnemios cortos- de la anatomía al tratamiento. Paris: Sauramps Medical; 2012.
45. De los Santos Real R, Morales MP, Payo RJ, Escalera AJ. Liberación proximal del gemelo medial por mínima incisión. Revista del pie y tobillo. 2011;XXV(1):42–6.
46. Uhl J-F, Gillot C. Anatomy of the veno-muscular pumps of the lower limb. Phlebology. 2015;30(3):180–93.
47. Apollonio A, et al. Epidemiology and healing of vascular ulcers in Italy. Acta Phlebologica. 2012;13(2): 101–3.

15 Compression Therapy for Venous Ulcer

Giovanni Mosti

15.1 Introduction

Leg ulcers have a venous pathophysiology in the vast majority of cases [1–4]. Superficial or deep venous insufficiency and deep vein obstruction produce ambulatory venous hypertension due to venous reflux and venous pumping function impairment. The impaired venous hemodynamics is the key pathophysiologic mechanism leading to skin damage through several intermediate steps.

Fibrin cuff formation around the microvessels leading to impaired gas (O_2, CO_2) exchange [5], white cell entrapment [6] causing skin necrosis, and growth factor inhibition [7] producing a stagnation of the healing process have been considered involved in ulcer onset and maintenance.

The treatment of venous leg ulcers (VLU) must be based on the correction of the hemodynamic impairment which can be achieved conservatively by means of compression therapy, walking, and leg elevation or by means of invasive procedures (open surgery, endovascular procedures as endovenous laser ablation, radiofrequency, foam sclerotherapy, conservative hemodynamic treatment).

G. Mosti
Angiology Department, MD Barbantini Clinic, Lucca, Italy

Compression therapy is frequently considered the first treatment option, and it is the only therapeutical procedure which achieved the grade 1A in most recent guidelines [8, 9]. The crucial point is choosing the most effective compression modality, which is still a matter of debate.

On one side there are clear evidences that inelastic is more effective than elastic material in counteracting the venous hemodynamic impairment [10–14]. This should "ensure" a superior effectiveness in promoting a higher healing rate of VLU, which are due to venous hemodynamic impairment. In addition we have some evidences that the higher the compression pressure, the higher the healing rate [9, 15, 16], and this is clearly in favor of inelastic bandages which exert a much higher pressure than elastic materials.

On the other side, we have many papers claiming a greater effectiveness of elastic stockings or elastic bandages compared with inelastic material [17–30].

Nevertheless studies comparing elastic and inelastic devices have so many flaws that their conclusions are hard to trust [31].

In this chapter we will try to provide updated information about compression therapy effects on venous hemodynamic and the most effective compression modality to achieve the best outcome in VLU treatment.

A. K. Khanna, R. Jindal (eds.), *Venous Disorders*, https://doi.org/10.1007/978-981-13-1108-6_15

15.2 Impaired Venous Hemodynamics

The venous pressure in the legs depends on body position: it is very low in supine position, it increases in the sitting position, and it is maximal in standing position. Actually in the sitting and standing position, the hydrostatic venous pressure results from the unbroken column of fluid that extends from the right heart to the foot which can be easily measured by calculating the distance from the right heart and the ankle in these different positions.

In the standing position, the venous pressure is about 70–80 mmHg both in normal individuals and in patients with venous disease. In the normal subjects, this pressure decreases significantly during active movements (e.g., walking) down to 20–30 mmHg due to venous pumping function and valvular function that fragment the blood column and reduce the hydrostatic venous pressure [32]. In patients with venous insufficiency, valves' failure causes the column of standing blood in the vein to remain unbroken even during ambulation, and a minimal hydrostatic pressure decrease occurs. In some clinical situations (e.g., venous obstruction), the hydrostatic pressure can even increase during and immediately after ambulation: this is what we call ambulatory venous hypertension (AVH) which causes venous congestion.

15.3 Effectiveness of Compression Therapy in Counteracting Ambulatory Venous Hypertension (AVH)

Compression therapy increases the transmural pressure increasing the extravenous pressure so narrowing or occluding the leg veins. This is the prerequisite for the hemodynamic effectiveness of compression therapy, but venous narrowing/occlusion can be possible only by applying an external pressure of the same magnitude or higher than intravenous pressure. Actually, it has been shown that due to different venous pressures in different body positions, a low external pressure in the range of 20 mmHg is able to narrow or occlude the veins in the supine position, but the compression pressure must rise to 50 mmHg in the sitting position and to close to 70–80 mmHg in the standing position [33] to exert the same effect. These data were confirmed by studies with magnetic resonance imaging (MRI) showing that in the standing position, a pressure of 40 mmHg is not able to occlude the veins that are completely occluded with a pressure of 80 mmHg [34] which was defined as very strong in a recent consensus paper [35].

Such high external pressure approaching or overcoming the intravenous pressure may produce a vein occlusion at every step during physical activity, so restoring a kind of valve mechanism. In this way compression reduces the AVH [14] by reducing the venous reflux [10, 11] and increasing the calf pumping function [12, 13].

15.4 Which Compression Material Is Able to Counteract AVH

All compression devices are basically made up with elastic or inelastic material. When wrapped on the leg, they exert a compression pressure which, according to the Laplace law, depends on the stretch applied to the bandage, the number of turns, and the radius of the leg segment [36].

The two materials have completely different physical characteristics.

The elastic or long-stretch material (represented by elastic stockings or elastic bandages with an extensibility higher than 100%) gives way to the muscle expansion, which occurs during standing and physical activity, resulting in a very low pressure difference between the resting and standing or walking conditions. The static stiffness index (SSI) which is the difference between the standing and the supine pressure is lower than 10 mmHg that characterizes the elastic range [37, 38]. Also the difference between diastolic and systolic pressure during muscular activity, responsible of these called "massaging effect" [39] of compression devices over the calf muscle, is very low. These characteristics are consistently maintained independently on applied pressure and material (if elastic stockings or elastic bandages). In conclusion elastic material exerts a quite sustained pressure. In addition it tends to regain its initial length when stretched, and this "return force" is directly related to the stretch applied to the bandage. The "squeezing effect" of a too stretched elastic material can be painful and not tolerated by the patients after a short time from application. As a consequence, when properly stretched, an elastic bandage will exert a supine pressure of 30–40 mmHg. This pressure will rise by 4–8 mmHg in a standing position and will never approach the intravenous pressure resulting unable to narrow or occlude the veins and to exert a hemodynamic effect (Figs. 15.1, 15.2, and 15.3). When we want to use elastic material to exert a very strong pressure in standing position, necessary to occlude the leg veins, elastic bandages must be applied with strong stretch, or several elastic stockings must be superimposed: in both these circumstances, the "squeezing effect" of these materials will be painful and poorly tolerated, as reported (Fig. 15.4).

An advantage of elastic materials is that they are easy to apply, usually as a single component.

The inelastic material (short stretch or inextensible bandages, Velcro devices, hybrid pumps) exerts its effect by resisting the increase of muscle volume during muscular contraction in standing position and during physical activity (the leg will give way) so producing higher peak pressures when standing or walking compared with elastic, long-stretch devices. Inelastic material doesn't have any elastic fiber and doesn't have any return force: it doesn't "squeeze" and can be applied with full stretch.

The modern composite, multilayer and multicomponent, inelastic bandages, including a padding layer with the inelastic material as a last component, exert a relatively low and

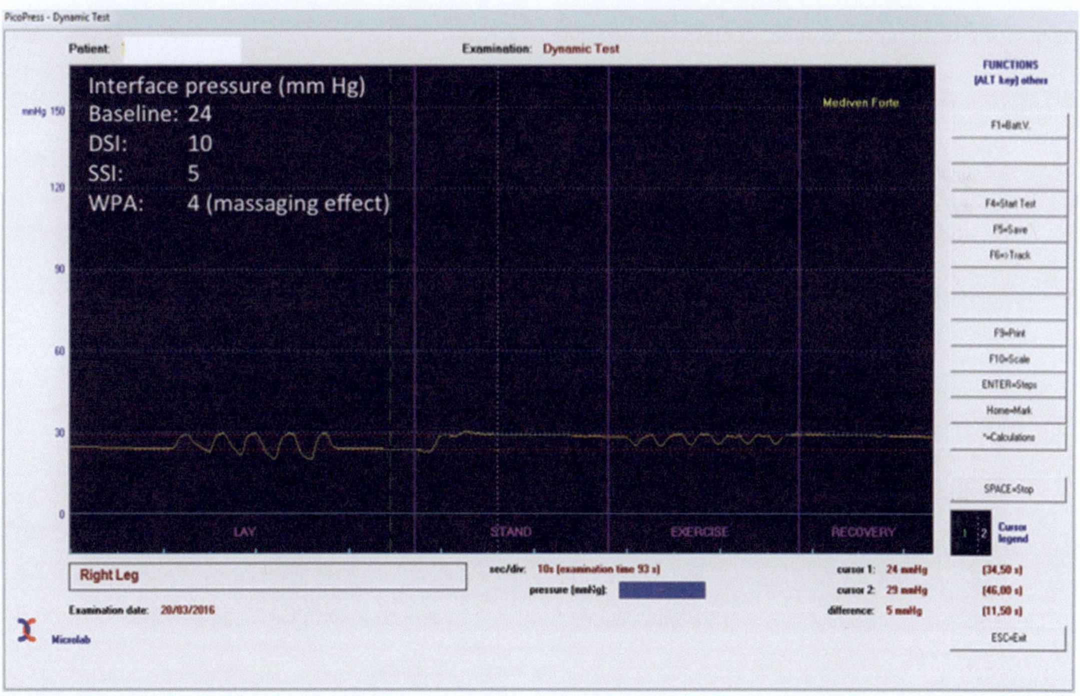

Fig. 15.1 Compression pressure tracings of an elastic stocking of the second class according to the RAL regulatory (mm 23–32 mmHg). Compression pressure increase by dorsiflexions, standing up, and walking is very small: sustained pressure. *DSI* (dynamic stiffness index) is the difference between diastolic and systolic pressure performing foot dorsiflexions in supine position; *SSI* (static stiffness index) is difference between standing and supine position. *WPA* (walking pressure amplitude) is the difference between systolic and diastolic pressure while walking

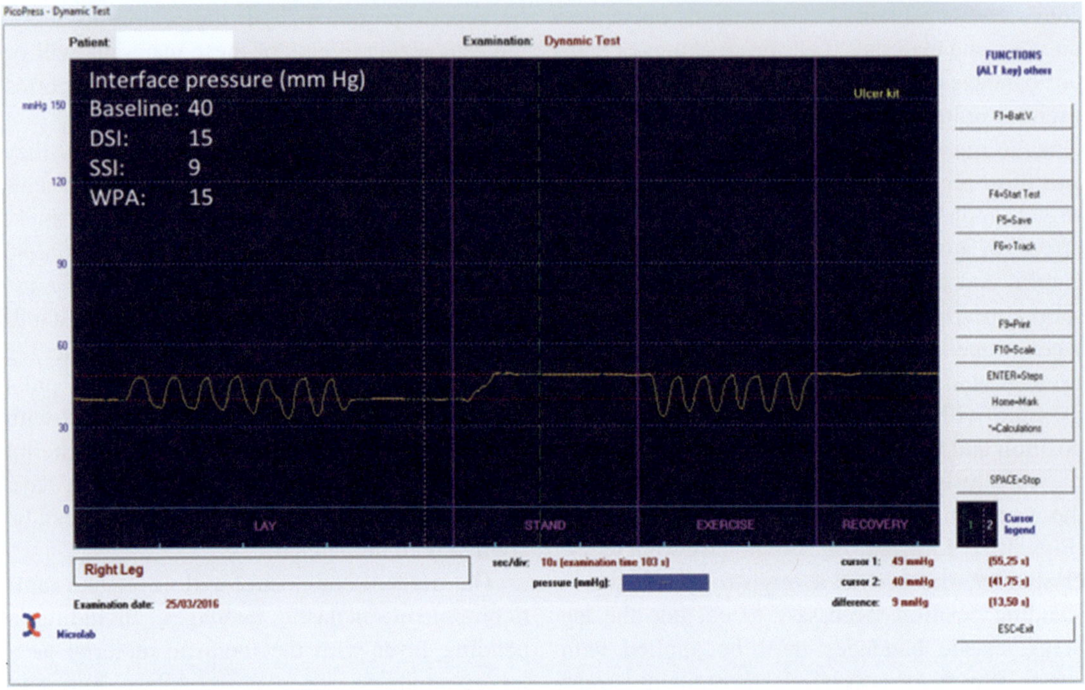

Fig. 15.2 Compression pressure tracings of an elastic kit made up of two superimposed elastic stockings exerting about 40 mmHg in supine position. Compression pressure increase by dorsiflexions, standing up, and walking is very small: sustained pressure despite of the resting pressure increase

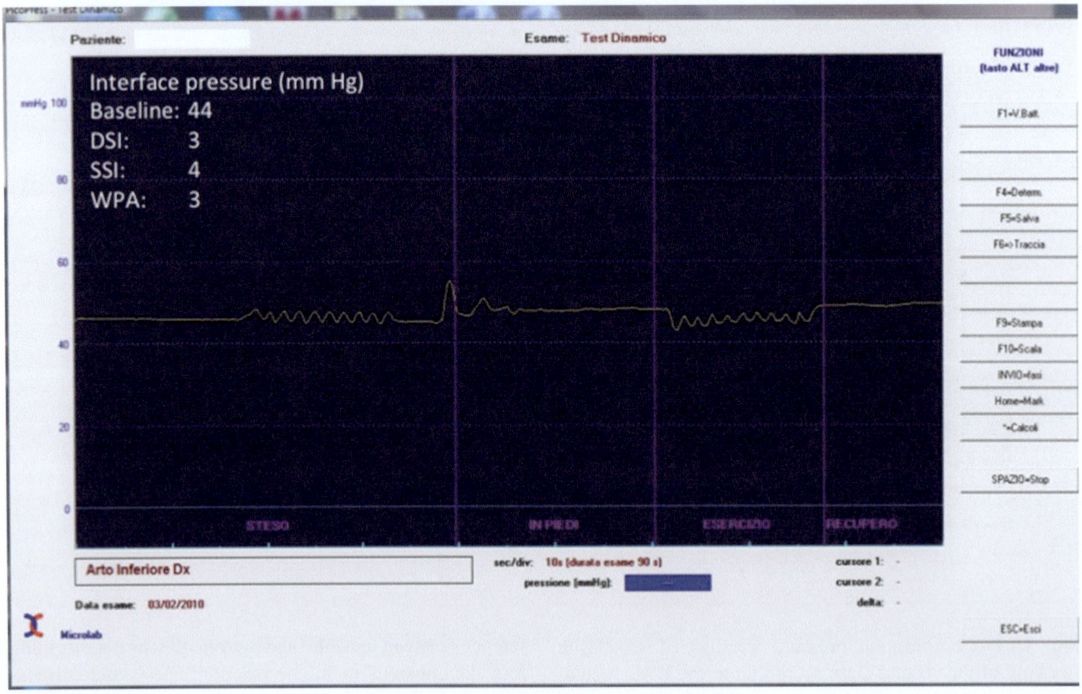

Fig. 15.3 Compression pressure tracings of an elastic bandage exerting about 40 mmHg in supine position. The dynamic characteristic is the same as with elastic stockings or kits

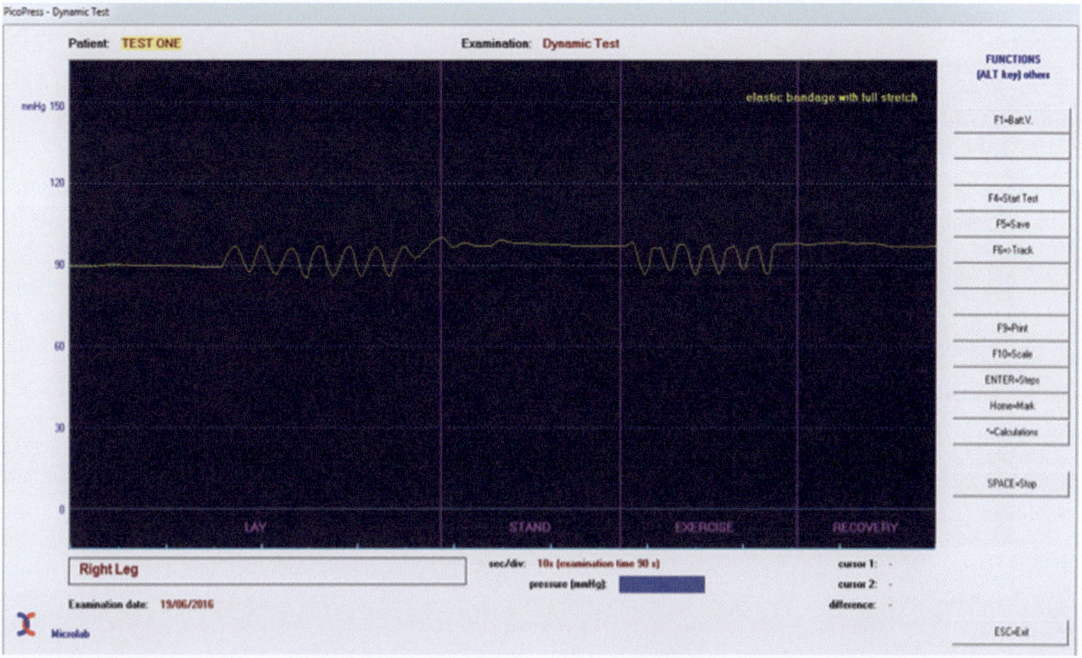

Fig. 15.4 Pressure curve of an elastic bandage applied with high stretch to exert a very strong standing pressure. It can be noticed that also the supine pressure must be very strong as the pressure increase by standing is very small with elastic material. This strong and sustained pressure can be painful

well-tolerated pressure at rest but a much higher pressure often higher than 70 mmHg during standing. The SSI is always >10 that characterizes the inelastic range. The intermittently strong or very strong pressure peaks during muscular exercise will overcome the intravenous pressure intermittently occluding the vein and so restoring a kind of valvular mechanism [14] (Figs. 15.5 and 15.6).

In a few words, the inelastic material is able to adapt to the body position by exerting a relatively low pressure in the resting position (comfortable) and a strong or very strong pressure in the standing position and during muscle activity (effective) coming close to an ideal compression device [40].

Unfortunately the multilayer, multicomponent inelastic bandages are difficult to apply and require expert and well-educated personnel. In a series of papers, it was demonstrated that only from 10 to 60% (depending on the paper) of health personnel treating venous ulcers were able to apply the target pressure with different inelastic bandages [41–45].

15.5 Hemodynamic Effects of Compression Materials

The different physical properties of elastic and inelastic materials result in completely different effects on venous hemodynamics.

Inelastic is significantly more effective than elastic material in:

- Reducing venous reflux both in patient with deep venous [10] and superficial venous incompetence [11]
- Improving the venous pumping function severely reduced in venous insufficiency [12, 13]
- Reducing AVH [14]

Inelastic material is able to reduce venous reflux and increase venous pumping function even at a low/mild pressure range of 20–40 mmHg [46] which has an important implication when inelastic compression necessary to improve venous hemodynamics must be applied with

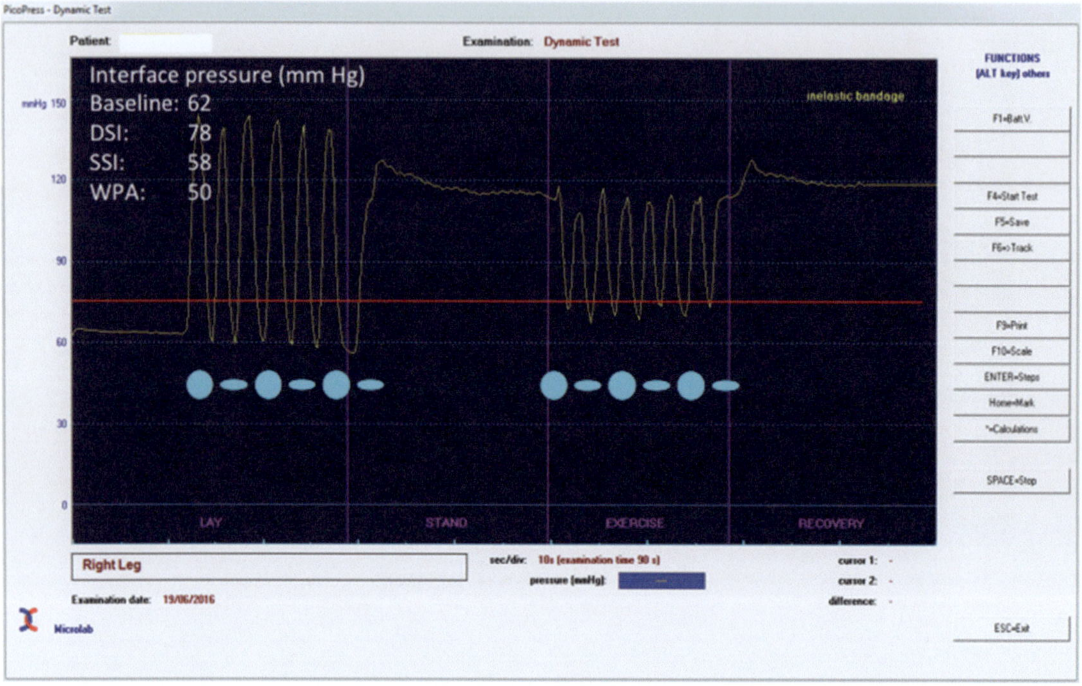

Fig. 15.5 Pressure curve of an inelastic bandage exerting a supine pressure of 60 mmHg. Compression pressure increase by dorsiflexions, standing up, and walking is very high: intermittent compression with high pressure peaks that overcome the intravenous pressure (represented by the red line) restoring a kind of valvular function

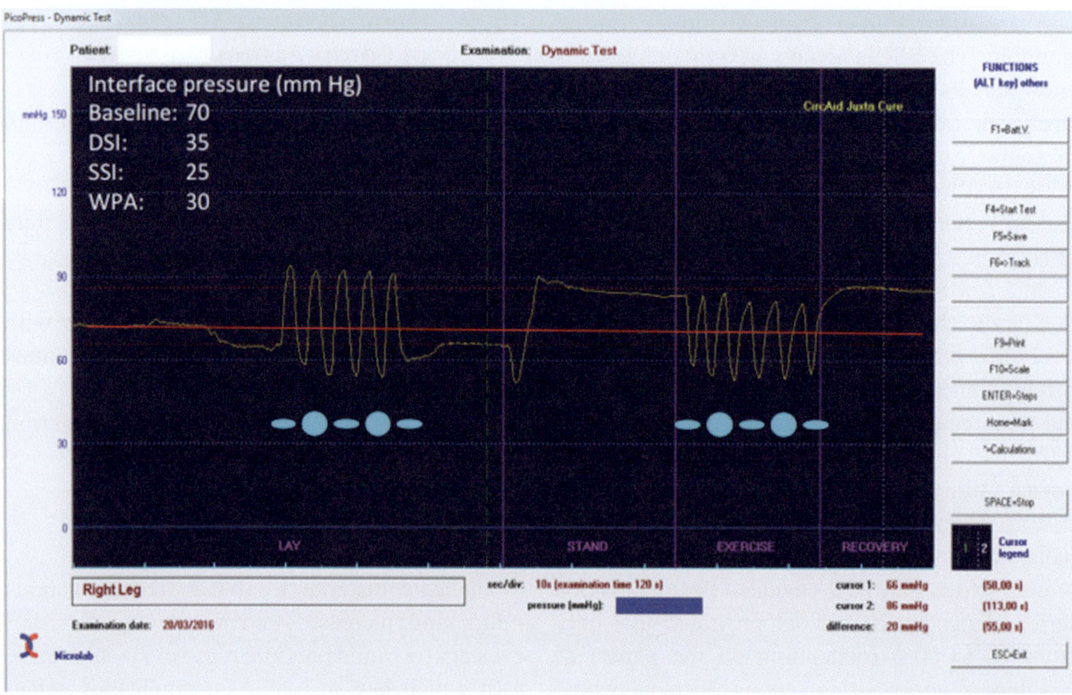

Fig. 15.6 Pressure curve exerted by a Velcro device designed for ulcer treatment. Also with this device, compression pressure increase by dorsiflexions, standing up, and walking is high overcoming the intravenous pressure and restoring a kind of valvular function

reduced pressure in patients with mixed arterio-venous ulcers.

Finally inelastic material maintains its hemodynamic effect overtime despite of a significant pressure drop as the stiffness of the bandage is well maintained as proved by the unchanged SSI and "massaging effect" [47].

15.6 Which Compression Material for VLU

No doubt that inelastic material, exerting strong or very strong pressure, is the most effective treatment modality to get the highest healing rate when looking for the best treatment option.

When correctly applied to exert a strong pressure, inelastic bandages can achieve an ulcer healing rate close to 100% in 3-month treatment [48].

Based on clinical and hemodynamic data, it is not easy to understand why many reports claim the superiority of elastic (both elastic stockings and elastic bandages) compared to inelastic material in improving the VLU healing rate [17–30]. Nevertheless it is important to underline many methodological flaws of these studies.

Compression therapy exerts its effects by providing compression pressure to the leg. Compression pressure is the dosage of compression therapy, but, contrary to any other field in medicine, the compression dosage has almost never been measured and reported when dealing with compression therapy even if the compression pressure measurement is easy to perform with accurate and cheap devices [49, 50].

Not measuring compression pressure, it is impossible to know if the bandages were correctly applied. They could have been applied too stretched, becoming painful and dangerous and forcing the patients to remove them, or too loose, becoming ineffective.

In addition not measuring the pressure or calculating the SSI produced an amazing mistake in almost all studies comparing elastic and inelastic bandages.

In these studies [17–24], the prototype of elastic material is the so-called four-layer bandage which was considered elastic by definition as it is made up of four different elastic components. Nevertheless measuring supine and standing pressure and calculating the SSI of the final bandage, it was possible to show that SSI is in the inelastic range. It may happen that the superimposition of different components and the friction between the layers change the elastic properties of the final bandage, making it inelastic [51]. In conclusion all these studies report a comparison between two different inelastic bandages, and the reported different outcomes in terms of healing rate may depend on the greater experience of dedicated personnel in applying the four-layer bandage.

Also the second comparison, inelastic bandages vs elastic stockings, has many major flaws.

First of all it has to be underlined that the elastic stockings taken into consideration for comparison are actually elastic kits or tubular devices exerting a high supine pressure of 40 mmHg or more and higher stiffness compared to a single stocking (although always in the range of elastic material) due to the friction between the two components [25–30]. In addition the subbandage pressure was, once again, not measured and the skillness of "bandagers" not reported. In these studies we may roughly know the pressure of elastic kits which is declared by the producer, but we do not have any information on the pressure of inelastic bandage that can be extremely variable [52, 53] as it only depends on the health personnel skillness which is usually poor [41–45]. As a consequence it could well be that a good elastic kit, also named "ulcer kit," was compared with a poorly applied bandage.

In a few studies where compression pressure is measured [15, 28, 29], it was demonstrated that the higher the pressure, the higher the healing rate, and this conclusion is in favor of inelastic bandages even despite the conclusion of author's papers. In fact, as well proved, inelastic bandages, when correctly applied, exert a compression pressure definitely higher than elastic material.

15.7 Inelastic Compression with Stiff Multicomponent Bandages for Ulcer Treatment: Always Mandatory?

When considering indications for compression in VLU treatment, it is also important to consider that compression therapy is largely underused even in the western countries, ranging from 15 to 53% of patients who would need compression [54, 55] and also that compression therapy by inelastic bandages is generally poorly applied. Many reasons can explain this lack of implementation of compression therapy in venous leg ulcer treatment, being lack of education in applying inelastic bandages, absence of self-confidence, and fear to produce further skin damages some of the most important reasons.

Nowadays we need to consider another treatment option: the adjustable Velcro® compression devices (AVCDs) or CircAid®(Medi, Bayreuth, Germany) which are becoming more and more widespread. These devices are quite inelastic and offer the advantages of inelastic material, already reported, in terms of improvement of the impaired venous hemodynamics [56, 57]. At the same time, they are very easy to use and can be applied and readjusted even by the patients themselves after a very short wearing and education time (about 2 h) [58]. Actually AVCDs have been proved more effective in achieving healing in patients with VLU when compared with four-layer bandages or with Unna Boot bandage even if with limited evidences [59, 60].

Also elastic kits offer an alternative option as they were shown to be effective in getting healing especially in small ulcers of recent onset. In fact, let us take for granted that the comparison between inelastic bandages and elastic kits is not trustable as it was burdened with major flaws, but just let us consider the effectiveness of elastic kits in getting ulcer healing. We can notice that elastic kits were able to achieve the ulcer healing in 36–96% of patients with small ulcers of recent onset in 3–4 months [25–30]. As Velcro® devices, elastic kits do not require expert personnel to be applied and allow self-management.

In conclusion when assessing the best treatment option for VLU compression therapy, inelastic materials are the most effective treatment modality. Therefore we may choose between inelastic composite bandages (difficult to apply) and Velcro® devices (easy to apply and allowing self-management).

When these options are not available, for different reasons (from lack to educated personnel to lack of suitable materials), elastic kits may offer an alternative effective solution especially in case of small ulcers of recent onset.

15.8 Ulcer Recurrence Prevention

VLUs may recur and the recurrence rate may be as high as 37% [61]. Surgical correction of superficial venous incompetence was shown to prevent ulcer recurrence significantly more effectively than compression therapy [62, 63]. Compression therapy is anyway effective in VLU recurrence prevention even if it must be considered as a second choice. Elastic stockings are used in this indication with the highest tolerable compression [64]. Compliance to compression by elastic stockings is considered even more important than compression pressure [65].

15.9 Special Circumstances

15.9.1 Inelastic Compression and Mixed Leg Ulcers

An arterial impairment affects about 15–20% of patients with venous leg ulcers [4, 66] causing a delayed healing. In these patients, compression improves venous hemodynamics, but it is considered possibly harmful for arterial inflow.

Actually some data confirm that compression therapy is possible in patients with mixed ulcers provided the patient is not affected by critical limb ischemia and that a reduced compression pressure is applied to these patients. In these circumstances it was shown that a reduced compression pressure, not higher than 40 mmHg, does not impair toe pressure [67], exerts beneficial effects on arterial flow both in the periwound skin and distally to the bandage [68], and is well tolerated [69]. In addition external compression up to 40 mmHg significantly increases arterial flow (even in patients with very low ABPI) and venous EF and may be considered as the basic treatment modality in managing patients with mixed ulceration.

15.9.2 Elastic or Inelastic Bandages in Patients with Leg Ulcers and Restricted Mobility?

An old dogma reports that inelastic material would work only during exercise so resulting ineffective in patients with restricted or absent mobility. In case of completely immobile and bedridden patient, a simple thrombo-prophylactic stocking exerting a pressure of about 20 mmHg is enough to occlude the veins. But in case the patient is able to perform a very minor physical activity and sit in a chair, a higher compression pressure is necessary to occlude the veins: around 50 mmHg in the sitting position and 70 mmHg in the standing position. In this case only inelastic material is able to exert this pressure without causing pain or any other skin damage.

In conclusion elastic compression is effective in completely immobile patients, but when they are partially immobile and still maintain some mobility, they would need inelastic compression [70, 71].

Conclusions

Compression therapy is extremely effective in promoting ulcer healing and improving quality of life in patients with venous leg ulcers.

There are convincing evidences that inelastic is more effective than elastic material in improving venous hemodynamics which is impaired in venous incompetence/obstruction. As a consequence they should be more effective in increasing the healing rate of ulcers whose pathophysiology is a venous hemodynamic impairment. Inelastic bandages are also very well tolerated as they exert a relatively low and tolerable pressure at rest and a much higher pressure in standing position and during walking.

In order to achieve the best results, compression therapy by inelastic bandages must be correctly applied and requires adequate education. It should be applied with strong pressure in patients with venous leg ulcers and with reduced pressure in patients with mixed ulcers or when pathophysiology does not involve a venous disease. Using Velcro® devices it is possible to achieve similar results as with inelastic bandages. Velcro ® devices offer the advantage to be easy to use, even by the patients themselves, but more extensive evidences on their effectiveness in achieving high ulcer healing rate are necessary.

Inelastic bandages are indicated also in patients with mixed ulcers provided they are applied with reduced compression pressure and in partially immobile patients.

Elastic stockings are effective in ulcer recurrence prevention, while elastic kits can be an effective treatment modality in small ulcer of recent onset.

References

1. Baker SR, Stacey MC, Singh G, Hoskin SE, Thompson PJ. Aetiology of chronic leg ulcers. Eur J Vasc Surg. 1992;6(3):245–51.
2. Shami SK, Sarin S, Cheatle TR, et al. Venous ulcers and the superficial venous system. J Vasc Surg. 1993;17:487–90.
3. Adam DJ, Naik J, Hartshorne T, Bello M, London NJ. The diagnosis and management of 689 chronic leg ulcers in a single-visit assessment clinic. Eur J Vasc Endovasc Surg. 2003;25(5):462–8.
4. Körber A, Klode J, Al-Benna S, et al. Etiology of chronic leg ulcers in 31,619 patients in Germany analyzed by an expert survey. J Dtsch Dermatol Ges. 2011;9(2):116–21.
5. Browse NL, Burnard KG. The cause of venous ulceration. Lancet. 1982;2(8292):243–5.
6. Coleridge Smith PD, Thomas P, Scurr JH, Dormandy JA. Causes of venous ulceration: a new hypothesis. Br Med J (Clin Res Ed). 1988;296:1726–7.
7. Falanga V, Eaglstein WH. The "trap" hypothesis of venous ulceration. Lancet. 1993;341(8851):1006–8.
8. O'Donnell TF, Passman MA, Marston WA, Ennis WJ, Dalsing M, Kistner RL, et al. Management of venous

leg ulcers: clinical practice guidelines of the Society for Vascular Surgery and the American Venous Forum. JVS. 2014;60:3S–59S.
9. Mosti G, De Maeseneer M, Cavezzi A, Parsi K, Morrison N, Nelzen O, et al. Society for Vascular Surgery and American Venous Forum Guidelines on the management of venous leg ulcers: the point of view of the International Union of Phlebology. Int Angiol. 2015;34(3):2012–218.
10. Partsch H, Menzinger G, Mostbeck A. Inelastic leg compression is more effective to reduce deep venous refluxes than elastic bandages. Dermatol Surg. 1999;25(9):695–700.
11. Mosti G, Partsch H. Duplex scanning to evaluate the effect of compression on venous reflux. Int Angiol. 2010;29(5):416–20.
12. Mosti G, Mattaliano V, Partsch H. Inelastic compression increases venous ejection fraction more than elastic bandages in patients with superficial venous reflux. Phlebology. 2008;23(6):287–94.
13. Mosti G, Partsch H. Measuring venous pumping function by strain-gauge plethysmography. Int Angiol. 2010;29(5):421–5.
14. Partsch B, Mayer W, Partsch H. Improvement of ambulatory venous hypertension by narrowing of the femoral vein in congenital absence of venous valves. Phlebology. 1992;7:101–4.
15. Milic DJ, Zivic SS, Bogdanovic DC, Jovanovic MM, Jankovic RJ, Milosevic ZD, Stamenkovic DM, Trenkic MS. The influence of different sub-bandage pressure values on venous leg ulcers healing when treated with compression therapy. J Vasc Surg. 2010;51(3):655–61.
16. Cullum N, Nelson EA, Fletcher AW, Sheldon TA. Compression for venous leg ulcers. Cochrane Database Syst Rev. 2001;2:CD000265.
17. Franks PJ, Moody M, Moffatt CJ, et al. Randomised trial of cohesive short-stretch versus four-layer bandaging in the management of venous ulceration. Wound Rep Reg. 2004;12:157–62.
18. Moffatt CJ, McCullagh L, O'Connor T, et al. Randomized trial of four-layer bandage systems in the management of chronic venous ulceration. Wound Rep Reg. 2003;11:166–71.
19. Fletcher A, Cullum N, Sheldon TA. A systematic review of compression treatment for venous leg ulcers. BMJ. 1997;315:576–80.
20. Callam MJ, Harper DR, Dale JJ, et al. Lothian Forth Valley leg ulcer healing trial—part 1: elastic versus non-elastic bandaging in the treatment of chronic leg ulceration. Phlebology. 1992;7:136–41.
21. Duby T, Hofman D, Cameron J, et al. A randomized trial in the treatment of venous leg ulcers comparing short stretch bandages, four layer bandage system, and a long stretch-paste bandage system. Wounds. 1993;5:276–9.
22. Ukat A, Konig M, Vanscheid W, et al. Short stretch versus multilayer compression for venous leg ulcers: a comparison of healing rates. JWC. 2003;12:139–43.
23. Scriven JM, Taylor LE, Wood AJ, et al. A prospective randomised trial of four-layer versus short stretch compression bandages for the treatment of venous leg ulcers. Ann R Coll Surg Engl. 1998;80:215–20.
24. Nelson EA, Iglesias CP, Cullum N, et al. Randomized clinical trial of four-layer and short-stretch compression bandages for venous leg ulcers. Br J Surg. 2004;91:1292–9.
25. Mariani F, Mattaliano V, Mosti G, Gasbarro V, Bucalossi M, Blättler W. The treatment of venous leg ulcers with a specifically designed compression stocking kit. Phlebologie. 2008;37:191–7.
26. Junger M, Partsch H, Ramelet AA, Zuccarelli F. Efficacy of a ready-made tubular compression device versus short stretch bandages in the treatment of venous leg ulcers. Wounds. 2004;16:313–20.
27. Jünger M, Wollina U, Kohnen R, Rabe E. Efficacy and tolerability of an ulcer compression stocking for therapy of chronic venous ulcer compared with a below-knee compression bandage: results from a prospective, randomized, multicentre trial. Curr Med Res Opin. 2004;20(10):1613–23.
28. Horakova MA, Partsch H. Compression stockings in treatment of lower leg venous ulcer. Wien Med Wochenschr. 1994;144(10–11):242–9.
29. Brizzio E, Amsler F, Lun B, Blättler W. Comparison of low-strength compression stockings with bandages for the treatment of recalcitrant venous ulcers. J Vasc Surg. 2010;51:410–6.
30. Amsler F, Willenberg T, Blättler W. Management of venous ulcer: a meta analysis of randomized studies comparing bandages to specifically designed stockings. J Vasc Surg. 2009;50:668–74.
31. Mosti G. Elastic stockings vs inelastic bandages for ulcer healing: a fair comparison? Phlebology. 2012;27(1):1–4.
32. Arnoldi CC. Venous pressure in the leg of healthy human subjects at rest and during muscular exercise in the nearly erect position. Acta Chir Scand. 1965;130(6):570–83.
33. Partsch B, Partsch H. Calf compression pressure required to achieve venous closure from supine to standing positions. J Vasc Surg. 2005;42:734–8.
34. Partsch H, Mosti G, Mosti F. Narrowing of leg veins under compression demonstrated by magnetic resonance imaging (MRI). Int Angiol. 2010;29(5):408–10.
35. Partsch H, Clark M, Mosti G, et al. Classification of compression bandages: practical aspects. Dermatol Surg. 2008;34:600–9.
36. Pellicer J, Garcia-Morales V, Hernandez MJ. On the demonstration of the young- Laplace equation in introductory physics courses. Phys Educ. 2000;35:126–9.
37. Partsch H. The static stiffness index: a simple method to assess the elastic property of compression material in vivo. Dermatol Surg. 2005;31:625–30.
38. Partsch H. The use of pressure change on standing as a surrogate measure of the stiffness of a compression bandage. Eur J Vasc Endovasc Surg. 2005;30:415–21.
39. Partsch H. Compression therapy in leg ulcers. Rev Vasc Med. 2013;1:9–14.

40. Partsch H. Compression therapy of venous ulcers. EWMA J. 2006;2:16–20.
41. Reynolds S. The impact of a bandage training programme. JWC. 1985;8:55–60.
42. Nelson EA, et al. Improvements in bandaging technique following training. JWC. 1995;4:181–4.
43. Keller A, Müller ML, Calow T, Kern IK, Schumann H. Bandage pressure measurement and training: simple interventions to improve efficacy in compression bandaging. Int Wound J. 2009;6:324–30.
44. Zarchi K, et al. Delivery of compression therapy for venous leg ulcers. JAMA Dermatol. 2014;150:730–6.
45. Protz K, et al. Compression therapy: scientific background and practical applications. JDDG. 2014;12(9):794–801.
46. Mosti G, Partsch H. Is low compression pressure able to improve venous pumping function in patients with venous insufficiency? Phlebology. 2010;25(3):145–50.
47. Mosti G, Partsch H. Inelastic bandages maintain their hemodynamic effectiveness over time despite significant pressure loss. J Vasc Surg. 2010;52(4):925–31.
48. Mosti G, Crespi A, Mattaliano V. Comparison between a new, two-component compression system with zinc paste bandages for leg ulcer healing: a prospective, multicenter, randomized, controlled trial monitoring sub-bandage pressures. Wounds. 2011;23(5):126–34.
49. Mosti G, Rossari S. L'importanza della misurazione della pressione sottobendaggio e presentazione di un nuovostrumento di misura. Acta Vulnol. 2008;6:31–6.
50. Partsch H, Mosti G. Comparison of three portable instruments to measure compression pressure. Int Angiol. 2010;29(5):426–30.
51. Mosti G, Mattaliano V, Partsch H. Influence of different materials in multicomponent bandages on pressure and stiffness of the final bandage. Dermatol Surg. 2008;34:631–9.
52. Partsch H. Variability of interface pressure exerted by compression bandages and standard size compression stockings. Proceedings of 20th Annual Meeting of American Venous Forum. Charleston; 20–23 February 2008.
53. Moffat C. Variability of pressure provided by sustained compression. Int Wound J. 2008;5(2):259–65.
54. Harding K et al. Simplifying venous leg ulcer management. Wound Int. 2015. Available at http://bit.ly/1r1uMdy.
55. Fife CE, et al. Why is it so hard to do the right thing in wound care? Wound Rep Reg. 2010;18:154–8.
56. Spence RK, Cahall E. Inelastic versus elastic leg compression in chronic venous insufficiency: a comparison of limb size and venous hemodynamics. J Vasc Surg. 1996;24(5):783–7.
57. Murthy G, Ballard RE, Breit GA, Watenpaugh DE, Hargens AR. Intramuscular pressures beneath elastic and inelastic leggings. Ann Vasc Surg. 1994;8(6):543–8.
58. Damstra R, Partsch H. Prospective, randomized, controlled trial comparing the effectiveness of adjustable compression Velcro wraps versus inelastic multicomponent compression bandages in the initial treatment of leg lymphedema. J Vasc Surg Venous Lymphat Disord. 2013;1:13–9.
59. Blecken SR, Villavicencio JL. Comparison of elastic versus nonelastic compression in bilateral venous ulcers: a randomized trial. J Vasc Surg. 2005;42:1150–5.
60. DePalma RG, Kowallek D, Spence RK, Caprini JA, Nehler MR, Jensen J, Goldman MP. Comparison of costs and healing rates of two forms of compression in treating venous ulcers. Vasc Surg. 1999;33:683–90.
61. McDaniel HB, Marston WA, Farber MA, Mendes RR, Owens LV, Young ML, et al. Recurrence of chronic venous ulcers on the basis of clinical, etiologic, anatomic, and pathophysiologic criteria and air plethysmography. J Vasc Surg. 2002;35:723–8.
62. Gohel MS, Barwell JR, Taylor M, Chant T, Foy C, Earnshaw JJ, et al. Long term results of compression therapy alone versus compression plus surgery in chronic venous ulceration (ESCHAR): randomised controlled trial. BMJ. 2007;335:83.
63. Howard DPJ, Howard A, Kothari A, Wales L, Guest M, Davies AH. The role of superficial venous surgery in the Management of Venous Ulcers: a systematic review. Eur J Vasc Endovasc Surg. 2008;36:458–65.
64. Nelson EA, Harper DR, Prescott RJ, Gibson B, Brown D, Ruckley CV. Prevention of recurrence of venous ulceration: randomized controlled trial of class 2 and class 3 elastic compression. J Vasc Surg. 2006;44(4):803–8.
65. Clarke-Moloney M, Keane N, O'Connor V, Ryan MA, Meagher H, Grace PA, Kavanagh E, Walsh SR, Burke PE. Randomised controlled trial comparing European standard class 1 to class 2 compression stockings for ulcer recurrence and patient compliance. Int Wound J. 2014;11(4):404–8.
66. Humphreys ML, Stewart AH, Gohel MS, Taylor M, Whyman MR, Poskitt KR. Management of mixed arterial and venous leg ulcers. Br J Surg. 2007;94(9):1104–7.
67. Top S, Arveschoug AK, Fogh K. Do short-stretch bandages affect distal blood pressure in patients with mixed aetiology leg ulcers? J Wound Care. 2009;18:439–42.
68. Mosti G, Iabichella ML, Partsch H. Compression therapy in mixed ulcers increases venous output and arterial perfusion. JVS. 2012;55(1):122–8.
69. Ladwig A, Haase H, Bichel J, Schuren J, Jünger M. Compression therapy of leg ulcers with PAOD. Phlebology. 2014;29(1S):7–12.
70. Mosti G. La terapia compressiva nel paziente con lesioni trofiche degli arti inferiori immobile o con mobilità limitata. Acta Vulnologica. 2009;7(4):197–205.
71. Partsch H. Quelle compression sur des patientsimmobiles: Allongement court ouallongement long? Geriatrie et Gerontologie. 2009;155:278–83.

Pelvic Congestion Syndrome 16

Devendra Dekiwadia, Birju Patel,
and Dilip Vaghasia

Pelvic congestion syndrome (pelvic vein incompetence) is a chronic disorder in which a persistent pelvic and lower abdominal pain occurs with a tendency to aggravate in standing posture. Women are affected more than men.

There are a number of "named" veins in the pelvis. But more than the named veins, there are un-named venous clusters in the pelvis. This makes pelvic venous pathology difficult to understand and make an analysis [1]. There are a few prominent names of the veins, e.g., iliac veins in all six iliac veins. Similarly each organ has a named vein draining out blood from its uterine or vesicular veins, etc. But all these organs rather have a common name attached, particularly in the pelvis. That is the "venous plexus," e.g., uterine venous plexus (Fig. 16.1). This signifies that any number of veins could exist around an organ draining it and forming a delta of veins meeting the main stream not unlike that of a river delta but vividly could join on any side of the stream due to multiple collateral pathways.

16.1 Various Factors That Could Affect Pelvic Venous System

16.1.1 Gravity

We often talk about the antigravity pathways of the lower limb veins and the calf pump. But we have no clear understanding of the pelvic antigravity venous flow. One could talk of the perennial muscles and the anterior abdominal wall contractions with the respiratory movements of the diaphragm causing the venous push in the former and the suction effect in the latter. Anatomically also the iliac veins are known for their none or least number of valves. Gravity may help in a "yogic" posture but not in the routine movements of the body like what happens in the legs.

16.1.2 Infection

The pelvic organs are known for chronic infections. Lower urinary tract infections, cervical and vaginal infections, prostatic infections, inguino-scrotal infections, and perineal and perianal infections are a few to name. These deep pelvic floor infections may cause maximum damage to the draining veins resulting in loss of their normal venous tones, leading to bidirectional flows: the refluxes. Over a period of time, a bidirectional flow may look for an alternative pathway and

D. Dekiwadia (✉) · B. Patel · D. Vaghasia
Dekiwadia Hospital, Rajkot, Gujarat, India

A. K. Khanna, R. Jindal (eds.), *Venous Disorders*, https://doi.org/10.1007/978-981-13-1108-6_16

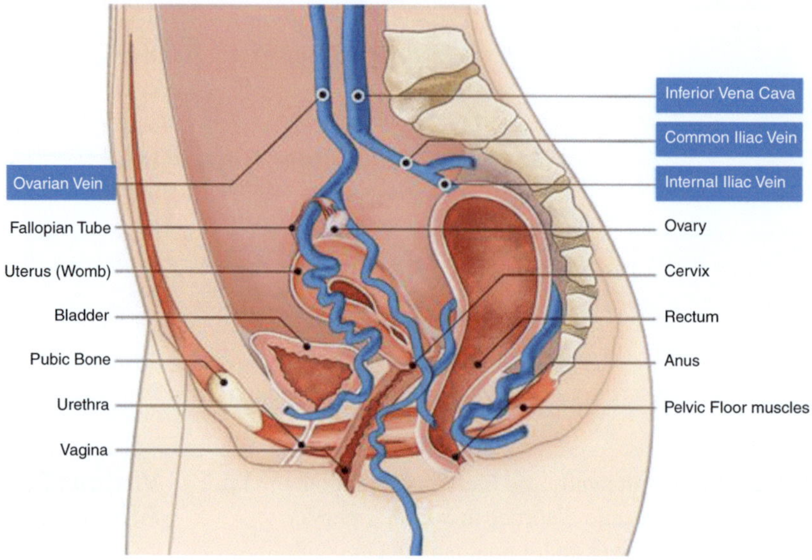

Fig. 16.1 Anatomy of pelvic veins

result in a route which may be caudal to the cardiac direction of venous flow.

16.1.3 Stretch and Damage to the Veins

The urinary bladder regularly and the uterus during pregnancy undergo a prolonged stretch leading to the venous plexus over its surface getting stretched and after repeated happenings (a full bladder during night times and surgeons performing prolonged surgical procedures) may cause a permanent alteration in the function of the draining veins.

16.1.4 Physiologic Venous Congestion

This occurs during immediate premenstrual phase, during premenopausal phase, and during normal intercourse. Hormone alterations occur during these. The impact of this may be different in different individuals and may be an additional cause for some to get pelvic vein disturbance.

16.1.5 Gravid Uterus

In females a hyperdynamic state of circulation selectively occurs around the gravid uterus. And the venous outflow is so much increased that a uterine hum of shuffle is audible with a stethoscope.

16.1.6 Vehicular Accidents

Pelvic injuries and surgery in the pelvic region can damage the veins, similarly resulting to what happens after infection. In the surgical world unless for the large named veins, any venous bleeding is not focused upon and a hemostasis is the goal during surgery. This may lead postoperatively to the acute need of alternative venous route to occur and a resultant congestion.

16.1.7 External Compression

The left renal vein (LRV) passes between the superior mesenteric artery anteriorly and the

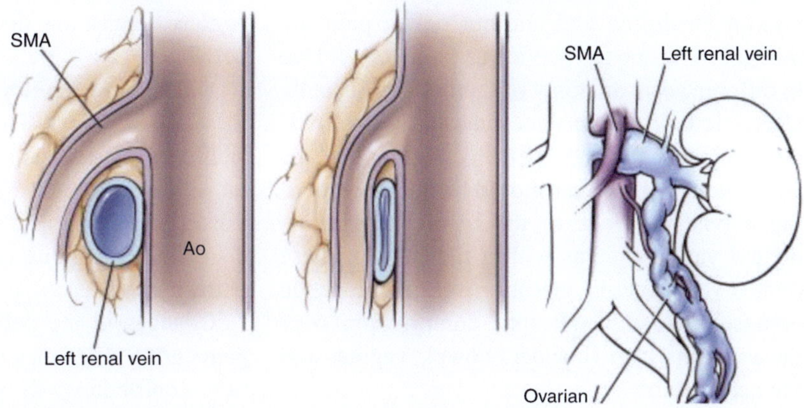

Fig. 16.2 Nutcracker syndrome

aorta posteriorly. Alternatively the vein may anatomically pass posterior to the aorta, i.e., between the aorta and the vertebral column. Compression of the left renal vein between these structures described is called the nutcracker syndrome. Compression of the LRV between the superior mesenteric artery and aorta is called anterior nutcracker syndrome and between the aorta and vertebral column is called posterior nutcracker syndrome.

The compression results in reflux in the left renal and gonadal vein due to prograde resistance (Fig. 16.2).

Similarly the left iliac vein compression by the right common iliac artery anteriorly and the sacral promontory or the vertebral column posteriorly is described as the May-Thurner syndrome.

Thirdly there may be compression over the iliac veins by the lymph nodes, in malignant growth, or in infections.

16.2 Clinical Diagnosis

Pelvic congestion syndrome (PCS) is a debilitating condition with delayed diagnosis even after laborious work-up. Little has been published in the literature. Recent guidelines about varicose veins associated with symptoms of PCS or suprapubic, vulval-perineal, or gluteal varices have been published. One in every ten patient with CVD has non-saphenous vein reflux. These patients have more often pelvic reflux particularly when vulvar and gluteal veins are present.

Pelvic congestion syndrome and pelvic vein congestion syndrome are synonymous, but in the former besides refluxing or congested venous drainage, there could be evidence of additional pathology, e.g., prostatitis associated with periprostatic venous congestion causing pelvic pain. Thus, two similar terminologies are used with almost the same meaning, the pelvic venous congestion syndrome and the pelvic congestion syndrome. PCS is defined as chronic pelvic pain resulting from reflux in or obstruction of the gonadal, gluteal, or periuterine veins. This may be associated with visible perineal or vulvar varicose veins [2, 3]. Pelvic pain may be due to many conditions in the pelvis, and the causes of pelvic venous congestion often are overlooked because many physicians evaluating and treating pelvic pain are unfamiliar with the pelvic venous syndromes. PCS is due to chronic pelvic venous hypertension, which usually is attributed to ovarian vein or internal iliac vein reflux. Aortomesenteric compression of the left renal vein with diversion of the renal vein outflow into the pelvis through the left ovarian vein is now recognized more frequently [4, 5]. Pelvic congestion syndrome and chronic pelvic pain are thought to be due to "pelvic varicose veins." Due to differences in anatomy of the pelvis, it usually affects females more than males. As with varicose veins in the legs, if the valves fail in the pelvic veins, blood that should be pumped out of the pelvis and back to the heart stays inside dilated varicose veins within the pelvis. These dilated veins cause congestion around the pelvic organs and can result into compression over these organs also (bladder, bowel, vagina, and the pelvic floor).

Though PCS is described commonly in the female gender, many observations are emerging demonstrating PCS in males also. Symptomatology and the organs affected will be described in two sections pertaining to males and females.

16.3 The Female PCS

Chronic pelvic pain, defined as noncyclic pelvic pain of greater than 6 months' duration, is a common presenting problem to the gynecologist. A third of all patients have no obvious etiology.

The exact proportion of females suffering from PCS is not known, but it is estimated as mentioned above that up to a third of patients in gynecology outpatients do not have anything wrong gynecologically, but a large number are reported to be having varicose veins in the pelvic areas aforementioned! This could be analogous to the male varicocele, but as the pelvic varicosities are not easily visible or palpable, the diagnosis is elusive. (One may not see what is unknown to him—an old medical saying.)

The symptoms can be understood as a result of gravity-related filling of the pelvic veins.

Four different types have been recognized: (1) asymptomatic vulvar varices, (2) insufficiency of the internal iliac vein and its tributaries, (3) gonadal vein reflux, and (4) obstruction and reflux of the left renal vein, nutcracker syndrome as described above.

Dull pelvic pain of PCS is thought to be due to venous congestion due to refluxing ovaries or pelvis.

During pregnancy intravascular volume increases occurs. The additional volume is stored in the venous system. The volume could be as high as 60%. This causes the veins to dilate, and this rapid dilatation may cause the distortion of venous valves and establish reflux pathways.

Changes in the pelvic structures and weight gain during pregnancy may cause venous obstruction contributing to pelvic pain. Estrogen is known to weaken the vein walls. A relationship between PCS and endogenous estrogen levels is suggested.

The common presentation includes degrees of pelvic and back pain. This is aggravated by standing and exercising. The severity is maximum at the end of the day. Relief in pain occurs after supine position, and most get relief upon awakening in the morning. It is often exacerbated with intercourse.

The pain may be intermittent or constant; it is often worse before or during menses. Some also experience postcoital pain lasting as long as a week or more associated with or without chronic low back pain, or symptoms of urinary tract infection. Many patients describe an aching, "full" or "heavy" sensation deep in the pelvis, a vulvodynia, or bulging of the veins of the labia. Vulvar and perineal varicosities may be a source of lower extremity varicosities in more than a quarter of women.

Most patients with PCS are between 25 and 50 years of age and are premenopausal. The pain has often been a problem for years, and many patients experience depression and personality changes commonly associated with chronic pain. The pain associated with intercourse results in some patient avoiding intercourse with secondary psychosocial stresses, which sometimes become major problem in their life.

PCS is seen in two clinicopathologic forms:

1. Related to the menstrual cycle: hormonal
2. Chronic pelvic congestion

Chronic pelvic congestion occurs with fibrous changes of the pelvic cellular tissues.

The common causes are unrecognized sepsis, obstetric trauma, and incompetence of the small pelvic veins. Dysmenorrhea, dyspareunia, postcoital pain, and recurrent chronic pelvic ache are the common presenting symptoms. The presence of varices of the pelvic veins has been shown to be the underlying etiology in a significant proportion of patients with PCS, caused by a combination of endocrine and mechanical factors. In patients with PCS, the severity and specific character of chronic pain syndrome were dependent on the diameter of maximal dilation and the site of varicose pelvic veins [6, 7].

The optimal diagnostic approach for PCS-related pelvic pain remains unclear.

Diagnosis in PCS can be supported by pelvic and transvaginal color Doppler ultrasound examination to demonstrate ovarian or pelvic varices. A vein diameter of 5 mm or more signifies reflux [8, 9].

It is important to note that a female would consult a gynecologist for her pelvic pain symptoms. But as the condition is not widely discussed or available as a single topic, not many are aware of it. Many women who are suffering from the symptoms of pelvic congestion syndrome are not having the appropriate investigations (transvaginal duplex ultrasound scan).

An MRI or a CT scan is commonly asked for, which does not show reflux or congestion.

16.4 Male PCS

The testicular veins originate from the testicles rather than inside the pelvis. Varicocele occurs when the valves fail and blood reflexes back to the testicular vein. This causes a different symptomatology. A refluxing internal iliac veins can cause prominent varicose veins in the gluteal and perineal area and even can cause hemorrhoids. An erectile dysfunction can also be secondary to PCS in male.

Unfortunately the area of pelvic venous congestion in males is commonly overlooked and difficult to diagnose or suspect clinically. In females, transvaginal duplex ultrasound scan can be readily performed and allows a quick glance of refluxing veins; however in males, a test is yet to be devised to understand this complex problem. Recent breakthrough in technologies such as IVUS (intravascular ultrasound) is granting a better insight in understanding the problem.

In patients with prostatodynia, intrapelvic venous congestion around the prostate is found quite predominantly. Insufficiency in venous circulation of the internal pudendal vessels is a characteristic sign observed in patients with intrapelvic venous congestion syndrome.

Prostatodynia or Chronic Pelvic Pain Syndrome (CPPS) Prostatodynia or chronic pelvic pain syndrome is an unexplained presentation of chronic pelvic pain associated with (1) nonspecific voiding symptoms and (2) pain located in the groin, genitalia, or perineum.

The lab test for urine microscopy shows no bacteria or pus cells.

Prostatitis Chronic nonbacterial prostatitis/chronic pelvic pain syndrome (CPPS)/pelvic myoneuropathy: Pain in the pelvic region or discomfort in the back, rectum, and/or penis. May be associated with urinary symptoms, sexual difficulties, and pain with sitting. Acute bacterial prostatitis is usually associated with UTI. Chronic bacterial prostatitis: Recurrent infections caused by incomplete urinary evacuation or prostatic stone can cause pelvic pain but is not related to congestion syndrome per se [10, 11].

Proctalgia Fugax Proctalgia fugax is a pelvic pain described as an "anal Charlie horse" that occurs after sexual activity, with a brief painful spasm.

Sexual Dysfunction Decreased libido is commonly caused by hormonal imbalance or medications (e.g., antidepressants). A decrease in blood flow can also be a cause for the loss of libido. Pain during sex or after can be experienced by both men and women.

Male Pelvic Congestion and Erectile Dysfunction Modification of lifestyle in the current scenario has led to higher occurrence of ED. With increase in age of men, testosterone deficiency can have a significant effect on their sexual and nonsexual symptoms. Younger age group are less likely to be affected in such fast scenarios [12].

Erectile function (EF) is induced by the release of nitric oxide (NO). Ratio of male having pelvic congestion with underlying sexual dysfunction has been documented in a study of cytokines in the pathophysiology of ED.

Phosphodiesterase-5 (PDE5) inhibitors such as sildenafil, tadalafil, and vardenafil are found to be effective in 80% of arterial ED, even with CVD. PDE5 inhibitors are safe and effective in the management of ED due to venous leak.

Post Prostate Cancer Treatment Chemotherapy or radiotherapy can result in fibrosis and periprostatic venous congestion.

Two syndromes are well-known clinical entities causing PCS or associated PCS with a post-thrombotic syndrome.

16.4.1 Nutcracker Syndrome

Nutcracker syndrome is caused by the compression of the *LRV* between the *SMA* and aorta (anterior nutcracker) or between the aorta and vertebral column (posterior nutcracker). This results in left renal congestion causing flank pain, hematuria, and unilateral renal venous hypertension and dysfunction due to back pressure. Further retrograde pressure falls on the left ovarian vein causing a severe PCS. (Ovarian vein reflux can occur due to other causes also, and therefore a refluxing ovarian vein should not be taken as a nutcracker syndrome.)

16.4.2 May-Thurner Syndrome

May-Thurner syndrome is caused by the compression of the left common iliac vein between the right common iliac artery anteriorly and the vertebral column posteriorly. This could result in a thrombotic outcome promoting a frank DVT or a large pelvic collateral pathway from the left EIV to right CIV via internal iliac veins. In a nonthrombotic outcome also over a period of time, a similar collateral pathway can be established causing pelvic venous congestion and PCS.

16.4.3 Musculoskeletal Dysfunction

Pain patterns are usually referral in nature, radiating to the lower back and thighs and into the suprapubic, abdominal, and pelvic region. Initially the pain may begin in a small area, and persisting pain can cause increased sensitivity in the local nerves leading to central sensitization.

16.4.4 Levator Ani Syndrome

Levator ani syndrome causes pain, pressure, or ache in the tailbone, rectum, and pelvis. Pain is intensified by prolonged sitting, sexual activity, defecation, and constipation. Presentation of pain may refer to the legs or buttocks. Burning micturition is also common. Unusual tension in the levator ani muscles is the cause for the syndrome.

16.4.5 Coccydynia

Pain in and around the region of the coccyx is called coccydynia. It may involve the pelvic floor muscles or the gluteal muscle.

16.4.6 Pudendal Neuralgia

The pudendal nerve starts from the sacral plexus and supplies motor and sensory control to the genital region. The rectum, perineum, vagina, labia, clitoris and urethra, male scrotum, and penis are supplied by the pudendal nerve. The motor branch of the nerve controls the sphincters of the rectum and urethra as well as the pelvic floor muscles. Irritation of the nerve is termed as neuralgia. In pudendal neuralgia, pain can be experienced in any of the abovementioned organ innervated by pudendal nerve. Muscle spasms are quite common. The symptoms could include itching, burning, tingling, cold sensations, and pain. The sensory symptoms may be referred into the groin, abdomen, legs, and buttocks [13].

16.5 *H. pylori* and PCS

Colonic *H. pylori* strains were found to be frequently associated with pelvic congestion, and they are considered as a possible underlying etiologic pathology in cases of pelvic pathology in general [14]. Migration of *H. pylori* to the colon under the influence of antibiotic violence leads to the accumulation of profuse amounts of ammonia unopposed or buffered by any acidity [15, 16]. This accumulation of ammonia in the colon is toxic and could also lead to pelvic congestion. The association of the colonic *H. pylori* strains with pelvic pathology and the role played by the inflammatory cytokines and the therapeutic effect of NO in ED may be useful to think "outside of the venous component of the PVCS".

16.6 Investigations for Imaging

Imagining modalities currently used for PCS workup are duplex ultrasound (DUS) (transabdominal or transvaginal), CT venography (CTV), and MR venography (MRV).

16.6.1 Ultrasonography

Transvaginal color Doppler ultrasound performed in a supine and upright position is the best screening modality. Valsalva is also considered while screening. An increase in pelvic venous channels is often revealed following the Doppler, thereby confirming that pelvic varices are affected by gravity-dependent filling. DUS is a dynamic test that can be performed in supine position and then in standing position to confirm PVR. DU also has the capability of detecting reflux and measuring the diameter of both ovarian veins and renal and iliac veins. Compression of the renal and iliac veins can also be imagined. DUS has a high sensitivity to identify abnormal ovarian vein diameter (Fig. 16.3). DU is also used to study PCS symptoms in cases of "prostatitis syndromes" and cryptogenic hematuria and/or with the prognosis of the infertile patients undergoing treatment of varicocele.

For the detection of prostatic capsular veins, a transperineal color Doppler flow imaging is used. Dilation of the prostatic capsular vein, pudendal plexus, plexus behind the bladder, and the prostatic capsular vein can be observed ultrasonically.

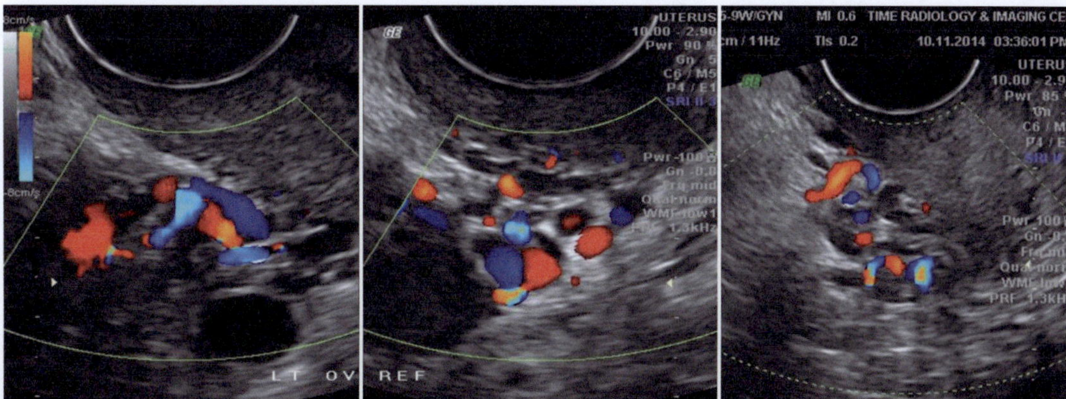

Fig. 16.3 Ovarian reflux, extensive varicose veins, and incompetent SFJ (left) and pelvic veins mild reflux with SFJ incompetence (right)

16.6.2 CTV, MRI, MRV, and Gadolinium Scans

MRV has moderate to high sensitivity (67%–100%) and specificity (67%–100%) for ovarian vein dilatation and reflux [17, 18].

CTV appears to be a good initial screening study and indicates CV with intention to treat. For the detection of large gonadal veins and associated varices, enhanced 3D magnetic resonance venography (MRV) is helpful. MRV combined with pelvic MRI allows us to exclude other common causes of pelvic pain such as fibroids, endometriosis, adenomyosis, ovarian masses, and lower lumbar intervertebral disc abnormities. It is thus an excellent modality for the information of chronic pelvic pain. The anatomic information gathered from the MRV also provides an excellent roadmap prior to venography and embolization.

16.6.3 Laparoscopy

Laparoscopy is usually unrewarding for the observation of pelvic varices.

16.6.4 Venography

Venography is used now as a therapeutic modality after the development of techniques of DUS, CTV, MRI, and MRV.

16.7 Treatment Options of PCS

There are very few options for the treatment of this condition.

16.7.1 Medical Treatment

If ED in males is indicated, antibiotic, anti-inflammatory, and phlebotonic drugs in general are used. Treatment modality is based upon hormone therapy which acts on venous receptors, venotonics which decrease the consequences of stasis. Also intermittent courses of anti-inflammatory agents and antibiotics are also prescribed if there is an inflammation secondary to local infection. Drugs that enhance venous tone could improve pelvic circulation and relieve pelvic pain [19].

16.7.2 Symptomatic Ovarian Vein Thrombosis

Information on ovarian vein thrombosis (OVT) is limited to some retrospective studies. Symptomatic OVT is rare. Patients fare well with anticoagulant: complete recanalization occurs in about two third of the patient.

Prevention by improving obstetrical exercise may be helpful.

16.7.3 Endovascular Treatment Options

Ovarian vein embolization is a safe and effective therapeutic method for the treatment of PCS. A clinical effectiveness ranging from 58% to 78% is achieved after transcatheter gonadal vein embolization. Recurrence is very unlikely, and majority of patients experience initial pain relief. An incomplete embolization of the varices and tributaries of the gonadal vein due to a pressure head is recreated through the remaining tributaries. Patients who present with atypical symptoms are those that tend to have partial relief of their pain post embolization and are the subset of patients that appear to have the most recurrences. A proper gonadal vein venogram together with interrogation of the internal iliac veins, to assess possible other/all refluxing pathways forming the pelvic varices, should be evaluated.

16.7.4 Venoplasty and Stenting

Venoplasty and stenting are the therapies used to improve venous outflow obstruction. The common procedures are for May-Thurner syndrome and nutcracker syndrome (Figs. 16.4 and 16.5).

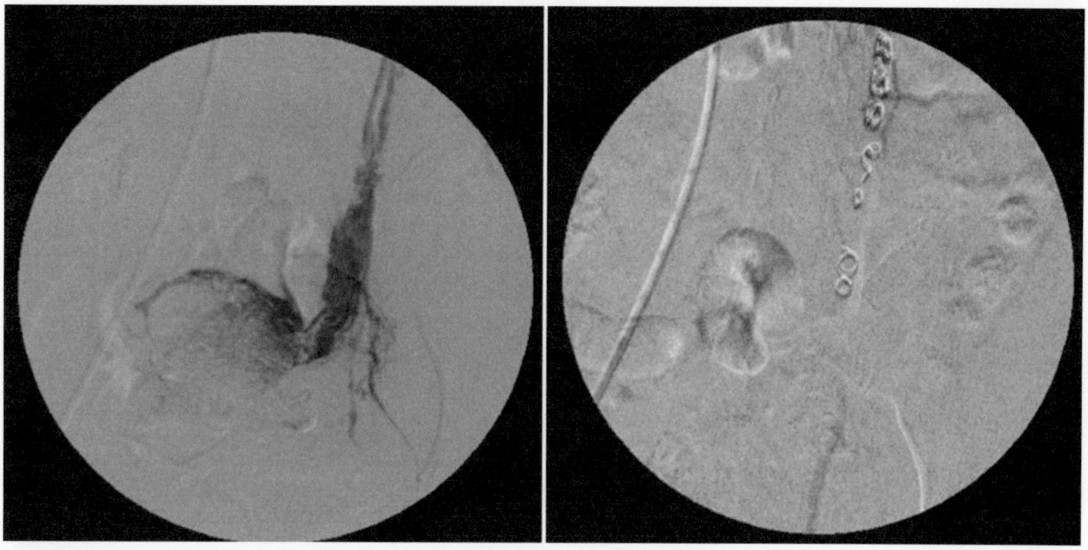

Fig. 16.4 Embolization of ovarian veins

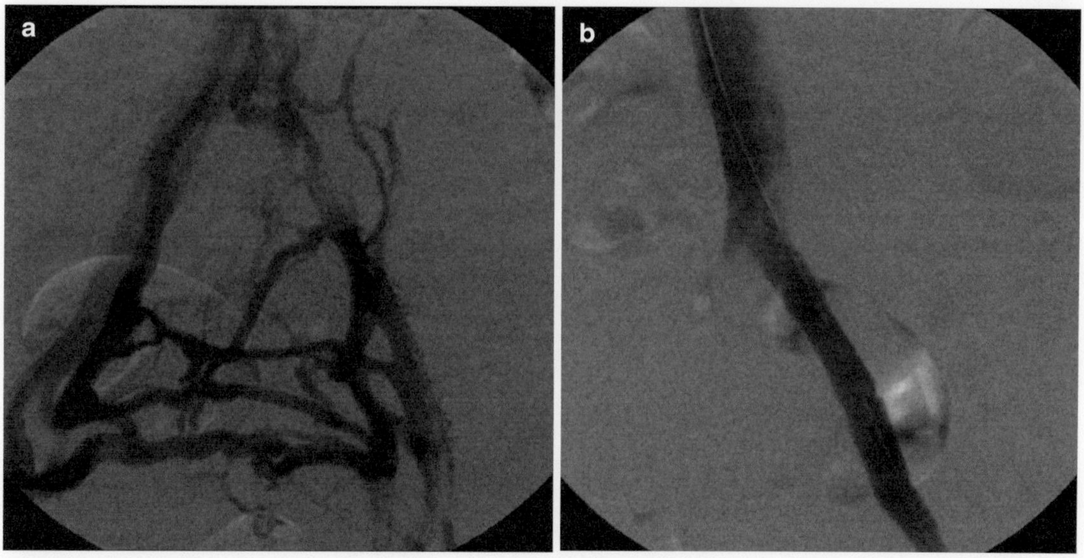

Fig. 16.5 Angioplasty. Stent deployed (**a**) before stenting, (**b**) after stenting

In May-Thurner syndrome, either postthrombotic or nonthrombotic compression of the left iliac vein, a balloon angioplasty helps alleviate the symptoms of PCS and PTs in younger individuals. Stents are usually reserved for elder patients as the long-term outcome of stents in the venous system is yet unknown, and it is observed that an occluded venous stent usually cannot be re-opened with balloon or a second stent like in the arterial system.

In nutcracker syndrome, temporary relief can occur after simple angioplasty or a stent deployment. However, long-term benefit comes from surgery.

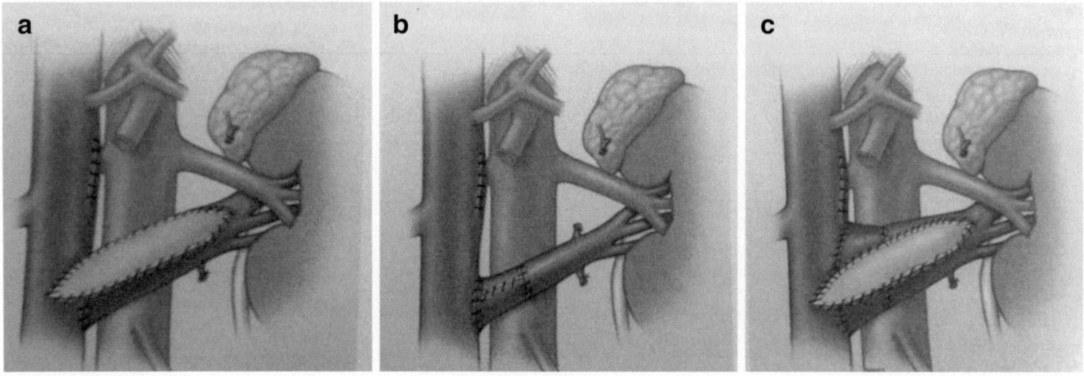

Fig. 16.6 Drawing of surgery in nutcracker syndrome: left renal (LRV) transposition to enlarge the renal vein (patch) or to decrease tension caused by the abdominal aorta and lack of retroperitoneal fat (cuff). (**a**) Vein patch, (**b**) vein cuff, (**c**) vein patch and cuff

16.7.5 Surgery

Most commonly described for surgery of PCS is the nutcracker syndrome. The following three types of surgical repairs are performed: left renal (LRV) transposition to enlarge the renal vein (patch) or to decrease tension caused by the abdominal aorta and lack of retroperitoneal fat (cuff), (a) vein patch, (b) vein cuff, and (c) vein patch and cuff [20] (Fig. 16.6).

Open surgery, mostly *LRV* transposition, is a safe and effective treatment of patient with nutcracker syndrome. However, one of the three patients after open repair required re-intervention, most frequently LRV stenting. An open reconstruction varies per patient in context to their anatomy and placement of vein patch or cuff can reduce restenosis. Renal vein stents, although they improve patency and durability, safety of the stents available currently need to be established.

PCS is treated medically after any specific pelvic pathology is ruled out. Surgical option is only considered if previous embolization proves to be ineffective. Therapeutic approach is pursued when a good preliminary result is obtained after embolization of the pelvic veins. But the patient should be routinely reassessed because of the nature of recurrent venous disorder. Patients are kept on regular follow-up post embolization and surgery.

Blood-Let Out Cupping Therapy in Female PCS: In the Arabic literature, PCS has been recognized long back, and a novel blood-let out cupping therapy is described [21].

Conclusion

Patients with PCS may present to general practitioners, phlebologists, surgeons, and gynecologists alike. Patients are to be partnered with regular opinions from gynecologists and urologists for females and males, respectively. It is necessary that patient undergoes a complete pelvic examination. The vascular specialist will only proceed with transcatheter embolization, endovascular balloon angioplasty, stent deployment, or open surgery. Due to the complexity in presentation of chronic pelvic pain, consultation with a neurologist, gastroenterologist, orthopedic surgeon, physiotherapist, and psychiatrist is often necessary.

References

1. Nicholson T, Basile A. Pelvic congestion syndrome, who should we treat and how? Tech Vasc Interv Radiol. 2006;9:19–23.
2. Lasry JL, Copp G, Balian E. Pelvi-perineal venous insufficiency and varicose veins of the lower limbs: duplex Doppler diagnosis and endoluminal treatment in thirty females. J Mal Vasc. 2007;32:23–31.

3. O'Brien M, Gillespie D. Diagnosis and treatment of the pelvic congestion syndrome. J Vasc Surg Venous Lymphat Disord. 2014;3:96–106.
4. Scultetus A, Villavicencio J, Gillespie D, Kao TR, Rich N. The pelvic venous syndromes: analysis of our experience with 57 patients. J Vasc Surg. 2002;36:881–8.
5. Hartung O, Grisoli D, Boufi M, Marani I, Hakam Z, Barthelemy P, et al. Endovascular stenting in the treatment of pelvic congestion syndrome caused by nutcracker syndrome: lessons learned from the first five cases. J Vasc Surg. 2005;42:275–80.
6. Loffredo V. Clinical aspects and complementary tests in pelvic congestive states. Rev Fr Gynecol Obstet. 1991;86:191–4.
7. Merchiers E, de Sutter P, Thiery L, Vandekerckhove D. Transvaginal ultrasonography: a profitable technic in the diagnosis and control of congestive pelvic syndrome. Phlebologie. 1991;44:395–400.
8. Tu FF, Hahn D, Steege JF. Pelvic congestion syndrome-associated pelvic pain: a systematic review of diagnosis and management. Obstet Gynecol Surv. 2010;65:332–40.
9. Gandini R, Chiocchi M, Konda D, Pampana E, Fabiano S, et al. Transcatheter foam sclerotherapy of symptomatic female varicocele with sodium-tetradecyl-sulfate foam. Cardiovasc Intervent Radiol. 2008;31:778–84.
10. Liddle AD, Davies AH. Pelvic congestion syndrome: chronic pelvic pain caused by ovarian and internal iliac varices. Phlebology. 2007;22:100–4.
11. Ganeshan A, Upponi S, Hon LQ, Uthappa MC, Warakaulle DR, et al. Chronic pelvic pain due to pelvic congestion syndrome: the role of diagnostic and interventional radiology. Cardiovasc Intervent Radiol. 2007;30:1105–11.
12. Mutha AS, Kulkarni VR, Bhagat S, et al. An observational study to evaluate the prevalence of erectile dysfunction (ED) and prescribing pattern of drugs and patients with ED visiting an Andrology Specialty Clinic, Mumbai: 2012-2014. J Clin Diagn Res. 2015;9(7):PC08–11.
13. Kamoi K. Pathologic significance of the internal pudendal vein in the development of intrapelvic venous congestion syndrome. Nippon Hinyokika Gakkai Zasshi. 1996;87:1214–20.
14. Nasrat AM, Nasrat SAM, Nasrat RM, Nasrat MM. Misconception and Misbehaviour towards Helicobacter pyloriis Leading to Major Spread of Illness. Gen Med (Los Angel). 2015 S1:002. doi:10.4172/2327-5146.1000S1-002.
15. Farinha P, Gascoyne RD. *Helicobacter pylori* and MALT lymphoma. Gastroenterology. 2005;128:1579–605.
16. Nasrat AM. The world misconception and misbehavior towards *Helicobacter pylori* is leading to major spread of illness. In: The 7th Anti-Aging Medicine World Congress, Monte-Carlo, Monaco; 2009.
17. Ascuitto G, Mumme A, Marpe B, Koster O, Ascuitto KC, Geier B. MR venography in the detection of pelvic venous congestion. Eur J Vasc Endovasc Surg. 2008;36:491–6.
18. Yand DM, Kim HC, Nam DH, Jahng GH, Huh CY, Lim JW. Time-resolved MR angiography for detecting and grading ovarian venous reflux: comparison with conventional venography. Br J Radiol. 2012;85:e117–22.
19. Charles G. Congestive pelvic syndromes. Rev Fr Gynecol Obstet. 1995;90:84–90.
20. Said SM, Gloviczki P, Kalra M, Oderich GS, Duncan AA, Fleming M, et al. Renal nutcracker syndrome: surgical options. Semin Vasc Surg. 2013;26:35–42.
21. Kwon SH, Oh JH, Ko KR, Park HC, Huh JY. Transcatheter ovarian vein embolization using coils for the treatment of pelvic congestion syndrome. Cardiovasc Intervent Radiol. 2007;30:655–61.

May-Thurner Syndrome

17

Soumya Khanna and Ajay K. Khanna

17.1 Introduction

May-Thurner syndrome (MTS) is a rarely diagnosed condition in which there is extrinsic venous compression by the arterial system against bony structure in the iliocaval territory. The condition is mostly asymptomatic in cases where there is partial obstruction, but progression with symptoms related to chronic venous hypertension or venous occlusion can occur, with or without venous thrombosis. This condition should always be kept in mind if a young woman comes with lower extremity swelling or deep vein thrombosis.

Though this syndrome was first described in 1851, a standard criterion to establish the diagnosis of MTS is yet to be established. The approach to diagnosis and treatment depends upon whether venous thrombosis is present or not. In previous years, MTS was diagnosed by the presence of pathologic features, but now the use of dynamic imaging techniques has led to a more radiologic based diagnosis. The definitive diagnosis is established by intravascular ultrasound (after removal of thrombosis, if necessary). The line of treatment includes minimally invasive treatment (angioplasty and stenting) of the venous lesion which opens up the obstruction thus providing immediate relief of symptoms with good long-term patency. In cases of venous thrombosis, endovascular treatment reduces rate of post-thrombotic syndrome.

S. Khanna (✉)
Institute of Medical Sciences,
Banaras Hindu University, Varanasi, India

A. K. Khanna
Department of General Surgery,
Institute of Medical Sciences,
Banaras Hindu University, Varanasi, India

17.2 Anatomy and Pathophysiology

May-Thurner syndrome is also known as iliocaval venous compression syndrome, iliac vein compression syndrome, Cockett syndrome, or venous spur. The most common variant of MTS is the compression of left iliac vein by the right common iliac artery over the fifth lumbar vertebrae [1] (Fig. 17.1).

In 1908, a cadaveric study on iliac veins was conducted by Mc Murrich, and he proposed that these obstructions were congenital in origin and were responsible for the increased incidence of deep vein thrombosis in left lower extremity [2]. In 1943, Ehrich and Krumbhaar contraindicated the findings of Mc Murrich by conducting a pathological study of the obstructed lesions and demonstrated that these obstructions comprised of collagen and elastin and are of acquired variety rather than congenital in nature [3]. It was in 1957 that a comprehensive understanding of the anatomic variants was made with the work of May and Thurner, after whom the syndrome is given its

A. K. Khanna, R. Jindal (eds.), *Venous Disorders*, https://doi.org/10.1007/978-981-13-1108-6_17

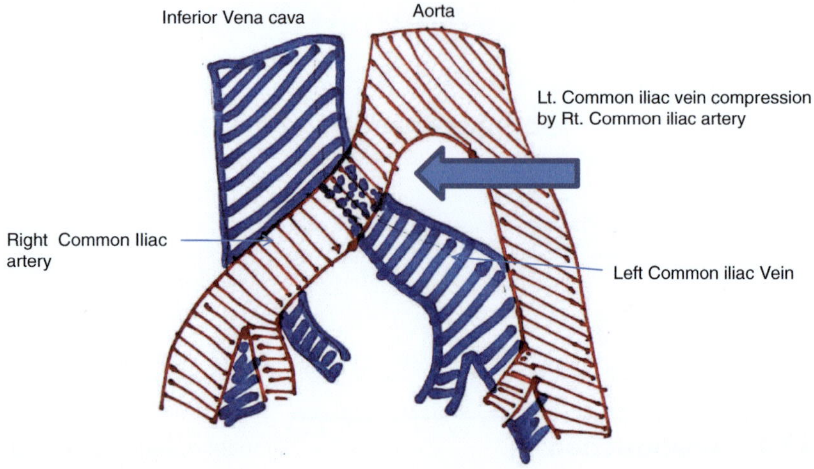

Fig. 17.1 May-Thurner syndrome

name. They found that 22% of 430 cadavers exhibited lesions in the left common iliac vein; these intraluminal thickenings were described as spurs and were postulated to arise from chronic expression of the left common iliac vein by the right common iliac artery. Three histologic types of spurs were described, namely, central, lateral, and fenestrated. Central spur occupied the anteroposterior plane and divided the lumen into two, lateral spur occurs along the sides of the left common iliac vein, and fenestrated spur results in lumen being covered in a lattice of spurs leading to decreased venous outflow [2, 3].

In 1967 Cockett illustrated the relationship between iliac vein compression and postthrombotic syndrome [4].

Other variants of MTS apart from the most common (the compression of LCIV by RCIA) are right-side MTS and compression of IVC by RCIA [4].

17.3 Epidemiology

The exact incidence and prevalence of MTS remain unknown and in fact underestimated since most of the cases are asymptomatic and require no treatment [5]. May-Thurner syndrome turned out to be the etiology in 2–5% of patients who came up with symptomatic lower extremity venous disorder [6].

17.4 Risk Factors

These factors might be directly associated with MTS or may convert asymptomatic MTS into a symptomatic one. They are female gender especially who are postpartum, multiparous, or using OCPs and have scoliosis, dehydration, and hypercoagulable disorder [7].

17.5 Clinical Features

The history of the patient and clinical presentation are the most important components required in formulating a diagnosis of MTS. It is particularly prevalent in younger and middle-aged women (mean age = 42), although men can also be affected [8].

Clinical presentation of symptomatic MTS includes left lower extremity swelling, pain, venous claudication, ulceration, and varicose veins. Rare symptoms include phlebitis, phlegmasia alba dolens, phlegmasia cerulea dolens, and bilateral or right-sided symptoms [2, 8].

The clinical stages of MTS can be classified as follows [9]:

Stage 1—asymptomatic left common iliac vein compression
Stage 2—formation of an intraluminal spur
Stage 3—occurrence of left iliac vein deep vein thrombosis

History of patient revealing recurrent DVT, unexplained edema, venous claudication, or varicosities should create a suspicion for MTS as an etiology. The findings can be further supported on physical examination indicating left lower extremity swelling, skin hyperpigmentation, varicose veins, telangiectasia, and ulceration on ankle [10].

17.6 Differential Diagnosis

Since May-Thurner syndrome is usually unilateral, the number of causes which need to be ruled out is limited. The other causes of iliac vein compression are pelvic mass like tumor, abscess, and hematoma, iliofemoral thrombosis as a result of trauma or surgery or immobilization or recent catheterization or radiation, and malignancies [11].

Uterine enlargement from fibroids, cancer, or pregnancy, aortoiliac aneurysm, retroperitoneal fibrosis, osteophytes, etc. are the other causes.

Some clinical presentations are rare but should not be missed as MTS associated with ruptured iliac vein and retroperitoneal hematoma, MTS occurring due to an iliac artery stent or endovascular stent graft, MTS secondary to prostate enlargement, and MTS presenting as hidden stroke in patients with a patent foramen ovale.

17.7 Diagnosis

Left common iliac vein compression is a normal anatomic variant and not necessarily a pathologic condition until the patient develops symptoms [12].

Moreover Mc Dermott et al. discovered that the extent of left common iliac vein compression in a single patient can vary over a short period of time; thus, the finding of extent of left common iliac vein compression by right common iliac artery in a single imaging study may just reflect the volume status of patient and may not be sufficient to suspect or confirm MTS [13].

A diagnostic imaging criterion is yet to be established for diagnosis of May-Thurner syndrome. It should exhibit persistent narrowing of the iliac vein due to the presence of permanent iliac spurs, regardless of patient positioning during imaging study. The patient can be placed in prone position as such position may demonstrate a decrease in collateral flow or reveal normal iliac vein competency [13]. More than 50% stenosis in the luminal diameter of the vein is considered an adequate indicator of left common iliac vein compression related to May-Thurner syndrome [14]. Other indicators of May-Thurner syndrome are the presence of venous collaterals, presence of intraluminal spurs, and changes in hemodynamic flow >2 mm Hg across the stenotic region with the patient in supine position [13, 14].

The diagnostic imaging modalities include:

1. Noninvasive venous imaging:
   (a) Duplex ultrasound
   (b) Plethysmography
   (c) CT/MR venography
2. Invasive venous imaging:
   (a) Catheter-based venography
3. Intravascular USG

17.8 Duplex USG

It is often the initial diagnostic modality in determining venous insufficiencies and deep vein thrombosis because it is noninvasive and easy to perform and is accurate in locating the lesion and determining the severity and cause of venous insufficiencies.

Although venous ultrasound has high sensitivity and specificity for the detection of proximal deep vein thrombosis using B mode using compressibility criterion, the deep location of the proximal iliac vein along with other factors (e.g., obesity, overlying gas) may limit ultrasound for making an accurate diagnosis of MTS [15].

Assessment of iliocaval stenosis can be done by measuring post-stenotic turbulence which gives out a mosaic appearance (noisy signal), an abnormal Doppler signal at the area of stenosis, and a sluggish and/or no spontaneous flow as well as very poor augmentation [16]. The contralateral vasculature serves as a control provided inferior vena cava thrombosis/occlusion is not present.

There are certain points which need to be kept in mind while performing Doppler. The angle of insonation should be <60°. For femoral vein evaluation, a 4–7 Mhz linear array transducer is used, whereas for iliac and caval vessels, the frequency should be 2–3 Mhz. B mode will help to compare decrease in vain diameter at the smallest lumen area to that of normal vein diameter.

Peak vein velocity is measured in the post-stenotic and compared to that of pre-stenotic segment. If the PVV gradient is more than 2.0, the finding is significant [16].

Limitations of ultrasound: It does not reveal specific anatomic characteristics of MTS such as iliac vein compression or intraluminal spurs [17], and since the iliac veins are located deeply, sometimes they get failed to visualize even by skilled sonographers.

17.9 Plethysmography

Air plethysmography determines the degree of venous reflux and evaluates any proximal obstructions [2]. According to Hurst et al., this modality has low sensitivity in confirming a diagnosis of MTS as it failed to detect any iliac vein obstructions in nine cases of venous occlusion. This technique can be used to assess the severity of venous symptoms, but using it as a diagnostic modality is questionable [8].

17.10 CT/MR Venography

It is a sensitive diagnostic modality for estimating the location and degree of stenosis in non-thrombosed veins, identifying venous collaterals, and identifying other anatomic variations.

Both CT and MR venograms have high sensitivity and specificity for diagnosing MTS (>95%) provided adequate technical protocols for image acquisition are followed [11].

A normal CT with 10 mm slices cannot always establish a diagnosis of MTS because iliac spurs are small and in addition to that they might be concealed by the fibrosis over the vasculature [18]. Thus if 3–5 mm slices are cut, then these lesions would not be missed.

The advantages of CT venography over compression Doppler US or traditional venography are lack of operator dependence, vivid imaging of the pelvic veins, and less time-consuming.

CT venography is contraindicated in pregnancy and renal impairment [18]. CT venography has advantage over MR venography as it may be better at identifying more severely stenotic lesions and identifying other causes of extrinsic venous compression as well [18].

MR venography (MRV) on the other hand provides better imaging of the pelvic and spinal structures including bulging or protruding intervertebral discs, lumbar vertebral degeneration, osteophytes, or spondylolisthesis [19]. The main advantages of MRV in the diagnosis of MTS include its noninvasiveness, ability to analyze all pelvic structures, and lack of operator dependence [11]. In addition to that, MRV can estimate the degree of venous collateral flow, which greatly assists in diagnosis of MTS [20].

Other benefit and advantage of MR venography over CT venography are that it can be performed without contrast; thus, it becomes a diagnostic imaging of choice in patients with contrast allergies or renal impairment [3]. The main drawbacks of MRV in the diagnosis of MTS are the vasculature above bifurcation has non-laminar flow which sometimes gives a confusing image [11]. It is expensive, time-consuming, and difficult to perform in severely ill patients [17]. Another limitation is that a single MRV study may not be sufficient to diagnose MTS since the degree of left iliac vein compression significantly differs in the same patient due to factors such as volume status or patient positioning [3].

17.11 Invasive Venous Imaging

Contrast venography/catheter-based venography has been widely considered as the gold standard modality to confirm a diagnosis of MTS [8]. Contrast dye must be injected in popliteal or femoral vein rather than veins on dorsum of the foot since injecting into dorsum of foot does not give sufficient exposure to iliac venous system [2] (Fig. 17.2).

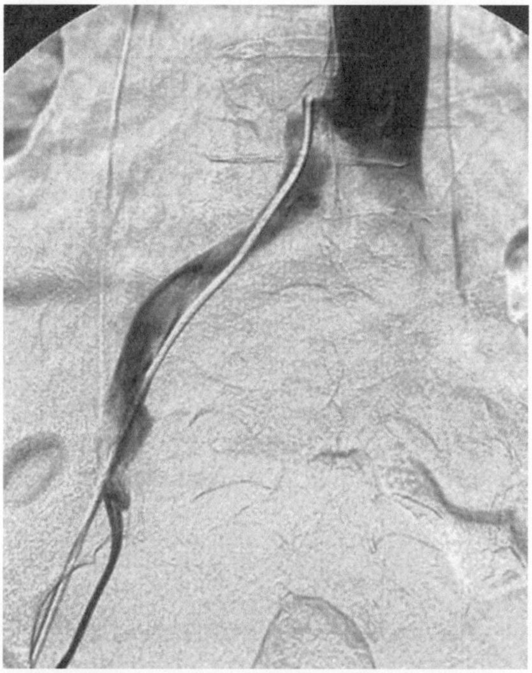

Fig. 17.2 Digital subtraction angiographic image showing non opacification of left common iliac vein subsequent to the level of common iliac arterial crossing due to venous thrombosis

Venography also helps in assessment of hemodynamic status of MTS through pressure gradient measurements. Iliofemoral stenosis is considered significant with a measurement of >2 mm Hg at rest and more than 3 mm Hg during strenuous work.

The main drawbacks of ascending venography are that it is time-consuming and invasive and cannot be performed in patients with widespread iliofemoral DVT, and post-procedural complications such as phlebitis may occur [17].

Venography also provides information toward chronicity of lesion as well as variable congenital features that may be associated, e.g., duplicated or rudimentary venous system [21].

The accuracy of this technique can be further improved by taking two or three projections during injection phase since in pancaked vein (i.e., externally compressed in anteroposterior plane), it will not exhibit diameter narrowing in the AP view [22]. It is equally effective to perform hand injection venography through the access sheath rather than using a power injector.

17.12 Intravascular Ultrasound

This modality can be used for diagnosis as well as a valuable adjunct for treatment of MTS. It has high sensitivity and specificity (>98%) [23]. It helps in detecting the precise morphology of the spur and thus can determine the severity and distribution of pathology. It is useful for determining vessel diameter, aiding stent placement, and ensuring full stent expansion.

17.13 Treatment

The treatment of MTS depends on whether deep vein thrombosis is present or not. If DVT is not present and patient is having mild symptoms, the treatment is conservative, and compression stockings are sufficient enough in relieving the symptoms.

For advanced non-thrombotic MTS with severe symptoms of chronic venous insufficiency, e.g., limb swelling, pain, and skin discoloration, treatment is focused toward reducing the severity of the stenotic venous lesion using angioplasty and stenting the affected segment. Angioplasty if done alone is associated with high recurrence rates [24]. Recurrence rates in case of stenting depends upon type of stent used [25].

If MTS is associated with venous thromboembolism, treatment is initiated with full therapeutic anticoagulation unless contraindicated. Further treatment requires decreasing the volume of thrombus using catheter-directed thrombolysis or pharmacomechanical thrombolysis. The underlying venous stenosis is evaluated, and if present, angioplasty and stenting of the given iliocaval segment are done.

With successful treatment, chances of post-thrombotic syndrome get reduced to <10%, but if no treatment is provided, the chances of occurrence of postthrombotic syndrome go as high as 80–90%. After successful intervention for symptomatic MTS, the patient is prescribed to use knee or thigh high compression stockings (30–40 mm Hg).

Patients having DVT, after intervention, are kept on therapeutic anticoagulation. The dosing, monitoring, and duration of anticoagulation are as per VTE guidelines [26]. If stenting has been performed and bleeding risk is low, then antiplatelet therapy is given [27]. If thrombolysis is contraindicated, a common femoral venotomy is performed to remove the thrombus [21]. If endovascular therapy fails, then open surgery is indicated [28].

The open surgery is done by dissection of the iliac vein from the overlying iliac artery, open thrombectomy, and possible patch angioplasty of the left iliac vein and may need adjunctive procedures, such as an arteriovenous fistula to enhance flow in the diseased vein [24].

If iliac vein is occluded, then surgical options include cross-femoral venous bypass (Palma-Dale procedure) [29] and femorofemoral or ileoileal prosthetic bypass, and femorocaval and aortic elevation may be done [30].

To assist long-term patency of the bypass grafts or reconstructed veins, an arteriovenous fistula is often created which is ligated after 6 weeks.

Complications of endovascular therapy may lead to jailing the contralateral common iliac vein which can cause thrombosis, rupture of iliac vein, migration or displacement of stent, and erosion of stent into overlying artery.

17.14 Efficacy of Endovenous Therapy

With the development of minimally invasive techniques and devices, the endovenous techniques have become treatment of choice in treating iliofemoral stenotic lesions and for decreasing the long-term consequences of venous outflow obstructions [31]. Even in cases with challenging anatomy, endovascular treatment has proved to be safer and has higher patency rates in cases of iliac vein stenosis [32].

It has been noted by reviewing of various studies that catheter-directed thrombolysis has shown to have more thrombus resolution and reduced risk for postthrombotic syndrome as compared to the anticoagulation treatment alone.

References

1. Virchow R. Ueber die Erweiterung kleinerer Gefäfse. Arch Pathol Anat Physiol Klin Med. 1851;3:427.
2. Shebel ND, Whalen CC. Diagnosis and management of iliac vein compression syndrome. J Vasc Nurs. 2005;23:10–7.; quiz 18–19. https://doi.org/10.1016/j.jvn.2004.12.001.
3. Brazeau NF, Harvey HB, Pinto EG, Deipolyi A, Hesketh RL, Oklu R. May-Thurner syndrome: diagnosis and management. Vasa. 2013;42:96–105. https://doi.org/10.1024/0301-1526/a000252.
4. Burke RM, Rayan SS, Kasirajan K, et al. Unusual case of right-sided May-Thurner syndrome and review of its management. Vascular. 2006;14:47.
5. Moudgill N, Hager E, Gonsalves C, et al. May-Thurner syndrome: case report and review of the literature involving modern endovascular therapy. Vascular. 2009;17:330.
6. May R, Thurner J. The cause of the predominantly sinistral occurrence of thrombosis of the pelvic veins. Angiology. 1957;8:419.
7. Marston W, Fish D, Unger J, Keagy B. Incidence of and risk factors for iliocaval venous obstruction in patients with active or healed venous leg ulcers. J Vasc Surg. 2011;53:1303.
8. Hurst DR, Forauer AR, Bloom JR, Greenfield LJ, Wakefield TW, Williams DM. Diagnosis and endovascular treatment of iliocaval compression syndrome. J Vasc Surg. 2001;34:106–13. https://doi.org/10.1067/mva.2001.114213.
9. Ibrahim W, Al Safran Z, Hasan H, Zeid WA. Endovascular management of May-Thurner syndrome. Ann Vasc Dis. 2012;5:217–21. https://doi.org/10.3400/avd.cr.12.00007.
10. Patel NH, Stookey KR, Ketcham DB, Cragg AH. Endovascular management of acute extensive iliofemoral deep venous thrombosis caused by May-Thurner syndrome. J Vasc Interv Radiol. 2000;11:1297–302. https://doi.org/10.1016/S1051-0443(07)61304-9.
11. Wolpert LM, Rahmani O, Stein B, Gallagher JJ, Drezner AD. Magnetic resonance venography in the diagnosis and management of May-Thurner syndrome. Vasc Endovasc Surg. 2002;36:51–7. https://doi.org/10.1177/153857440203600109.
12. Kibbe MR, Ujiki M, Goodwin AL, Eskandari M, Yao J, Matsumura J. Iliac vein compression in an asymptomatic patient population. J Vasc Surg. 2004;39:937–43. https://doi.org/10.1016/j.jvs.2003.12.032.
13. McDermott S, Oliveira G, Ergül E, Brazeau N, Wicky S, Oklu R. May-Thurner syndrome: can it be diagnosed by a single MR venography study? Diagn Interv Radiol. 2013;19:44–8. https://doi.org/10.4261/1305-3825.DIR.5939-12.1.
14. Liu Z, Gao N, Shen L, Yang J, Zhu Y, Li Z, Si Y. Endovascular treatment for symptomatic iliac vein compression syndrome: a prospective consecutive

series of 48 patients. Ann Vasc Surg. 2014;28:695–704. https://doi.org/10.1016/j.avsg.2013.05.019.
15. Lensing AW, Prandoni P, Brandjes D, et al. Detection of deep-vein thrombosis by real-time B-mode ultrasonography. N Engl J Med. 1989;320:342.
16. Labropoulos N, Borge M, Pierce K, Pappas PJ. Criteria for defining significant central vein stenosis with duplex ultrasound. J Vasc Surg. 2007;46:101.
17. Lamba R, Tanner DT, Sekhon S, McGahan JP, Corwin MT, Lall CG. Multidetector CT of vascular compression syndromes in the abdomen and pelvis. Radiographics. 2014;34:93–115. https://doi.org/10.1148/rg.341125010.
18. Chung JW, Yoon CJ, Jung SI, Kim HC, Lee W, Kim YI, Jae HJ, Park JH. Acute iliofemoral deep vein thrombosis: evaluation of underlying anatomic abnormalities by spiral CT venography. J Vasc Interv Radiol. 2004;15:249–56. https://doi.org/10.1097/01.RVI.0000109402.52762.8D.
19. Oguzkurt L, Tercan F, Pourbagher MA, Kizilkilic O, Turkoz R, Boyvat F. Computed tomography findings in 10 cases of iliac vein compression (May-Thurner) syndrome. Eur J Radiol. 2005;55:421–5. https://doi.org/10.1016/j.ejrad.2004.11.002.
20. Gurel K, Gurel S, Karavas E, Buharalıoglu Y, Daglar B. Direct contrast-enhanced MR venography in the diagnosis of May-Thurner syndrome. Eur J Radiol. 2011;80:533–6. https://doi.org/10.1016/j.ejrad.2010.04.033.
21. Meissner MH, Gloviczki P, Comerota AJ, et al. Early thrombus removal strategies for acute deep venous thrombosis: clinical practice guidelines of the Society for Vascular Surgery and the American Venous Forum. J Vasc Surg. 2012;55:1449.
22. Birn J, Vedantham S. May-Thurner syndrome and other obstructive iliac vein lesions: meaning, myth, and mystery. Vasc Med. 2015;20:74.
23. DeRubertis BG, Lew W, Jabori S, et al. Importance of intravascular ultrasound imaging during percutaneous treatment of May-Thurner syndrome. J Vasc Surg. 2012;56:580.
24. Mickley V, Schwagierek R, Rilinger N, et al. Left iliac venous thrombosis caused by venous spur: treatment with thrombectomy and stent implantation. J Vasc Surg. 1998;28:492.
25. Gloviczki P, Lawrence PF. Iliac vein stenting and contralateral deep vein thrombosis. J Vasc Surg Venous Lymphat Disord. 2017;5:5.
26. Jaff MR, McMurtry MS, Archer SL, et al. Management of massive and submassive pulmonary embolism, iliofemoral deep vein thrombosis, and chronic thromboembolic pulmonary hypertension: a scientific statement from the American Heart Association. Circulation. 2011;123:1788.
27. Kearon C, Akl EA, Comerota AJ, et al. Antithrombotic therapy for VTE disease: antithrombotic therapy and prevention of thrombosis, 9th ed: American college of chest physicians evidence-based clinical practice guidelines. Chest. 2012;141:e419S.
28. Hartung O, Benmiloud F, Barthelemy P, et al. Late results of surgical venous thrombectomy with iliocaval stenting. J Vasc Surg. 2008;47:381.
29. Palma EC, Esperon R. Vein transplants and grafts in the surgical treatment of the postphlebitic syndrome. J Cardiovasc Surg (Torino). 1960;1:94.
30. Dale WA, Harris J. Cross-over vein grafts for iliac and femoral venous occlusion. J Cardiovasc Surg (Torino). 1969;10:458.
31. Binkert CA, Schoch E, Stuckmann G, et al. Treatment of pelvic venous spur (May-Thurner syndrome) with self-expanding metallic endoprostheses. Cardiovasc Intervent Radiol. 1998;21:22.
32. O'Sullivan GJ, Semba CP, Bittner CA, et al. Endovascular management of iliac vein compression (May-Thurner) syndrome. J Vasc Interv Radiol. 2000;11:823.

18 Nutcracker Syndrome

Ajay Savlania and Shivanesan Pitchai

18.1 Introduction

Left renal vein (LRV) compression between the superior mesenteric artery (SMA) and abdominal aorta is referred to as the nutcracker phenomenon (NCP) or LRV entrapment and was first described by anatomist Grant in 1937 [1]. Abdominal aorta and superior mesenteric artery (SMA) act as two arms of a 'nutcracker' that can potentially compress the left renal vein [2]. The term nutcracker syndrome (NCS) is the clinical presentation of this phenomenon which is assigned to those patients who present with signs or symptoms of left renal venous congestion and have the anatomical LRV compression [3]. De Schepper, a Belgian physician named this phenomenon as 'nutcracker syndrome' [4]. Anatomically classical anterior nutcracker syndrome, in which there is compression of distal LRV between aorta and proximal SMA, is analogous to superior mesenteric artery syndrome (Wilkie's syndrome) wherein the third part of duodenum gets compressed anteriorly by SMA and posteriorly by aorta [5–10]. The retroaortic or circumaortic renal vein may get compressed between the aorta and the vertebral body causing symptom which is called posterior nutcracker syndrome [11]. NCP on the right side, due to compression of large veins by the gravid uterus, has been also reported [12].

A case of concurrent anterior and posterior NCS affecting circumaortic left renal vein (collar) where the anterior tributary of LRV compressed between the aorta and the SMA, while the posterior tributary of LRV compressed between the aorta and the vertebral column has been described [13].

18.2 Anatomy in Relation to Nutcracker Compression of Renal Vein

The left-sided renal vein is 5–9 cm long and 2.5–3 times the length of the right renal vein. It starts from the left renal hilum and receives tributaries of the left adrenal gland and left gonadal, ureteral and sometimes lumbar veins before draining into the inferior vena cava between T12 and L2 [14–16].

The angle of origin normally between the superior mesenteric artery and the abdominal aorta is approximately 90°. The left renal vein (LRV) usually passes in front of the aorta through the crotch formed by superior mesenteric artery and the abdominal aorta. Superior mesenteric artery origin from the aorta makes a unique configuration, so that SMA has a 4–5 mm course in the anterior direction before taking downward

A. Savlania (✉)
Postgraduate Institute of Medical Education and Research, Trivandrum, India

S. Pitchai
Sree Chitra Tirunal Institute for Medical Sciences and Technology, Trivandrum, India

A. K. Khanna, R. Jindal (eds.), *Venous Disorders*, https://doi.org/10.1007/978-981-13-1108-6_18

direction thus forming configuration of an inverted J. This distinctive anatomy prevents compression of the left renal vein in the aorto-mesenteric window. In contrast, patients with nutcracker syndrome have superior mesenteric artery origin from aorta at angle less than 90°, which makes aortomesenteric window narrow due to steep descent of SMA from aorta leading to compression of the LRV distally and left renal vein hypertension proximally. This is termed as anterior nutcracker syndrome [17]. The retroaortic left renal vein is an anatomical variant which makes LRV susceptible to compression between the aorta and the vertebral column leading to left renal venous hypertension. This is termed as posterior nutcracker syndrome [18].

18.3 Pathophysiology

The anomalies of both superior mesenteric artery and left renal vein have been implicated in causation of NCS. Anatomically critical factors in relation to the superior mesenteric artery include acute angle associated with abnormally low or anterolateral origin from the abdominal aorta. Venous anatomical variants noted in cases of NCS include retroaortic course of the left renal vein or circumaortic left renal vein. Abnormal dorsal ptosis of the left kidney with secondary stretching of the left renal vein over the aorta and high course of the left renal vein has also been cited as possible factors which can contribute to compression of LRV [19]. Excessive fibrotic tissue around the origin of the SMA can also contribute to the compression of the left renal vein [20]. LRV compression is aggravated by the standing position because of the weight of the bowel and may be underestimated in imaging carried out in the supine position (CT, MR angiography). Lower body mass index has been shown to correlate with increased incidence of NCP probably due to reduced retroperitoneal fat which in turn reduces the angle between SMA takeoff and aorta [13].

Venous compression induces LRV hypertension and development of collateral pathways with variceal dilatation of tributaries, which causes the symptoms. Beinart et al. described normal gradient of pressure between LRV and inferior vena cava is less than 1 mmHg [21]. The gradient of pressure between the LRV and inferior vena cava may increase up to 3 mmHg due to compression by the SMA leading to rupture of thin-walled septum between the small veins and the collecting system in the renal fornix leading to haematuria [22]. It has also been postulated that haematuria may be the result of communication between dilated venous sinuses and adjacent renal calices [23].

18.4 Clinical Features

Nutcracker syndrome occurs more commonly in females, and age group affected ranges from childhood to seventh decade, but most cases are reported in second to fourth decades of their lives.

The most commonly reported symptom is haematuria and is due to elevated venous pressure which leads to rupture of thin-walled varices into the collecting system. It varies from micro- to macro-haematuria, occasionally resulting in anaemia that may require blood transfusions [24, 25].

Abdominal or flank pain is the second most common symptom, which may radiate to the posteromedial region of the thigh or gluteal region. The pain can be exacerbated by sitting position, standing position, walking or riding on a bicycle [26, 27]. Flank pain due to left ureteric colic can occur because of the passage of clots in the ureter.

Left renal vein hypertension is the usual cause of varicoceles [28]. The compression of LRV is noticed in 50–100% of patients with varicocele, although not every patient with varicocele will have distended LRV [29, 30] . Varicosities in relation with distended LRV can be noticed around the renal calyces, renal pelvis and ureter and sometimes at the gluteal or vulvar region [31, 32]. Large variceal veins can be picked up on pelvic and abdominal duplex or venography [33]. Symptoms that changes with position change are hallmark of NCS and should be correlated with duplex sonography [34–37]. Nutcracker phenomenon usually becomes more prominent in standing than supine positions because of visceral proptosis and acute angulation of aortomesenteric angle (the angle between the aorta and the SMA) [38].

Orthostatic proteinuria is seen in some 14% of patients where albumin in urine appears in standing position and minimal to no protein excretion seen in supine position [39]. Nutcracker syndrome has also been reported to be associated with chronic fatigue syndrome in few patients [40].

Nutcracker syndrome with venous reflux in pelvic collaterals may lead to pelvic congestion. This group of patients may have dysuria, dyspareunia, dysmenorrhoea, increased polycystic changes in the ovaries and variations in venous duplex waveform while performing Valsalva manoeuver. Most patients have associated pelvic varicoceles. Patients of pelvic congestion syndrome up to 10% were found to have nutcracker syndrome. In some patients, gonadal vein flow interruption improves symptoms, but gonadal veins may act as main outflow vessels, and so their flow interruption may increase NCS symptoms [26, 30, 31].

It is not clear why some patients with NCP which are incidentally detected on imaging, and in cases with even ligated LRV [15], remain asymptomatic, whereas others have symptoms.

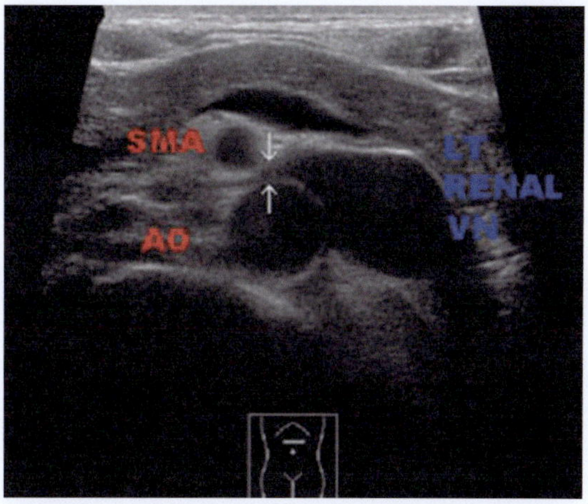

Fig. 18.1 Ultrasonography of the upper abdomen in transverse section showing the classical compression of LRV in aortomesenteric window (white arrows), and size of proximal LRV is almost five times that of narrowed portion

18.5 Diagnosis

18.5.1 Duplex Scanning

Duplex assessment should be the first choice for evaluation, as it is a noninvasive modality. A duplex scan (Fig. 18.1) should be performed after overnight fasting and fibre-free diet on the previous day of imaging. The viscerorenal arteries bearing segment of abdominal aorta must be examined via horizontal, sagittal sections, and most importantly LRV diameter and peak systolic velocity in LRV should be measured in transverse section. In nutcracker syndrome, left renal vein stenosis at the aortomesenteric window is considered significant only if the diameter specifically anteroposterior of the LRV on the left side of the aorta is five times than that of stenotic region and if the peak systolic velocity (PSV) at the stenotic segment is five time higher than the PSV measured at the hilum of the left kidney [41] (Fig. 18.1). The examiner should also look for collateral pathways, particularly for reflux in the left gonadic vein in the cases of associated pelvic congestion syndrome. Duplex scan has sensitivity and specificity of 78% and 100%, respectively, when flow reversal in the collateral veins is included in the diagnostic criteria. In NCS both distended and non-distended left renal vein can exist, and even normal flow can also exist in distended LRV. The ability to assess colour flow in collateral veins also aids in diagnosis of the nutcracker syndrome [33].

18.5.2 Computerised Tomographic and Magnetic Resonance Angiography

Computerised tomography angiogram is a noninvasive imaging modality, which offers multiplanar imaging for assessment. Portal venous phase of CT angiography should be used, which clearly shows the status of left renal vein and delineates its relationship with the surrounding structures. Magnetic resonance angiography (MRA) can provide the same information and has the advantage of avoiding exposure to radiation.

CT angiogram (CTA) findings can include LRV compression between the SMA and the abdominal aorta (aortomesenteric window) with proximal dilatation of the vein (Fig. 18.2) and the presence of left kidney hilar region varicose veins

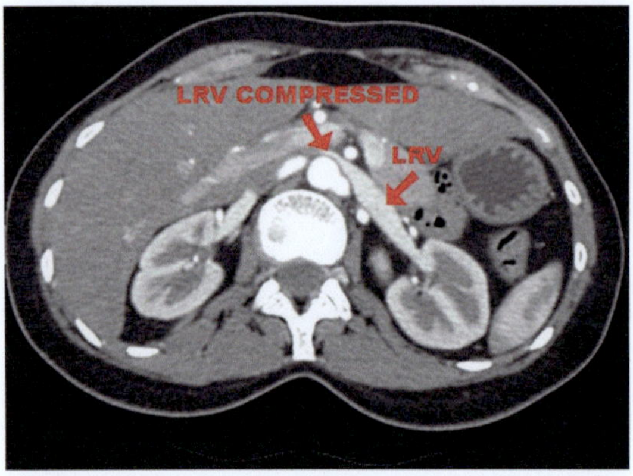

Fig. 18.2 CT angiogram abdomen, transverse section, reveals the compression of LRV between SMA anteriorly and aorta posteriorly. Red arrows marking the compressed area

and collateral pathways. In posterior nutcracker syndrome, the vein follows a posterior course to aorta (retroaortic), and CTA may show compression of LRV between aorta and lumbar vertebra. CTA can show acute angle takeoff by SMA from the aorta and can have a relatively low or anterolateral origin, and the space between the SMA and the aorta at the level of the left renal vein crossing is reduced [42]. A classical triangular narrowing of the LRV at the aortomesenteric portion, named beak sign of the LRV, can be useful in diagnosis of the noncompensated nutcracker syndrome [43].

18.5.3 Phlebography and Renocaval Gradient

Left renal vein phlebography can be performed by percutaneous technique using femoral vein or brachial vein access under local anaesthesia. Phlebography with renocaval pressure gradient assessment is considered as propitious in establishing the final diagnosis of NCS. Left renal venous phlebography allows visualisation of the point of LRV compression at the mesoaortic window with stasis of dye or delayed clearance of dye and also shows venous collaterals in perirenal and periureteral region with reflux into the gonadal and adrenal tributaries. The renocaval pressure gradient by pullback technique between the left renal vein and vena cava should be >3 mmHg to clinch the diagnosis of NCS which is otherwise in normal situation is <1 mmHg [21].

18.6 Urology Evaluation for Haematuria

Haematuria in NCS, which is often microscopic in presentation, mandates urological evaluation. Urine microscopy and urine culture should be performed to rule out glomerular cause and infectious aetiology of haematuria. Urologic assessment can include cystoscopy to locate haematuria to left ureter and flexible ureterorenoscopy or even renal biopsy. Andrianne et al. described a preoperative technique, in which clamping of the renal vein is followed by appearance of immediate reversible gross haematuria. Haematuria provocation test by percutaneous technique has also been proposed, which can be performed during conventional phlebography by temporarily occluding LRV in preoperative evaluation for formal diagnosis of this syndrome in suspected patients [44].

18.7 Other Investigations

The platelet counts and coagulation profile should be checked. Other causes of haematuria as urinary tract, tuberculosis and bilharziasis should be ruled out.

18.8 Differential Diagnosis

It is often challenging to diagnose NCS; all other causes of haematuria and flank pain should be ruled out before diagnosing NCS. Differential diagnosis includes glomerulonephritis, urinary tract infection, renal calculi, primary varicocele, pelvic congestion syndrome due to other causes, vascular malformation, endometriosis and musculoskeletal problems causing flank pain.

18.9 Indications for Intervention

The proper correlation between the degree of the LRV compression and severity of the symptoms is lacking. Hence for optimal results of endovascular or surgical management of NCS, selection of the patient for intervention is of prime importance. The interventions are considered only if there is severe and intractable symptoms or failure to respond after conservative management, which some authors recommend a period of 2 years of conservative approach for patients aged <18 years and for a duration of 6 months in case of adults [17, 45, 46] .

18.10 Treatment

Management of the nutcracker syndrome has evolved over the last five decades. The available options can be categorised as:

1. Surveillance
2. Endovascular management:
   (a) Stenting
   (b) Embolisation of gonadal veins
3. Surgical management:
   (a) Renal vein transpositioning/reimplantation
   (b) Other procedures—renal autotransplantation, renal vein bypass, etc.

18.10.1 Surveillance

Conservative management is generally advocated in young patients (<18 years) especially when patients present with microscopic haematuria, short-lived intermittent episode of painless gross haematuria, insignificant pain or atypical symptoms. General advice is to encourage weight gain so that the retroperitoneal fat increases which may decrease the posterior renal ptosis thereby reducing the tension over the renal vein. With physical growth, an increase in fibrofatty tissue around the takeoff of the SMA may also relieve the LRV compression. The conservative approach should be favoured up to a period of 2 years following detection of problem in young patients below 18 years. Nearly 75% of patients respond to conservative approach probably due to physical development [47]. In another series from Mayo Clinic, Reed et al. reported a 30% success in decreasing LRV compression by non-intervention approach with stress given on weight gain to increase the fat in retroperitoneum [48]. Angiotensin-converting enzyme (ACE) inhibitors have been shown to be beneficial in patients with NCS having orthostatic proteinuria [49].

18.10.2 Endovascular Treatment

Endovascular management of NCS is gaining acceptance recently mainly due to advantage of being minimally invasive and associated with least morbidity and mortality. With experience gained in treating various venous occlusive conditions such as May-Thurner syndrome, Budd-Chiari syndrome and superior vena caval obstruction, the same principle is applied in treating NCS. First described by Neste et al. in 1996, it has become more appealing than the traditional open surgical treatment [50]. The procedure is done via femoral access. A wide and long self-expanding stent (10–20 mm in diameter and 40–70 mm in length) is preferable. The stent is deployed from the first division of the renal vein and extended into IVC, to reduce the chance of stent migration. Post-procedural gradient is measured. Around 3–6-month period of dual antiplatelet followed by single-antiplatelet therapy is usually advised although few authors prefer initial treatment with anticoagulation.

Other endovascular options include embolisation of the left gonadal vein or other tributaries of the LRV especially in patients presenting with isolated varicocele or pelvic congestion syndrome. In patients with pelvic congestion syndrome and demonstrable pelvic varicoceles, embolisation of ovarian veins may provide significant symptomatic improvement in 56–98% of patients [27]. Although good results have been reported in the literature [51], this technique occludes the main (and symptomatic) collateral outflow pathways and thus could lead to worsening of the obstruction with resultant aggravation of renal symptoms.

18.10.3 Surgical Management

Surgical treatment should be guided by symptomatic nature of disease entity rather than mere presence of nutcracker phenomenon, because of the poor correlation between imaging evidence of NCP and symptoms [17, 46]. Since the basic pathology is compression of the LRV, any direct procedures on the LRV are likely to be most efficacious with least risk to other structures.

Ever since the first procedure reported by Pastershank [9], multiple techniques of surgical management have been reported of varying surgical complexity to resolve the problem, but the most commonly used procedure is left renal vein direct reimplantation into the inferior vena cava below the normal anatomical opening to prevent direct compression in acute angle of aortomesenteric window. To date, LRV reimplantation is the surgical method of choice as reported by Mayo Clinic group [52].

Procedure of LRV Transposition

The surgical procedure of choice has been transposition of the LRV caudally into the inferior vena cava. The procedure is performed through a midline laparotomy, transperitoneal approach. The small and large bowels are packed away, and retroperitoneum is opened in midline, inferior to the transverse mesocolon between duodenum on right side and inferior mesenteric vein on left side. The LRV is completely mobilised after dissecting from fibrofatty tissue all around. The left adrenal vein is routinely ligated and divided to facilitate LRV mobilisation. The gonadal vein can be ligated in patients with varicocele, and descending lumbar vein can be ligated selectively, if necessary. The patient is systemically heparinised by unfractionated heparin 1 mg/kg dose with target activated clotting time of 250 s, a side-biting clamp applied on the IVC across the LRV confluence and the LRV transected with a mini-cuff of IVC and re-anastomosed to the left lateral aspect of the caudal portion of IVC in an end-to-side tension-free manner with continuous or interrupted sutures of 4.0 or 5.0 polypropylene (Fig. 18.3). The proximal opening in the IVC is

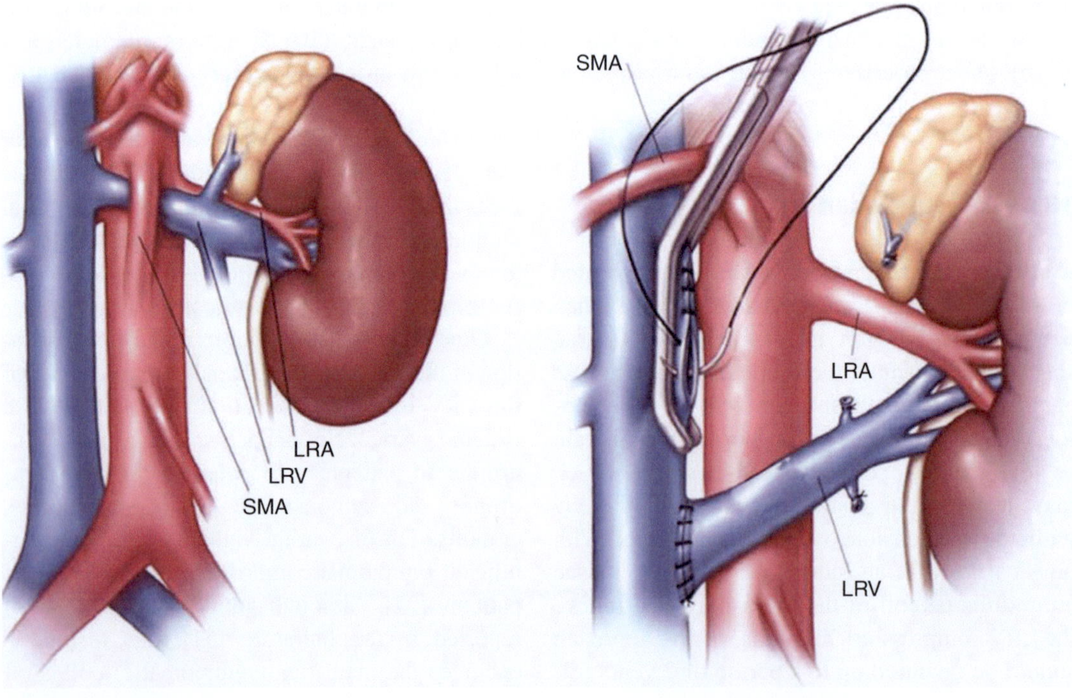

Fig. 18.3 Image showing the most commonly done surgery in NCS, the reimplantation of left renal vein in caudal segment of inferior vena cava in end-to-side fashion

oversewn with continuous sutures of 4.0 or 5.0 polypropylene. Other adjuncts used in this procedure include saphenous vein patch, vein cuff or combination of patch and cuff. These adjuncts either enlarge the renal vein (e.g. vein patch) thereby reducing anastomotic narrowing or lengthen the vein (e.g. vein cuff) thereby facilitating tension-free anastomosis [52]. LRV transposition can also be done via laparoscopy as reported by Hartung et al. [53]. But being a technically difficult procedure and requiring a significant learning curve, laparoscopic repair did not gain widespread acceptance and is limited to centres of excellency. Early complications of the LRV transposition are thrombosis of the LRV, bleeding, chylous ascites and postoperative ileus. Delayed complications of anastomotic stenosis and recurrence of symptoms have been reported.

Other Surgical Procedures

Various other surgical procedure have been described for treating NCS, which includes renal autotransplantation, SMA transposition, gonado-caval bypass, spleno-renal bypass, aortic transposition, renopexy, external stenting, nephrectomy, etc. Renal autotransplantation involves nephrectomy and transplantation of the kidney into either ipsilateral or contralateral iliac fossa as in live donors. It offers maximum efficacy in terms of normalisation of renal venous congestion, but it is a more invasive and complex surgery (requiring three anastomosis) when compared with the other procedures [54, 55].

In gonadal vein transposition technique, the left gonadal vein is transected and reimplanted into IVC. It drains not only the left kidney but also decompresses the pelvic congestion, so especially indicated when associated with pelvic varices with high-pressure gradient. But this procedure did not receive much appreciation, and only a limited literature is available [26]. Superior mesenteric artery transposition entails transection of the SMA at its junction with the abdominal aorta and re-anastomosis to the abdominal aorta at a lower level away from the left renal vein. But since this procedure entails high risk for mesenteric ischemia, it is generally not preferred [56]. Laparoscopic spleno-renal bypass was reported by Chung and Gill in a symptomatic young female with NCS with complete resolution of the symptoms [57]. Barnes et al. described an external stenting procedure wherein an externally supported PTFE graft was wrapped around the LRV [58]. But due to lesser invasive endovascular stenting, this procedure is no longer performed now.

18.10.4 Long-Term Results

Gloviczki et al. from Mayo Clinic in their experience with LRV transposition (with or without adjuncts) in 36 patients showed complete resolution of symptoms in 87% of them. Primary, primary assisted, and secondary patencies at 2 years were 74%, 97% and 100%, respectively. Freedom from reintervention at 1 and 2 years were 76% and 68%, respectively [52]. Hohenfellner et al. reported 88% success after the open surgical treatment, but the reintervention was required in 24% patients because of stenosis/occlusion. However secondary patency was 100% in this series [59].

Chen et al. published the largest series of endovascular treatment of NCS which included 61 patients with midterm and long-term outcomes. In their series almost majority of the patients showed resolution of symptoms with follow-up ranging from 6 months to 72 months [60]. Similarly Wang et al. reported near-complete resolution of symptoms in 30 patients with NCS managed with endovascular stenting with mean follow-up of 3 years [61].

Even though the results are attractive, the main complications associated with LRV stenting are stent migration, in-stent stenosis, erosion and vein occlusion resulting from fibromuscular hyperplasia, thrombosis or fracture. The reported incidence of these complications is very rare [19]. Stent migration into right atrium requiring open surgical management has been reported [60]. Cohen et al. reported one case of stent compression by the SMA at 18-month follow-up which needed an open surgical reconstruction [62]. Despite the fact that this technique is minimally invasive, further studies will be required to establish its role in the management of nutcracker syndrome.

18.11 Summary

Renal nutcracker syndrome is very rare entity to diagnose, which can afflict patients from childhood to late adulthood. Diagnosis of NCS can be made in patients who present with micro- to macroscopic haematuria and left side flank pain, and radiological evaluation confirms the haemodynamically significant LRV compression. It is unclear why LRV compression results in symptoms in some patients and many remain asymptomatic in spite of imaging showing classical compression of LRV. Continued disabling symptoms require intervention after period of conservative management has failed. Over the time multiple surgical procedures have been described for its management, but most commonly used procedure is left renal vein transposition which has shown durable and consistent results. Recent data favours the endovascular stenting as acceptable and preferred line of management over the surgery, although more data on long-term result is awaited considering durability of procedure.

References

1. Grant JCB. Methods of anatomy. Baltimore: Williams & Wilkins; 1937. p. 158.
2. Shin JI, Lee JS. Nutcracker phenomenon or nutcracker syndrome? Nephrol Dial Transplant. 2005;20:2015.
3. El Sadr AR, Mina E. Anatomical and surgical aspects of the operative management of varicoceles. Urol Cutan Rev. 1950;54:257–62.
4. De Schepper A. Nutcracker phenomenon of the renal vein causing left renal vein pathology. J Belg Radiol. 1972;55:507–11.
5. Barsoum MK, Shepherd RF, Welch TJ. Patient with both Wilkie syndrome and nutcracker syndrome. Vasc Med. 2008;13(3):247–50.
6. Bedoya R, Lagman SM, Pennington GP, et al. Clinical and radiological aspects of the superior mesenteric artery syndrome. J Fla Med Assoc. 1986;73(9):686–9.
7. Cohen LB, Field SP, Sachar DB. The superior mesenteric artery syndrome: the disease that isn't, or is it? J Clin Gastroenterol. 1985;7(2):113–6.
8. Hearin JB. Duodenal ileus with special reference to superior mesenteric artery compression. Radiology. 1966;86(2):305–10.
9. Pastershank SP. Left renal vein obstruction by a superior mesenteric artery. J Can Assoc Radiol. 1974;25(1):52–4.
10. Wilson-Storey D, MacKinlay GA. The superior mesenteric artery syndrome. J R Coll Surg Edinb. 1986;31(3):175–8.
11. Ali-El-Dein B, Osman Y, Shehab El-Din AB, et al. Anterior and posterior nutcracker syndrome: a report on 11 cases. Transplant Proc. 2003;35(2):851–3.
12. Radisic MV, Feldman D, Diaz C, et al. Unexplained hematuria during pregnancy: right-sided nutcracker phenomenon. Int Urol Nephrol. 2007;39(3):709–11.
13. Sharper KRL, Jackson JE, Williams G. The nutcracker syndrome: an uncommon cause of haematuria. Br J Urol. 1994;74:144–6.
14. Satyapal KS. The renal veins: a review. Eur J Anat. 2003;7(Suppl 1):43–52.
15. Savlania A, Sashidhar K, Sidharth V, et al. Collateral venous drainage of solitary functioning left kidney with occluded renal vein following juxtarenal aortic aneurysm repair. J Vasc Surg Venous Lymphat Disord. 2015;3(3):325.
16. Urban BA, Ratner LE, Fishman EK. Three-dimensional volume-rendered CT angiography of the renal arteries and veins: normal anatomy, variants, and clinical applications. Radiographics. 2001;21(2):373–86.
17. Hohenfellner M, Steinbach F, Schultz-Lampel D, et al. Nutcracker syndrome: new aspects of pathophysiology, diagnosis and treatment. J Urol. 1991;146:685–8.
18. Lau JLT, Lo R, Chan FL, et al. The posterior nutcracker. Haematuria secondary to retroaortic left renal vein. Urology. 1986;28:437–8.
19. Wei SM, Chen ZD, Zhou M. Intravenous stent placement for treatment of nutcracker syndrome. J Urol. 2003;170:1934–5.
20. Zhang HK, Shen LG, Li M, et al. Diagnosis and treatment of left renal venal entrapment syndrome. Chin J Gener Surg. 2001;16:511.
21. Beinart C, Sniderman KW, Tamura S, et al. Left renal vein to inferior vena cava pressure relationship in humans. J Urol. 1982;127:1070–1.
22. Nishimura Y, Fushiki M, Yoshida M, et al. Left renal vein hypertension in patients with left renal bleeding of unknown origin. Radiology. 1986;59:663–7.
23. Buschi AJ, Harrison RB, Norman A, et al. Distended left renal vein: CT/sonographic normal variant. AJR Am J Roentgenol. 1980;135:339–42.
24. Beinart C, Sniderman KW, Saddekni S, et al. Left renal vein hypertension: a cause of occult hematuria. Radiology. 1982;145(3):647–50.
25. Stewart BH, Reiman G. Left renal venous hypertension "nutcracker" syndrome: managed by direct renocaval reimplantation. Urology. 1982;20(4):365–9.
26. Scultetus AH, Villavicencio JL, Gillespie DL. The nutcracker syndrome: its role in the pelvic venous disorders. J Vasc Surg. 2001;34(5):812–9.
27. Maleux G, Stockx L, Wilms G, et al. Ovarian vein embolization for the treatment of pelvic congestion syndrome: long-term technical and clinical results. J Vasc Interv Radiol. 2000;11(7):859–64.
28. Zerhouni EA, Siegelman SS, Walsh PC, et al. Elevated pressure in the left renal vein in patients

with varicocele: preliminary observations. J Urol. 1980;123(4):512–3.
29. Unlu M, Orguc S, Serter S, et al. Anatomic and hemodynamic evaluation of renal venous flow in varicocele formation using color Doppler sonography with emphasis on renal vein entrapment syndrome. Scand J Urol Nephrol. 2007;41(1):42–6.
30. Park SJ, Lim JW, Ko YT, et al. Diagnosis of pelvic congestion syndrome using transabdominal and transvaginal sonography. AJR Am J Roentgenol. 2004;182(3):683–8.
31. Rogers A, Beech A, Braithwaite B. Transperitoneal laparoscopic left gonadal vein ligation can be the right treatment option for pelvic congestion symptoms secondary to nutcracker syndrome. Vascular. 2007;15(4):238–40.
32. Wendel RG, Crawford ED, Hehman KN. The "nutcracker" phenomenon: an unusual cause for renal varicosities with haematuria. J Urol. 1980;123(5):761–3.
33. Takebayashi S, Ueki T, Ikeda N, et al. Diagnosis of the nutcracker syndrome with color Doppler sonography: correlation with flow patterns on retrograde left renal venography. AJR Am J Roentgenol. 1999;172:39–43.
34. Braedel HU, Schindler E, Polsky MS. Selective renal phlebography in the diagnosis of renal pelvic and ureteric varices. Br J Urol. 1977;49(5):365–70.
35. Fitoz S, Ekim M, Ozcakar ZB, et al. Nutcracker syndrome in children: the role of upright position examination and superior mesenteric artery angle measurement in the diagnosis. J Ultrasound Med. 2007;26(5):573–80.
36. Stavros AT, Sickler KJ, Menter RR. Color duplex sonography of the nutcracker syndrome (aortomesenteric left renal vein compression). J Ultrasound Med. 1994;13(7):569–74.
37. Zhang H, Li M, Jin W, et al. The left renal entrapment syndrome: diagnosis and treatment. Ann Vasc Surg. 2007;21(2):198–203.
38. Sayfan J, Halevy A, Oland J, et al. Varicocele and left renal vein compression. Fertil Steril. 1984;41(3):411–7.
39. Takahashi Y, Sano A, Matsuo M. An ultrasonographic classification for diverse clinical symptoms of pediatric nutcracker phenomenon. Clin Nephrol. 2005;64(1):47–54.
40. Takahashi Y, Sano A, Matsuo M. An effective "transluminal balloon angioplasty" therapy for pediatric chronic fatigue syndrome with nutcracker phenomenon. Clin Nephrol. 2000;53(1):77–8.
41. Kim SH, Cho SW, Kim HD, et al. Nutcracker syndrome: diagnosis with Doppler US. Radiology. 1996;198:93–7.
42. Fu W, et al. Diagnosis of the nutcracker phenomenon by multislice helical computed tomography angiography. Chin Med J. 2004;117:1873–5.
43. Kim KW, Cho JY, Kim SH, et al. Diagnostic value of computed tomographic findings of nutcracker syndrome: correlation with renal venography and renocaval pressure gradients. Eur J Radiol. 2011;80(3):648–54.
44. Andrianne R, Limet R, Waltregny D, et al. Hematuria caused by nutcracker syndrome: preoperative confirmation of its presence. Prog Urol. 2002;12:1323–6.
45. He Y, Wu Z, Chen S, et al. Nutcracker syndrome—how well do we know it? Urology. 2014;83(1):12–7.
46. Shokeir AA, el-Diasty TA, Ghoneim MA. The nutcracker syndrome: new methods of diagnosis and treatment. Br J Urol. 1994;74(2):139–43.
47. Tanaka H, Waga S. Spontaneous remission of persistent severe haematuria in an adolescent with nutcracker syndrome: seven years' observation. Clin Exp Nephrol. 2004;8(1):68–70.
48. Reed NR, Kalra M, Bower TC, et al. Left renal vein transposition for nutcracker syndrome. J Vasc Surg. 2009;49:386–93; discussion: 393-4.
49. Ha T-S, Lee E-J. ACE inhibition can improve orthostatic proteinuria associated with nutcracker syndrome. Pediatr Nephrol. 2006;21(11):1765–8.
50. Neste MG, Narasimham DL, Belcher KK. Endovascular stent placement as a treatment for renal venous hypertension. J Vasc Interv Radiol. 1996;7:859.
51. d'Archambeau O, Maes M, De Schepper AM. The pelvic congestion syndrome: role of the "nutcracker phenomenon" and results of endovascular treatment. JBR-BTR. 2004;87:1–8.
52. Erben Y, Gloviczki P, Kalra M, et al. Treatment of nutcracker syndrome with open and endovascular interventions. J Vasc Surg Venous Lymphat Disord. 2015;3(4):389–96.
53. Hartung O, Azghari A, Barthelemy P, et al. Laparoscopic transposition of the left renal vein into the inferior vena cava for nutcracker syndrome. J Vasc Surg. 2010;52:738–41.
54. Chuang CK, et al. The nutcracker syndrome managed by autotransplantation. J Urol. 1997;157:1833–4.
55. Salehipour M, et al. The role of renal autotransplantation in treatment of nutcracker syndrome. Saudi J Kidney Dis Transpl. 2010;21:237–41.
56. Thompson PN, Darling RC 3rd, Chang BB, et al. A case of nutcracker syndrome: treatment by mesoaortic transposition. J Vasc Surg. 1992;16:663–5.
57. Chung BI, Gill IS. Laparoscopic splenorenal venous bypass for nutcracker syndrome. J Vasc Surg. 2009;49(5):1319–23.
58. Barnes RW, Fleisher HL 3rd, Redman JF, et al. Mesoaortic compression of the left renal vein (the so-called nutcracker syndrome): repair by a new stenting procedure. J Vasc Surg. 1988;8:415–21.
59. Hohenfellner M, D'Elia G, Hampel C, et al. Transposition of the left renal vein for treatment of the nutcracker phenomenon: long-term follow-up. Urology. 2002;59:354–7.
60. Chen S, Zhang H, Shi H, et al. Endovascular stenting for treatment of nutcracker syndrome: report of 61 cases with long-term follow up. J Urol. 2011;186:570–5.
61. Wang X, Zhang Y, Li C, et al. Results of endovascular treatment for patients with nutcracker syndrome. J Vasc Surg. 2012;56:142–8.
62. Cohen F, Amabile P, Varoquaux A, et al. Endovascular treatment of circumaortic nutcracker syndrome. J Vasc Interv Radiol. 2009;20:1255–6.

Venous Trauma

19

Arvind Kohli and Gurjit Singh

19.1 Introduction

There has been an ever-increasing incidence of vascular trauma all over the world. Extremity injuries contribute for 80% of all cases of vascular injuries, and out of them, lower extremities are involved in two thirds of these patients. Males are affected in 90% and females in 10% cases. The true incidence of isolated venous trauma is underreported. Quan et al. [1] reported that only 25% of extremity vascular trauma had isolated venous injury. Despite the variability in magnitude of trauma, most of venous injuries (75%) occur concomitantly with arterial injury.

19.2 Challenges of Vascular Injuries

These injuries are the most dramatic challenges facing trauma surgeons because the repair is often urgent. Gaining control of and reconstructing a major vascular injury can be technically demanding. The fundamental difference between elective vascular surgery and vascular trauma is the physiology of the wounded patient. A lacerated major vessel is typically only one component of the multi-trauma complex that includes injuries to other organs and systems. These patients are often critically ill and rapidly approaching a point of physiologic irreversibility. In these dramatic clinical circumstances, the key to a favorable outcome is maintaining correct priorities [2].

19.3 Etiology

The leading cause of vascular injury in general and venous injuries in particular continues to be penetrating wounds, out of which *gunshot wounds* contribute to 70–80% of all cases requiring intervention, whereas stab *wounds* are the next common cause (5–10%) of cases requiring intervention. Blunt trauma occurs in (5-10%)of cases subsequent to road traffic accidents along with presence of fracture of long bones of dislocation of joints therebyincresing the risk of venous injury. Iatrogenic injury accounts for 5% of cases, that includes Endovascular procedures like central line placement and endovascular and venous cardiac interventions [3].

19.4 Distribution of Venous Trauma

Majority of vein injuries (90%) affect the extremities with almost similar distribution in upper and lower extremitiy. Clouse et al. [4] have described

A. Kohli
Department of CTVS, GMC, Jammu, India

G. Singh (✉)
Division of CTVS, JK Medicity Hospital, Jammu, India

A. K. Khanna, R. Jindal (eds.), *Venous Disorders*, https://doi.org/10.1007/978-981-13-1108-6_19

the incidence of venous injuries as femoral (17%), IVC (15%), jugular (15%), brachial (14%), and popliteal vein (8%).

19.5 Diagnosis

Diagnosis of venous injuries may not be obvious on clinical examination as they in most of cases form part of the polytrauma. Patients present with a growing hematoma, or blood discharge from a penetrating wound. In most of the cases, the venous injuries are detected during exploration of a major arterial injury.

Color Doppler ultrasound scan detects intimal tears, thrombosis, contusion, pseudoaneurysms, and arteriovenous fistulae. Although the color doppler scan is operator dependent, it has sensitivity of 95% and specificity of 99% with overall accuracy of 98%.

19.6 Angiography

Angiography is the premium procedure for diagnosis of vascular injuries both arterial and venous. Where hybrid operating suits are available, angiography can be performed in the operating room enabling the surgeon to identify the injury and manage expeditiously. Angiography has sensitivity of 92–96%, specificity of above 96%, and accuracy of 98%.

19.7 CT VenoGram (CTV)

With the advent of improved CT scan, detection of venous injuries has greatly improved. In fact CTV is becoming a viable alternative to angiography. Occasionally CTV can be nondiagnostic due to significant artifact from bullet fragments or other foreign bodies. It has to be complemented with DSA which gives sensitivity of 90–100% and specificity of 98–100%.

19.8 Magnetic Resonance Venography (MRV)

MRV is used less frequently in acute settings. Metal implants such as cerebral aneurysm clips and cardiac pacemakers preclude the use of MRI, or it is difficult to ascertain whether the patient have such devices in emergency situation [2, 3, 5].

19.9 Treatment of Venous Injuries

19.9.1 Immediate Treatment

Although the controversy continues in polytrauma with profound hemorrhage and severe venous injuries, ligation of the injured vein is a life-saving procedure. Nevertheless, ligation may not be an appropriate solution in all patients, and it appears that there is merit in repair of many injured lower extremity veins, particularly the popliteal vein when it is a single return conduit, assuming that the patient's general condition will permit, in an attempt to prevent acute venous hypertension initially and chronic venous hypertension and phlegmasia of the leg subsequently.

Various modalities for operative management of venous trauma have been advocated keeping in view the nature of injury. The aim is to save the limb and prevent long-term venous dysfunction. Operative procedures include ligation of the injured vein, lateral venorrhaphy, end-to-end anastomosis, venous patch angioplasty, and venous interposition graft. Many reports suggest that lateral venorrhaphy produces good patency rates; however, more complex repairs are also known to give optimal long-term results. Venous ligation is indicated in polytrauma with profuse hemorrhage and associated injuries which necessitates priority and in cases where there are complex venous lacerations. Time consumed for performing these repairs is worrying factor for outcome.

Venous repair using interposition prosthetic or vein graft is debatable keeping in view the post-operative patency; however, if interposed, reverse saphenous vein graft is considered to have better outcome than prosthetic graft. The use of temporary shunts both in repair of venous and arterial injuries is recommended, and use of shunts maintains patency without the use of systemic anticoagulation in the short term [6].

Endovascular management of venous injuries has been described like the use of endovascular balloon inserted through the femoral vein for control of unrelenting venous hemorrhage from injured iliac vein thereby enabling the surgeons to repair that segment in good time. In addition in selected patients, use of venous stents for managing venous injuries of the iliac, IVC, and axillary vein has been described.

Conclusion

Aggressive management after vein ligation can minimize complications by implementation of limb elevation, compression, and early fasciotomy when indicated. Repair of venous injuries is not mandatory for limb salvage or prevention of long-term morbidity. However, aggressive approach to venous repair specifically with injury to popliteal vein should be followed.

References

1. Quan RW, Adams ED, Cox MW, et al. The management of trauma venous injury: civilian and wartime experiences. Perspect Vasc Surg Endovasc Ther. 2006;18(2):149–56.
2. Gillespie D, Quan RW. The management of extremity venous trauma. In: Gloviczki P, editor. Handbook of venous disorders: guidelines of the American venous forum. 3rd ed. Chap. 51. London: Hodder Arnold; 2009. p. 569–72.
3. Rich NM. Management of venous trauma. Surg Clin North Am. 1988;68:809–21.
4. Clouse WD, et al. In-theater management of vascular injury: 2 years of the Balad Vascular Registry. J Am Coll Surg. 2007;204:625–32.
5. Qi Y, Gillespie DL. Venous trauma: new lessons and old debates. Perspect Vasc Surg Endovasc Ther. 2011;23(2):74–792.
6. Quan RW, Gillespie DL, Stuart RP, Chang AS, Whittaker DR. The effect of vein repair on the risk of venous thromboembolic events: a review of more than 100 traumatic military venous injuries. J Vasc Surg. 2008;47(3):571–7.

20 Therapeutic Options in Lymphedema

Waldemer Lech Olszewski
and Marzanna Teresa Zaleska

20.1 Introduction

Lymphedema of limbs characteristically means increase in the volume of extremity caused by accumulation of tissue fluid, proliferation of fibroblasts and adipocytes, and excessive production of collagen. There is also increase in infiltrating immune cell mass. Bacterial colonization ensues as the result of lack of lymphatic transport away of microbes penetrating the foot and palm skin. Under physiological conditions capillary filtrate-tissue fluid flows into the lymphatics and is transported via the collecting lymphatic trunks to the blood circulation. The transported calculated volume for one lower limb ranges from 20 to over 200 ml in some cases during 24 h [1]. Obliteration of the transport lymphatic channels and sinuses of regional lymph nodes causes stasis of intercellular water, proteins, and migrating immune cells. Contractility of the lymphatics disappears. Tissue changes are hyperkeratosis, fibrosis, and accumulation of tissue fluid/lymph under the epidermis with occasional lymphorrhea [2]. The most common complication of tissue fluid stasis is bacterial dermato-lymphangio-adenitis (DLA) [3]. For a long time, there was no awareness of the progressive tissue changes leading to the development of elephantiasis, and accumulation of mobile fluid was considered as the main event in increased volume of the limb.

W. L. Olszewski (✉)
Central Clinical Hospital, Ministry of Internal Affairs, Warsaw, Poland

M. T. Zaleska
Deptartment of Applied Physiology, Mossakowski Medical Research Center, Polish Academy of Sciences, Warsaw, Poland

20.2 How Important Is Restoration of Tissue Fluid Outflow from Limb Tissues?

For centuries lymphedema was considered as an accumulation of excess water with proteins that should be treated by total excision of the diseased tissue or drainage procedures as various types of bridging tissue flaps between the lymphedematous and healthy regions. Operations designed by Charles [4], Sistrunk [5], Thompson [6], or Goldsmith [7] were widely applied with rather unsatisfactory results. Delayed wound healing, leakage of tissue fluid from the denuded surfaces, and chronic inflammation of foot tissues, continuously penetrated by environmental microbes, were the common events.

The actual understanding of the pathomechanism of development of lymphedema and tissue changes, based on the contemporary human studies, drastically changed the surgical approach to therapy of lymphedema. Modern techniques of imaging of the lymphatic vascular system (X-ray contrast lymphography, lymphoscintigraphy, near-infrared lymphography, angiography, CT,

A. K. Khanna, R. Jindal (eds.), *Venous Disorders*, https://doi.org/10.1007/978-981-13-1108-6_20

and MRI), discovery of spontaneous lymphatic contractility, visualization of sites of accumulation of stagnant tissue fluid, and evidence for the presence of bacterial flora in stagnant tissue fluid/lymph allowed not only to redesign old types of surgery but also to propose procedures restoring lymph flow by microsurgical anastomoses [8–11]. This has been further possible by the improvement of optics of operating microscopes and production of ultrathin traumatic sutures. Additional impact on the development of microsurgical procedures had also the long-term lymphangiographic observations of gradual obliteration of peripheral segments of collecting trunks after skin infections (erysipelas) and/or their proximal obliteration after lymphadenectomy, the so-called die-back phenomenon [12]. They prompted surgeons to early surgical intervention by performing anastomoses of the still patent collectors with the neighboring veins.

Furthermore, debulking surgery, still indicated for millions of patients, has become more satisfactory due to pretreatment with antibiotics controlling colonizing microbes resulting in fast healing of surgical wounds. Moreover, antibiotic prophylaxis saved foot tissues, deprived of lymphatic drainage, from chronic inflammation [3]. High-efficiency diathermy scalpels facilitated tissue resection without using ligatures frequently being expulsed from the debulking wounds for months. Various types of external compression as bandages, stockings, and intermittent pneumatic compression devices have improved the long-term results of surgery, forcing tissue fluid flow through newly formed pathways either to the veins or the non-swollen parts of the body.

20.3 Physiological Operations

20.3.1 Lymphonodo- and/or Lymphatico-Venous Microsurgical Shunts

With the developing technique of microsurgery in the 1960, we thought of using microsurgical methods for the creation of artificial lymphovenous shunts [8–11]. The operation of microsurgical lymphovenous was designed for decompressing the lymphedematous limb of the accumulated lymph and directing its flow to the venous system distally to the site of lymphatic obstruction. The operation mimicked the natural anastomosis of the thoracic duct with the subclavian vein, by with the creation of microsurgical shunts between the lymphatics and veins. The physiological principles of the operation were based on the observations of natural anatomical lymphovenous communications in the retroperitoneal space in animals and in humans in cases of obstruction of the thoracic duct. In our project, the lymph node was cut transversely, and lymph oozing started from the cortical sinuses (Fig. 20.1). Then, the node was implanted end-to-side into an excised wall window of the neighboring vein. First experimental operations were performed on dogs, and the mesenteric lymph node after transection and its distal part with afferent lymphatics were implanted into the inferior vena cava. Lymph flowed freely into the vein because pressure in the vena cava was slightly negative at inspiration. These shunts created in dogs remained patent throughout their life.

In 1966, we carried out the first five operations of microsurgical lymphovenous shunts in humans, directing the stream of stagnant lymph of the lymphedematous lower limbs to the femoral vein [8–11]. Over the course of time, various modifications of the lymphovenous shunt operations have been introduced and tried by us and other authors. The number of operations around the world cannot at present be accurately estimated; however, more than 100 thousand should have been performed. The worldwide experience in indications, technique, and results was described in abundant literature [13–43] (Fig. 20.2).

20.3.2 Microsurgical Inguinal Lymphovenous Shunts

Two types of shunts are performed, the lymph node-saphenous vein (LNSV) and afferent lymphatics-saphenous vein (LVSV) or other superficial veins.

Detailed Indications

Lymphedema at an early stage (I and II) of postinflammatory, postsurgical, and hyperplastic type

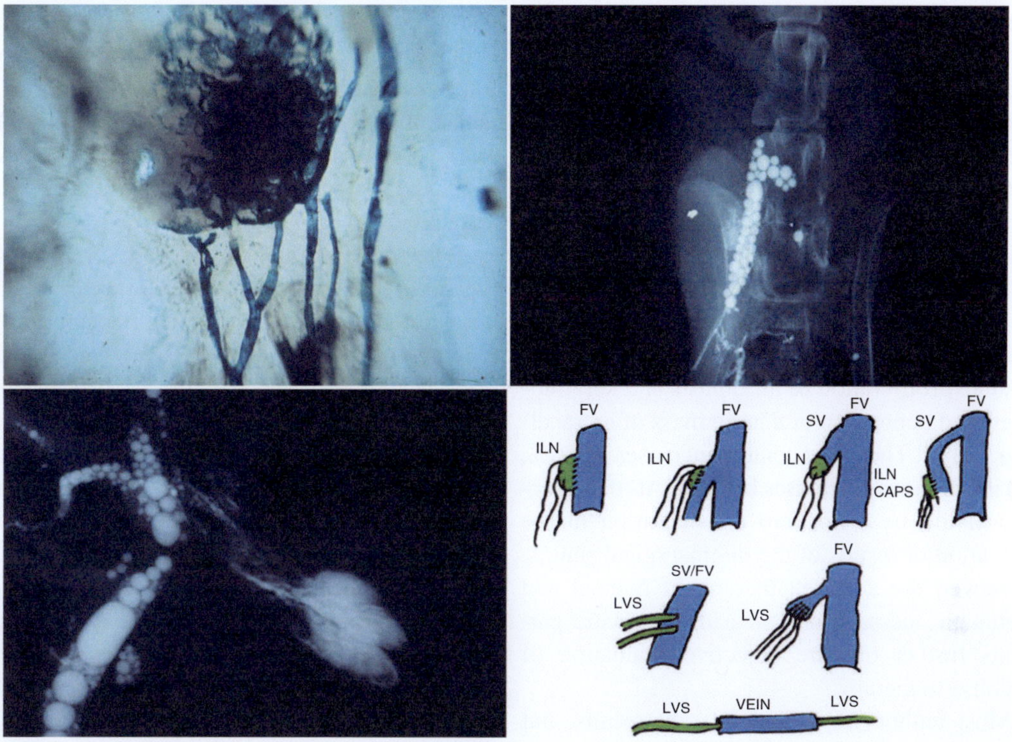

Fig. 20.1 Pictures illustrating the first lymphovenous microsurgical shunts performed in dogs in 1966. Upper left – lymph node with afferent lymphatics and node sinuses. Lower left – transverse section of the node and implantation to the vein and contrast medium injected into the node flowed to the vein. Upper right – contrast medium injected into the vein implanted mesenteric node flows to the IVC. Lower right – various modifications of microsurgical lymph node and lymphatic–vein anastomoses. *FV* femoral vein, *ILN* inguinal lymph node, *SV* saphenous vein, *LVS* lymphatic vessels, *ILN caps* inguinal lymph node capsule (no parenchyma)

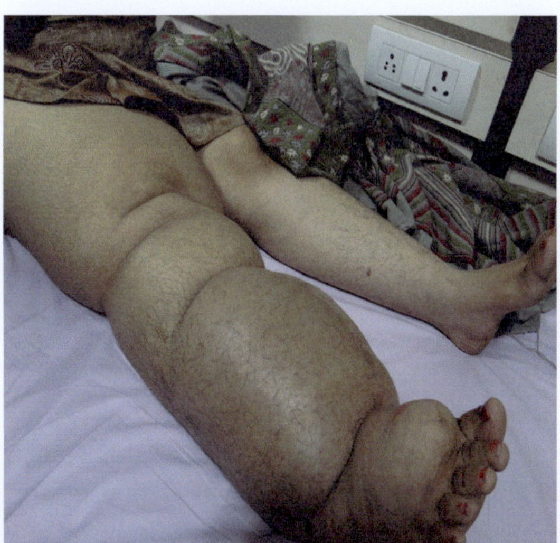

Fig. 20.2 Typical picture of obstructive lymphedema of the lower limb for surgical treatment. Conservative therapy unsuccessful

with at least one calf or thigh lymphatic and a single inguinal or iliac lymph node is visible on the functional lymphoscintigraphy (performed during limb pneumatic massage or after standard time walking). Surgical lymphovenous shunts should be performed as soon as obstructive lymphedema is diagnosed. Also preventive shunts at the time of inguinal or axillary lymphadenectomy are highly recommended. The long-term follow-up would show the efficacy of the early intervention.

Lack of indications: (a) stages III and IV with no lymphatics or nodes on lymphoscintigraphy, (b) idiopathic lymphedema with soft skin, pitting edema, but no lymphatic structures on lymphoscintigraphy

Contraindications: (a) recent attacks of dermato-lymphangio-adenitis (DLA) and (b) skin ulcer

Postoperative Clinical Evaluation Criteria

They include (a) decrease in leg circumference, (b) improved flexion in the ankle (to 80°) and knee joints (minimum 90°), (c) increase in the softness (compliance) of tissues, and (d) subsidence of limb pain during long-lasting upright position. The volume of the limb will never be the same as it was before the lymphatic injury. Lymphedema is a condition characterized by an increase in extravascular fluid and protein volume, proliferation of fibroblasts and keratinocytes, and deposition of a large mass of extracellular matrix. The water content increases by 50%, and the dry mass increases by 20%. All these factors should be taken into consideration in the evaluation of results of the microsurgical shunts. Moreover, the adjuvant therapy as manual and pneumatic massage and wearing of elastic garments further obscure objective evaluation of response to therapy.

Most authors report good early results, but subsequent deterioration may occur as early as 6 months after the operation [11–34]. There are, however, exceptions with cases observed with permanent improvement after 10–40 years.

20.3.3 Microsurgical Lymphatico-Venous Shunts at Different Levels of the Lower and Upper Limb

A number of modifications of surgical lymphatico-venous shunts have been developed since the publication of our technique in 1967 and 1968 [13–38]. They included end-to-end and end-to-side anastomoses and interposition of vein fragments bridging the ends of severed lymphatics.

20.3.4 Super-Microsurgical Lymphatico-Venous Shunts

Development of high-dissolving power optics and superfine atraumatic sutures as well as infrared lymphography opened the way for performing multiple anastomoses between the small superficial lymphatics and the neighboring veins. Various technical modifications of anastomoses have been proposed [39–43]. The early results seem to be satisfactory; however, only the long-term follow-up will prove their effectiveness.

The microsurgical lymph node or lymphatic vessel to vein shunts have their established position among the therapy modalities for lymphedema of lower limbs. Our and others' long-lasting experience indicates that (a) only patients with lymphedema with local segmental obstruction but still partly patent and contracting distal lymphatics and without an active inflammatory process in the skin, subcutaneous tissue, and lymph vessels present satisfactory results; (b) classified according to the etiology of lymphedema, the best results are obtained in cases of hyperplastic, followed by postsurgical and postinflammatory types; and (c) primary idiopathic lymphedema of non-genetic type should be treated with conservative means.

20.4 Creation of Artificial Lymph (Edema Fluid) Flow Pathways by Implantation of Hydrophobic Silicone Tubings

None of the so far applied conservative and surgical methods proved to restore the shape and function of the limbs to normal conditions. In advanced cases of lymphedema, all main lymphatics are obstructed, and tissue fluid accumulates in the interstitial spaces, spontaneously forming "blind channels" or "lakes" (Figs. 20.3, 20.4, 20.5, and 20.6). The only solution would be to drain these spaces by creating artificial pathways for edema fluid to flow away to the non-obstructed regions where absorption of fluid can take place. This can be achieved by the formation of artificial pathways for edema fluid to flow by subcutaneous implantation of silicone tubings "lymphatics" placed along the limb from the most distal parts to its root and continue to more proximal regions with fluid

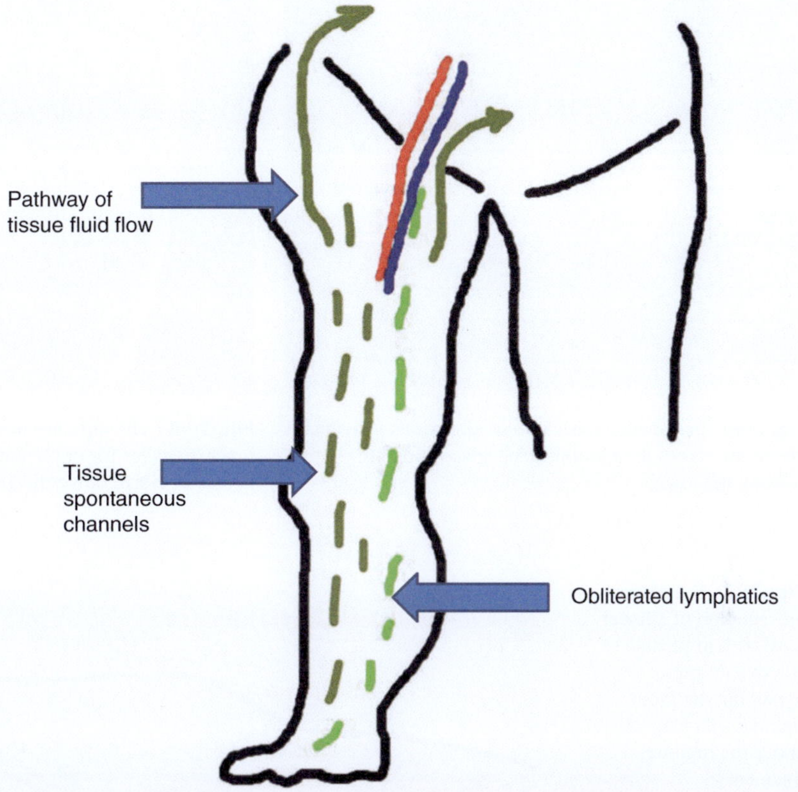

Fig. 20.3 Schematic presentation of tissue changes in a lymphedematous limb. Collecting trunks are obstructed. Tissue fluid forms spontaneous tissue lakes and channels. It finds its way to the femoral canal and to the buttock and lumbar region. To facilitate flow away, artificial channels bypassing the inguinal obstruction site should be constructed

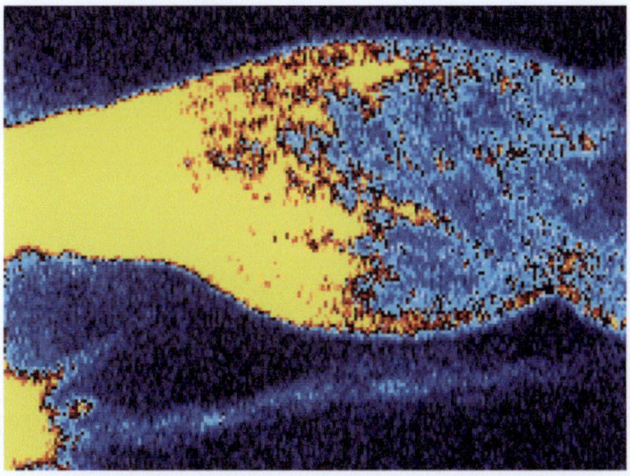

Fig. 20.4 The tissue fluid channels and subepidermal dilated microlymphatics are shown on a lymphoscintigram (yellow and light blue shadows)

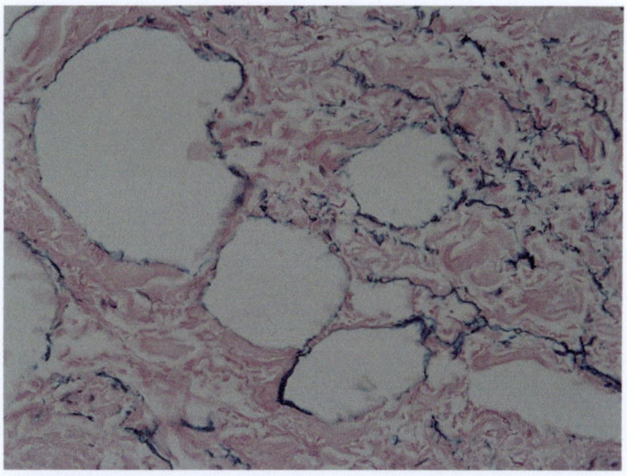

Fig. 20.5 Histological picture of tissue fluid channels in lymphedema

absorption capacity (Fig. 20.7). In the lower limbs, this is an implant from the foot to the hypogastrium or lumbar region and in the upper limbs from the hand dorsum to the scapular area [44, 45]. This is a three-modality procedure: (1) silicone tubing implantation, (2) intermittent pneumatic compression and elastic support, and (3) prophylactic antibiotics to prevent bacterial colonization.

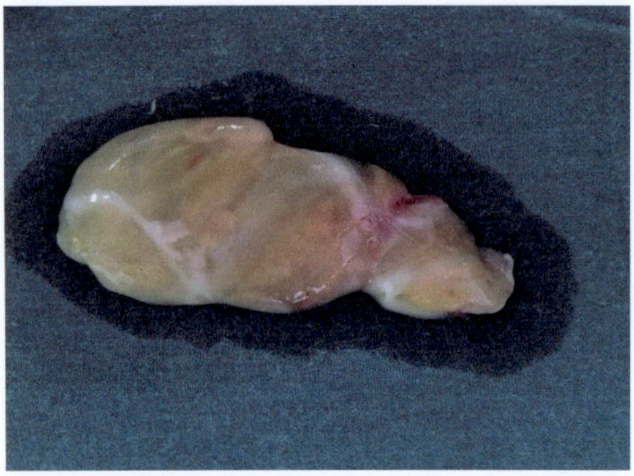

Fig. 20.6 Fragment excised from edematous subcutaneous tissue shows fluid in the tissue spaces flowing out and soaking the towel

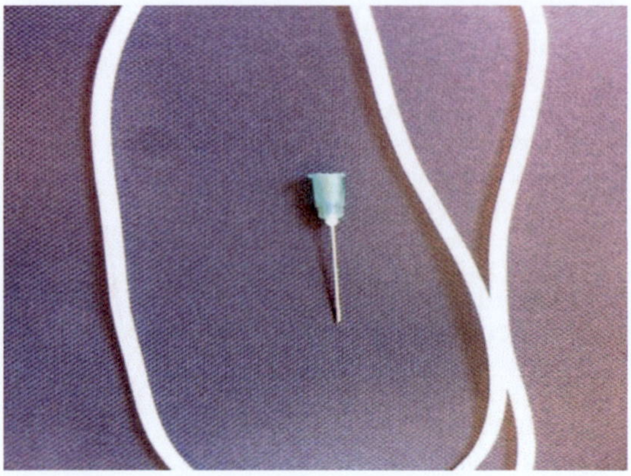

Fig. 20.8 The silicone tubing 3 mm outer and 1.8 mm inner diameter for implantation. For comparison injection needle of a size of a collecting lymphatic trunk

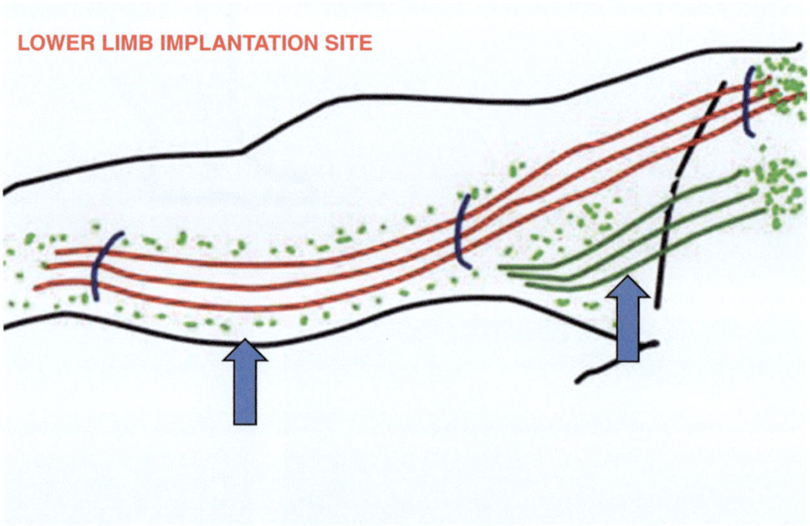

Fig. 20.7 Schematic presentation of a lower limb with implanted silicone tubings bypassing the groin running subcutaneously above the inguinal ligament

20.4.1 Implantation Technique of Silicone Tubings

Briefly, a 2-cm-long incision is made in the hypogastrium or lumbar region 10 cm above the inguinal crease or scapular area. A 1.5-cm-wide and 100-cm-long metal tunneler is introduced under the skin and bluntly moved in the subcutaneous tissue toward the thigh and internal aspect of the calf or forearm and hand dorsum. Other 2-cm-long incisions are made in the groin, calf, or forearm, and the lower end of the conductor is exteriorized. Three silicone tubings with lateral holes at 5 cm distance each are introduced into its lumen and moved upward (Fig. 20.8). Tunneler is then removed. No fixing of tubings is necessary. Silicone is hydrophobic, and there is no adhesion and ingrowth of tissue cells. Moreover, elasticity of silicone prevents kinking, twisting, or obstruction of the lumen (Fig. 20.9). Patent tubings were seen on lymphoscintigraphy (Figs. 20.10 and 20.11) and accumulation of fluid on ultrasound images (Fig. 20.12) and "angiography" (Fig. 20.13).

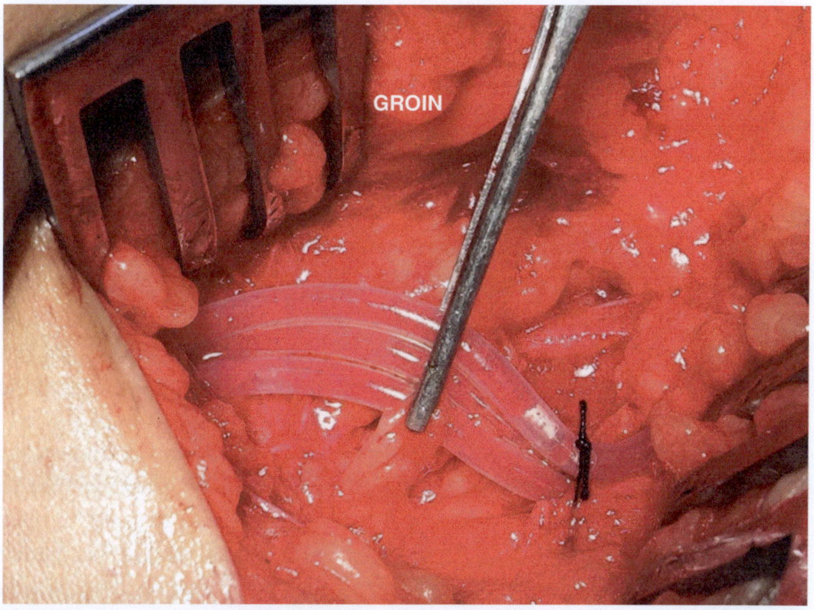

Fig. 20.9 Subcutaneously implanted silicone tubings in the groin. Upper end in the lumbar region, lower above the internal ankle. See tissue fluid in their lumen

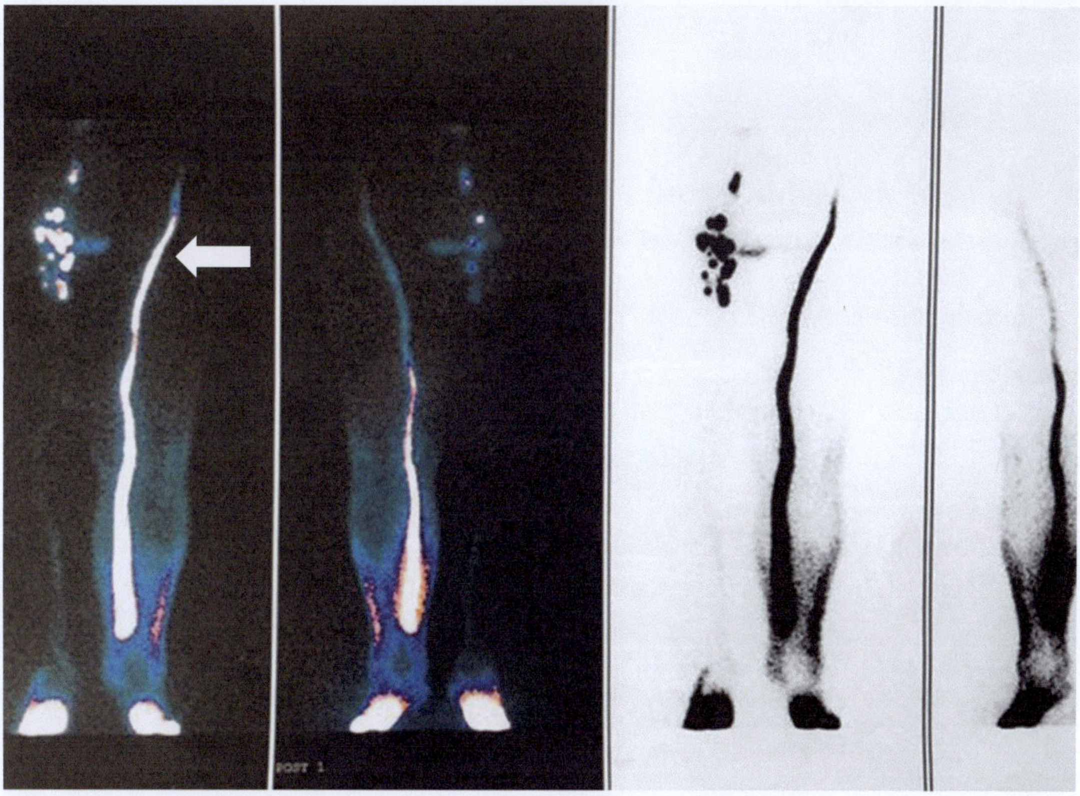

Fig. 20.10 Lymphoscintigram 6 months after subcutaneous implantation in the lower lymphedematous limb (arrow). Implant bypassing the site of obstruction at the inguinal level

20.4.2 Postimplant Therapy

Patients are put on daily 1 h intermittent pneumatic compression for 14 days in OPD and continued as home care. Elastic stockings of second degree of compression are used before surgery. Limb circumference measurements are made at five levels daily for the first 14 days in the OPD and then weekly at home at the same time of the day and the same limb position.

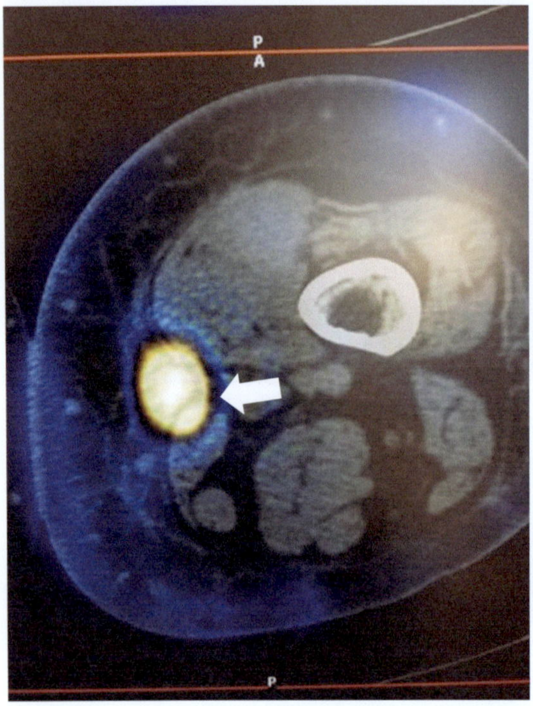

Fig. 20.11 SPECT–CT lymphoscintigram of the thigh with implanted silicone tubings (arrow)

20.4.3 Results

So far, 80 patients divided into 2 groups with lymphedema of lower [46] limbs after hysterectomy and upper limbs [30] after mastectomy stages II and III underwent implantation of silicone. The follow-up of 15 patients is now reaching 4 years. A fast decrease of limb circumference was observed already during the first days after implantation lasting for 2 weeks to become slower thereafter (Fig. 20.14). The mean decrease in circumference in the mid-calf was 4% with range of 3–17% (Fig. 20.15) and in the forearm 10% in the mid-forearm and 5% in the mid-arm during week 1 to reach 15 and 10% after 4 months, respectively ($p < 0.05$) (Figs. 20.16, 20.17, 20.18, 20.19, and 20.20).

The accumulating tissue fluid cannot flow along the tubings by itself and requires a propelling force (Figs. 20.21 and 20.22). This can be provided by the application of intermittent pneumatic compression as well as walking in short-stretch bandages or stockings. Tissue edema fluid is drained from the swollen tissues to the hypogastrium or lumbar or

Fig. 20.12 Ultrasound picture of implanted silicone tubings with fluid around them (arrow – lower inlet)

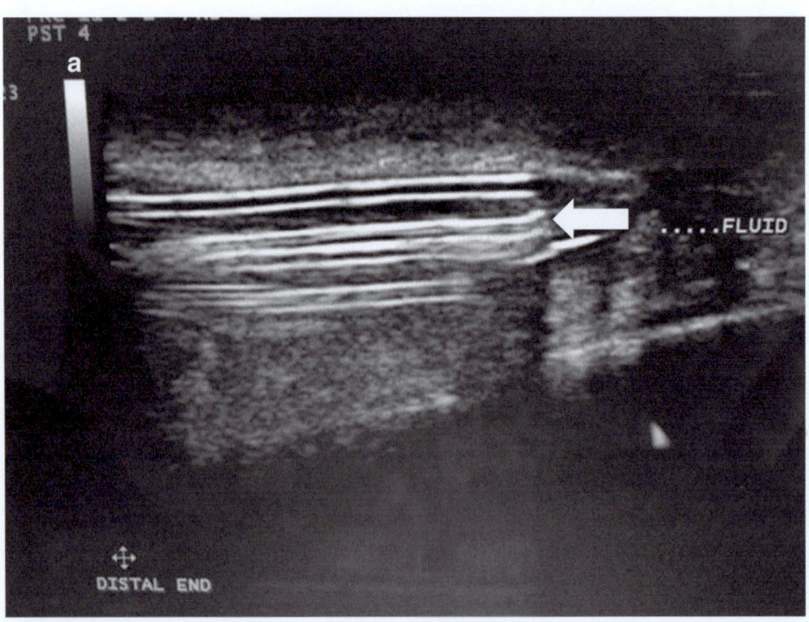

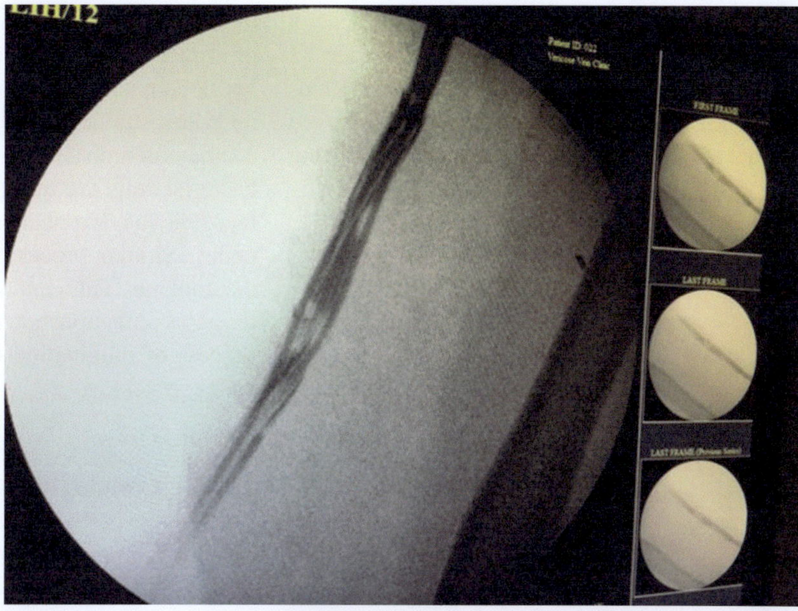

Fig. 20.13 Contrasted silicone tubings injected with arterial nonionic medium 1 year after implantation. Contrast medium in and around tubings with visible lateral openings

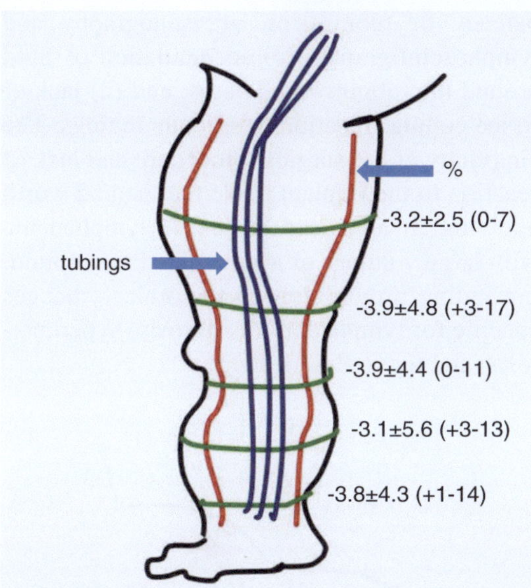

Fig. 20.14 Three-year follow-up results. Decrease in circumference is similar at all levels. This means there was equal evacuation of edema fluid from all parts of the limb. Follow-up 45 pts. 12–36 months, mean percentage ± SD, range

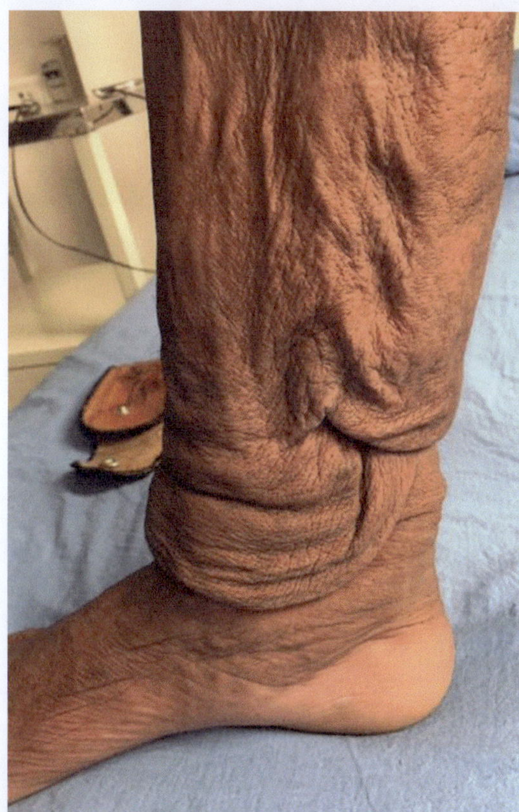

Fig. 20.15 Lower limb 3 weeks after silicone tubings implantation. See redundant skin requiring plastic operation

scapular regions. The question remains open about the absorption capacity of healthy tissues at the outlet of tubings. We observed a low-degree edema developing in this region during the day activities subsiding during the night rest. This could be accounted for by sufficient absorption capacity from the hypogastrium.

There were no major inflammatory reactions to the implanted tubing in 95% of observed patients. In four patients a several days lasting inflammation was seen in the leg at the upper end of implants and was easily controlled by antibiotics. This reaction was most likely caused by the microbes drained from the foot of the lymphedematous limb. Under normal conditions single bacterial cells are transported from the skin surface via the lymphatics to the regional lymph nodes. Similar process should take place along the implants. This cannot be considered in clinical terms as infection but rather as a physiological process of elimination of microbes by the lymphatic system.

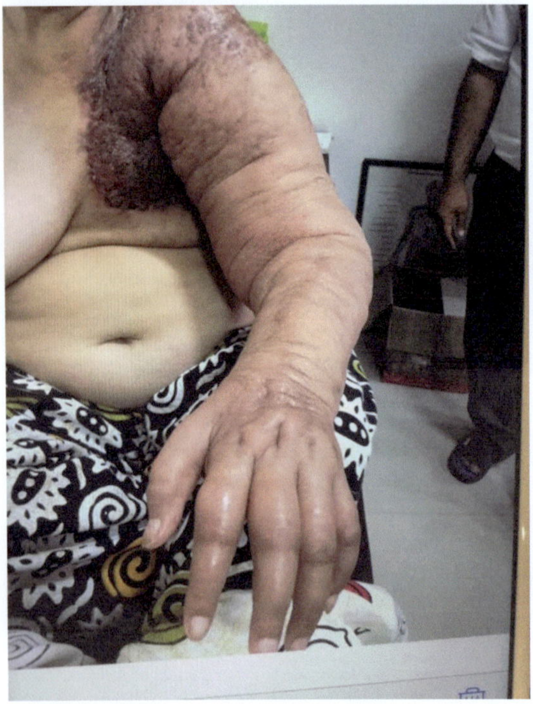

Fig. 20.16 Picture of typical postmastectomy advanced lymphedema requiring fast decompression of tissues by implantation of silicone tubings

20.4.4 Conclusions

Taken together, this study showed (a) evident fast decrease of calf circumference from the day of implantation and stabilization after weeks when excess fluid was evacuated, (b) patency of tubings on ultrasonography and lymphoscintigraphy, (c) accumulation of fluid around the tubings in all cases, and (d) lack of tissue cellular reaction to silicone tubings. The simplicity of the surgical procedure and lack of reaction to the implant make the method worth applying in advanced stages of lymphedema with large volumes of accumulated tissue fluid, preventing progression of anatomical changes specific for lymphedema as fibrosis, hyperkeratosis, and tissue fluid leakage.

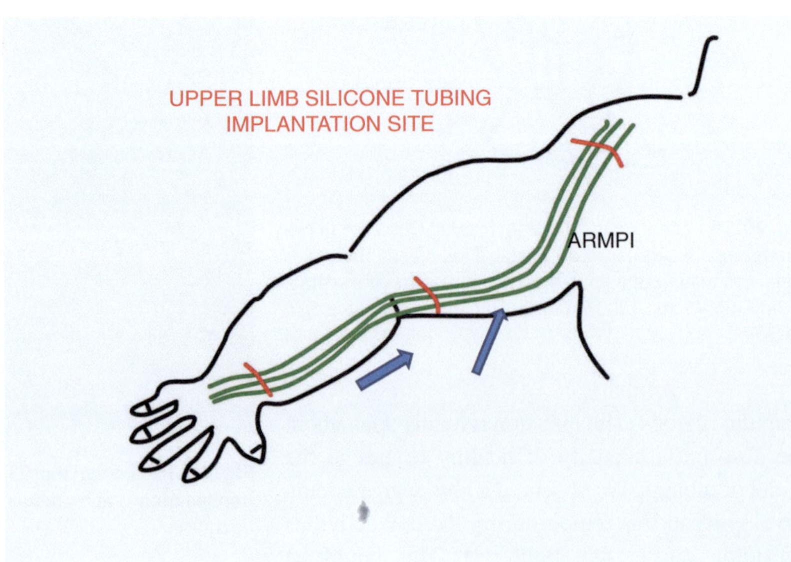

Fig. 20.17 Schematic presentation of silicone implants in the upper limb bypassing the axillary pit

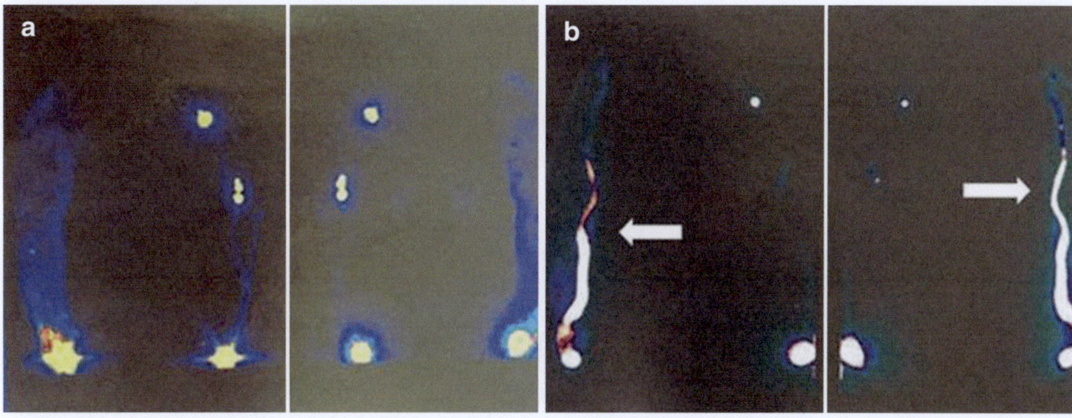

Fig. 20.18 SPECT–CT lymphoscintigram of silicone tubing before (left) and after (right) implantation of silicone tubings (arrow)

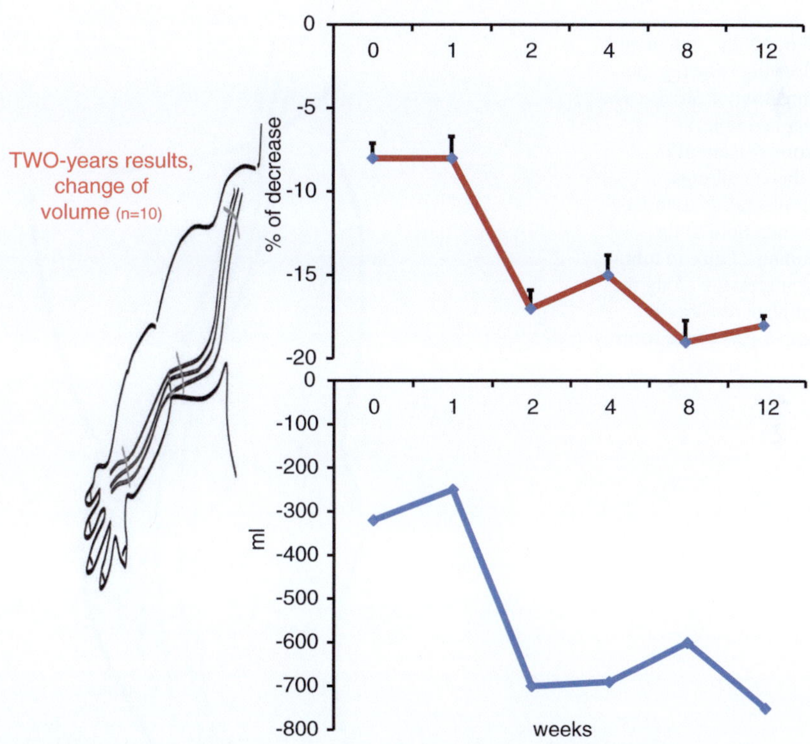

Fig. 20.19 Two-year follow-up after implantation to postmastectomy lymphedema limbs. Volume change data from the first 3 months show rapid decrease of limb size within 2–3 weeks and then maintenance phase with same limb circumferences. Studies showed lack of mobile edema fluid and increase in fibrosis

20.5 Debulking Procedures

This operation holds strong its established position in the lymphatic surgery in lymphedema of the lower limbs stage IV, previously known as elephantiasis. The number of patients in this advanced stage can be counted in millions, especially in the developing countries. It is still not uncommon in the western hemisphere.

20.5.1 The Morphological Changes of Advanced Stage IV Lymphedema

These comprise (1) hyperkeratosis and fibrosis of skin, (2) fibrosis of subcutis, (3) lack of lymphatic collectors in the subcutaneous tissue with formation of numerous tissue fluid lakes, (4) tissue fluid subepidermal blisters

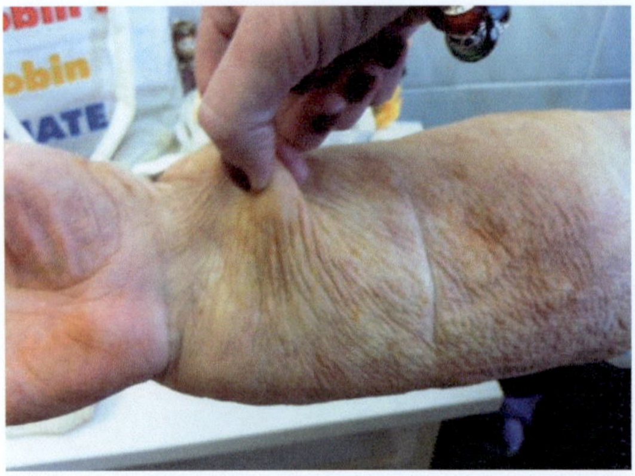

Fig. 20.20 Skin fold 5 days after implantation showing rapid evacuation of edema fluid. Note thick skin fold due to tissue fibrosis

with leakage, (5) growth of fat tissue, (6) fibrosis of muscular fascia, (7) lack of immune cells in tissue fluid due to limited capillary filtration and cell extravasation, (8) superficial skin ulcers, (9) bacterial colonization of deep tissues, (10) frequent episodes of dermato-lymphangio-adenitis (DLA) (previously called cellulitis) attacks and sepsis, and (11) doubling or tripling limb weight with destruction of the hip and knee joints. These tissue changes totally immobilize patients and make them prone to septic attacks. The only solution is multistage partial debulking.

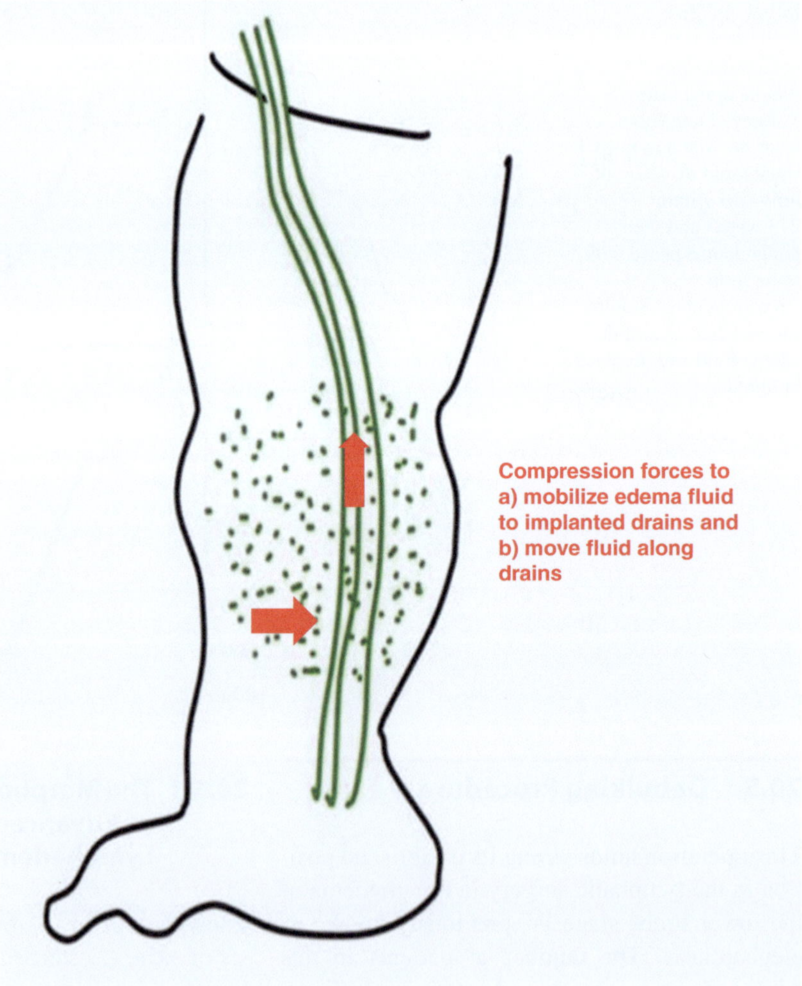

Fig. 20.21 Schematic drawing showing the direction of forces to be applied in limb compression after silicone tubings implantation to move edema fluid to the tubings. Once in tubings compression along the implant toward the upper part of the limb should be used

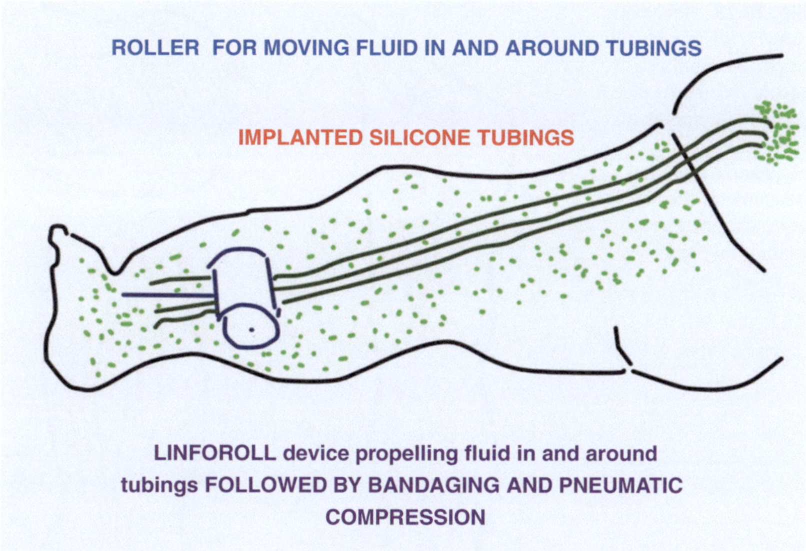

Fig. 20.22 Special device used for massaging out fluid from the limb with implanted tubings. The Linforoll roller is moved along the implant under pressure of 80–120 mmHg

20.5.2 Surgical Procedures

The classic radical operations as total denuding of the limb down to fascia and covering with epidermal grafts turned to be unsatisfactory because of subsequent acute infections of the remaining foot skin, epidermal ulcerations, and plasma and tissue fluid leakage from the uncovered surfaces.

The author redesigned the surgical procedures by introducing new elements in debulking surgery, as (1) long-term systemic antibiotic preparation (3 months), (2) resection of longitudinal strips of redundant skin and subcutaneous tissue (with fibrotic lymphatics) in the calf and thigh and covering the denuded surface with pedunculated flaps (Fig. 20.23), (3) and excision of the thickened fibrotic fascia. A routine debulking operation in the calf is illustrated in Fig. 20.24 a–d. It shows that the calf should remain covered by pedunculated skin flaps.

The contemporary protocol includes:

1. Antibiotic preparation (amoxiclav 1.0 g or ciprofloxacin 0.5 g daily orally for 2–3 months)
2. Daily disinfection of the skin with antimicrobial soap containing phenol or similar chemical for 14 days before operation
3. Two-week limb elevation in bed or intensive pneumatic compression
4. Surgery divided into three stages: (a) removal of fibrotic inguinal lymph nodes and vessels, (b) 3–4 weeks later surgical excision of fibrotic lymphatics down to the knee level together with the neighboring fibrous infected tissues, and (c) debulking of the calf and dorsum of the foot by three longitudinal vertical strips (medial, lateral, and posterior) of the skin, subcutis, and fascia, performed in three stages at 6 weeks intervals
5. Night bed-confined limb elevation and continuation of 1.0 g of amoxiclav or 0.5 g cipro for another month and later administration of long-lasting penicillin 1,200,000 unit every 3 weeks for years
6. Elastic support (pressure grade III)
7. Intermittent pneumatic compression daily for 1 h

20.5.3 Results

Results are generally satisfactory with fast uneventful healing, sometimes marginal necrosis of the flaps. In the course of healing, hard longitudinal scars are formed preventing tissue expansion by the accumulating tissue (edema) fluid. Usually no recurrent edema is seen in the calf, but it is partly remaining on the dorsum of the foot. There is a decrease of frequency of recurrent DLA

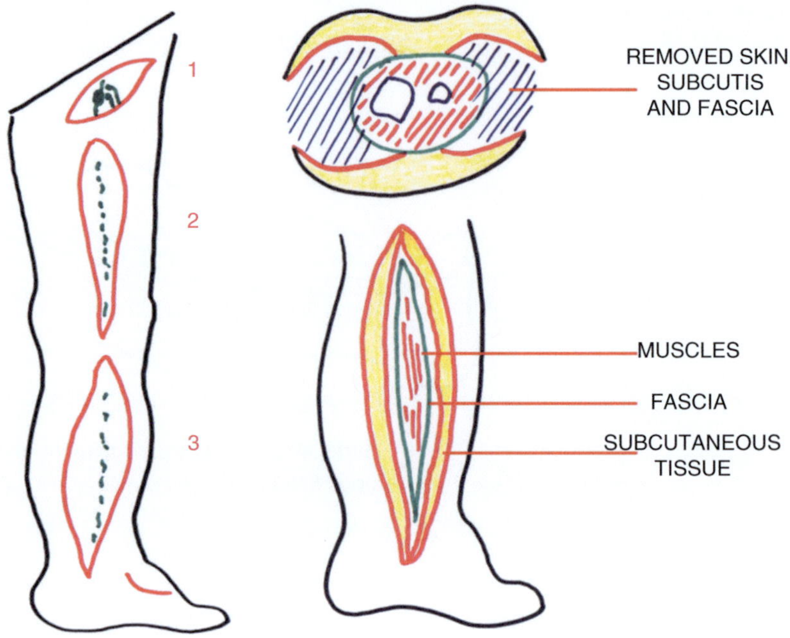

Fig. 20.23 Schematic drawing of various types of partial debulking operations in advanced stage IV lymphedema (previously elephantiasis). Total denuding of the calf is not more practiced (details in text)

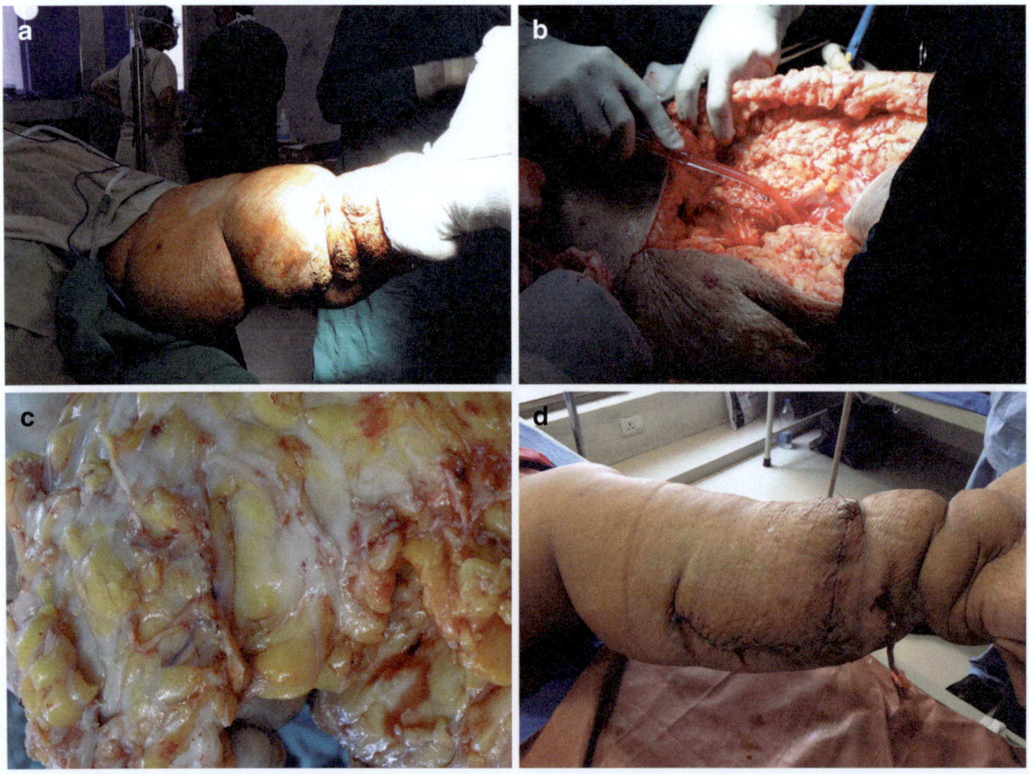

Fig. 20.24 Pictures presenting sequential stages of debulking. Subcutaneous tissue and underlying fascia together with skin strip are removed. (**a**) Lymphedematous leg stage IV lymphedema. (**b**) Exposed deep tissues. (**c**) Excised specimen. Note fat globules and fibrous strands, little free fluid, (**d**) after operation. Note that debulking should be done in stages and calf should be covered by pedunculated but not free flaps

attacks, although it may be partly attributed to the administration of long-term penicillin.

Lymphatic ulcers should be removed with excess of tissue as there is no healing of the surface because of continuous leakage of tissue fluid.

20.6 Excision of Fibrotic Inguinal Lymphatics and Nodes Causing Lymph Stasis with Patent Peripheral Lymphatics

There is a group of patients with lymphedema with hard swollen tissues but no major changes in the foot and calf skin with some few lymphatics in the calf but no visible nodes on lymphoscintigraphy. This group may be resistant to any conventional conservative therapy. The main reason for lymph stasis seems to be fibrotic (postinflammatory) inguinal lymph nodes. The author performs in these cases revision of the inguinal fossa and removes the "what was a lymph node" with obliterated afferent lymphatics.

20.6.1 Indications

The indications are (1) lymphedema stages III and IV, (2) lack of thigh lymphatics and inguinal nodes on lymphoscintigrams with visible rudimentary calf lymphatics, (3) rapidly increasing size (volume) of the entire limb limiting movements, (4) frequent attacks of DLA (>5/year), and (5) fibrotic nodes and lymphatics upon groin surgical revision. Operations are done only when all the criteria are met. The operation brings about decrease in thigh volume and softening of its tissues in over 80% of cases. It is also performed as the first stage before major debulking of the calf and thigh.

20.7 Liposuction

The technique of liposuction of lymphedematous tissues has been transferred from plastic surgery treating local fat deposits disfiguring the limbs, neck, breast, abdomen, and other regions of the body. The technique has been adapted to therapy of lymphedema by many authors [47–50]. According to the published literature, satisfactory results are obtained in postmastectomy lymphedema and some types of lipoedema of the lower limbs in females. In these cases the dominant tissue in the subcutis is fat which cannot be decreased in volume using the compression garments and intermittent pneumatic compression. The limitation of the method are difficulties in the suction of fibrous tissue dominating in advanced stages of lower limb lymphedema, large internal wound surface, formation of hematoma, and redundancy of the skin. The late follow-up data will prove the efficacy of the procedure. The net results of liposuction are difficult to evaluate because of elastic garments worn by patients from the first moment after surgery. Nevertheless, this method has an established position in the therapy of selected cases of lipoedema.

20.8 The Pre- and Postoperative Pharmacological Support for Lymphatic Surgery

Lymphedematous tissues and edema fluid contain a large mass of *Staphylococcus epidermidis* and *Staphylococcus aureus* sensitive to antibiotics [46]. These microorganisms are responsible for the attacks of DLA [3]. Before operation of lymphovenous shunts, implantation of silicone tubings, liposuction, and debulking, patients should receive 1 g of amoxicillin for 1–3 months, depending on the degree of tissue inflammatory changes, and this protocol is continued postoperatively for another month. Then, long-lasting penicillin administration should be given in a dose of 1,200,000 IU i.m. every 3 weeks for years, which is now a routine procedure in the prevention of dermato-lymphangio-adenitis (DLA, previously "cellulitis"). This low dose of antibiotic controls the growth of bacteria normally present in lymph and edema tissue fluid, especially in the presence of a foreign body as implants and nonabsorbable sutures. The maintenance dose of penicillin fulfills the body requirement for antibacterials under the condition of high bacterial mass in the lymphedematous tissues.

20.9 Postoperative Physiotherapy Propelling Edema Fluid to Site of Absorption

This is usually (a) sequential intermittent pneumatic massage with sleeve pressure of 80–120 mmHg, 1 h twice a day, for 10–30 days followed immediately by (b) elastic stocking or pentahose of II or III degree compression or elastic bandaging (40 mmHg) and (c) intensive walking.

20.10 Surgical Methods in the Stage of Clinical Experiment

These are (1) transplantation of lymphatic trunks and (2) lymph nodes with afferent lymphatics bridging the site of mechanical barriers for lymph flow.

20.10.1 Free Transplants of Lymphatics

They were developed by Baumeister and served mainly as the therapy of the postmastectomy lymphedema [51]. The effectiveness of these methods has been proved in some cases on lymphoscintigrams. Again, as with other surgical methods of treatment of lymphedema, with exception of debulking, the net results have been overshadowed by the parallel physiotherapy and administration of antibiotics.

20.10.2 Transplantation of Vascularized Lymph Nodes

The microvascular lymph node transfer (LNT) is the recent promising method for the treatment of postmastectomy lymphedema, especially in its early stage [52–56]. The recipient sites are the wrist, axilla, and forearm. A groin flap containing lymph nodes based on the superficial circumflex iliac vessels and the anastomoses to the superficial radial artery and cephalic vein were performed. Others used similar groin flaps but as recipient vessels the circumflex scapular vessels. The superficial branch of the superficial circumflex iliac artery as the dominant vessel responsible for the vascularization of the lymph nodes was reported with the wrist and the anastomosis to the radial artery. Combined breast reconstruction using abdominal flaps with the transfer of vascularized inguinal lymph nodes based on the superficial circumflex iliac vessels or the superficial inferior epigastric vessels and the anastomoses performed from the deep inferior epigastric vessels end-to-end to the thoracodorsal vessels was reported. Different criteria for staging do not allow objective evaluation of results, especially the anatomical site with the maximum improvement. Altogether, authors claim 70% cases had satisfactory results in terms of decrease of circumference and relief of neuropathic pains.

20.10.3 Conclusions

Taken together, lymph node transfer is able to alleviate postmastectomy upper extremity lymphedema. However, the improvement is variable, and no conclusions have been drawn regarding which technique, group of donor lymph nodes, or recipient site can ensure the maximum reduction of the affected limb. Furthermore, the mechanism of putative regrowth of lymphatic collectors both afferent and efferent should be proved. Stimulation of this process by VEGFs seems to be promising; however, only lymphatic capillarogenesis and not vasculogenesis has so far been documented. Formation of lymphoid cell aggregates is secondary and dependent on the existing lymphatic trunks. The question remains open whether there might be a signal from the nodes for its lymph vessels budding off and joining the recipient vessels. Absorption of excess tissue fluid in the node and its diffusion to the node blood capillaries have not been proved, and it is not expected to explain eventual good results in humans.

20.11 General Conclusions

Taken together, an evident progress has been made since mid of the twentieth century in the therapy of lymphedema. Elephantiasis has practically disappeared in the western hemisphere. This has been the effect of combined manual drainage, pneumatic compression, elastic garments, and administration of long-term antibiotics for the prevention of chronic and recurrent acute dermato-lymphangio-adenitis (DLA), as well as surgical procedures with first of all lymphovenous shunts, followed by novel types of debulking. The search for methods for restoration of lymphatic drainage by transplantation of lymphatics and lymph nodes is a promising effort in regenerative medicine. The indications for surgical treatment of lymphedema should be diversified depending on the etiology of this condition. The majority of lymphedema cases around the world are of postinflammatory (post-infective?) type with gradual obliteration of the peripheral lymphatics. The inflammatory causative factor remains and adversely affects patency of the constructed anastomoses. The posttraumatic type of lymphedema has at least two pathological components as prolonged healing of damaged tissues like bones and muscles and wound infection that may gradually damage the draining lymphatics and nodes. The postsurgical oncological cases are the most favorable for early microsurgical shunts as the peripheral lymphatic trunks are healthy and retain their contractility for years. Lymphoscintigraphic and infrared lymphographic functional pictures decide upon the site and expected effectiveness of the microsurgical shunts. The most promising new approach of implantation of silicone tubings, which replaces the nonfunctioning (obliterated or excised) lymphatics, is easy to perform in millions of patients, has an operation lasting for 30 min, and is valued at 300–500 USD only, should be widely applied to evaluate its effectiveness. Early surgical intervention has now become a must, taking into consideration that lymphedema is an ongoing process of fibrosis of subcutis and muscular fascia and in advanced stages fibrous and fat tissues dominate in volume over the excess of stagnant tissue fluid. All surgical procedures should be followed by external compression of the limbs and administration of long-term low-dose penicillin controlling bacteria present in the stagnant tissue fluid.

References

1. Olszewski WL, Engeset A, Sokolowski J. Lymph flow and protein in the normal male leg during lying, getting up, and walking. Lymphology. 1977;10:178–83.
2. Olszewski WL, Jamal S, Manokaran G, et al. Skin changes in filarial and non-filarial lymphoedema of the lower extremities. Trop Med Parasitol. 1993;44:40–4.
3. Olszewski WL. Episodic dermatolymphangioadenitis (DLA) in patients with lymphedema of the lower extremities before and after administration of benzathine penicillin: a preliminary study. Lymphology. 1996;29:126–31.
4. Charles H. Elephantiasis of the leg. In: Latham A, English TC, editors. A system of treatment, vol. 3. London: Churchill; 1912.
5. Sistrunk WE. Contribution to plastic surgery: removal of scars by stages; an open operation for extensive laceration of the anal sphincter; the Kondoleon operation for elephantiasis. Ann Surg. 1927;85:185–93.
6. Thompson N. The surgical treatment of chronic lymphedema of the extremities. Surg Clin North Am. 1967;47:445–503.
7. Goldsmith HS, De los Santos L, Beattie EJ. Relief of chronic lymph-edema by omental transposition. Ann Surg. 1967;166:573–85.
8. Olszewski WL. Experimental lympho-venous anastomoses. In: Proceedings of the congress. Lodz: Polish Society of Surgeons; 1966. p. 62.
9. Nielubowicz J, Olszewski WL. Surgical lymphaticovenous anastomosis. (Preliminary note). Minerva Cardioangiol. 1967;15:254–6.
10. Nielubowicz J, Olszewski W. Experimental lymphovenous anastomosis. Br J Surg. 1968;55:449–51.
11. Nielubowicz J, Olszewski W. Surgical lympho-venous shunts in patients with secondary lymphedema. Br J Surg. 1968;55:440.
12. Fyfe NC, Wolfe JH, Kinmonth JB. "Die-back" in primary lymphedema – lymphographic and clinical correlations. Lymphology. 1982;15:66–72.
13. Degni M. New technique of lymphatic-venous anastomosis (buried type) for the treatment of lymphedema. VASA. 1974;3:479–83.
14. Guseva LI. Lympho-venous anastomosis in the treatment of lymphatic edema of the lower extremities

(clinico-experimental study). Eksp Khir Anesteziol. 1976;(6):26–8. In Russian
15. Gilbert A, O'Brien BM, Vorrath JW, et al. Lymphaticovenous anastomosis by microvascular technique. Br J Plast Surg. 1976;29:355–60.
16. Bresadola F, Mannella P, Sortini A, et al. Peripheral lymphatico-venous anastomosis. New surgical technic. Minerva Chir. 1978;33(23–24):1711–8.
17. Gloviczki P, Kadar A, Soltesz L. Factors determining the patency of experimental anastomoses between lymphatic vessels and veins. MorpholIgazságügyi Orv Sz. 1980;20:250–5. In Hungarian
18. Politowski M, Bartkowski S, Dynowski J. Lymphovenous fistula for treatment of primary lymphedema of extremities. Pol Med J. 1970;9:438–44.
19. Pokrovskij AV, Spiridonov AA, Thkor SN. Indications and technique of creating lymphovenous anastomosis in lymphedema of the extremities. Klin Khir. 1971;9:11–5.
20. O'Brien BM. Microlymphaticovenous surgery for obstructive lymph-oedema. ANZ J Surg. 1977;47:284–91.
21. Kerstein MD, Licalzi L. Microvascular procedures in the management of lymphedema. Vasc Surg. 1977;11:188–95.
22. Fox U, Montorsi M, Romagnoli G. Treatment of lymphedema of the extremities with lymphatico-venous anastomosis. Minerva Chir. 1980; 35(19):1455–60.
23. Gong-Kang H, Ru-Qi H, Zong-Zhao L, et al. Microlymphaticovenous anastomosis for treating lymphedema of the extremities and external genitalia. J Microsurg. 1981;3:32–9.
24. Huang GK, Hu RQ, Liu ZZ, et al. Microlymphati covenous anastomosis in the treatment of lower limb obstructive lymphedema: analysis of 91 cases. Plast Reconstr Surg. 1985;76:671–85.
25. Olszewski WL. Physiology and microsurgery of lymphatic vessels in man. Lymphology. 1981;14:44–60.
26. Jacobson JH 2nd. Microlymphaticovenous anastomosis for lymph-edema. J Microsurg. 1982;3:255–7.
27. Krylov VS, Milanov NO, Abalmasov KG, et al. Reconstructive micro- surgery in treatment of lymphoedema in extremities. Int Angiol. 1985;4:171–5.
28. Campisi C, Tosatti E, Casaccia M, et al. Microsurgery of the lymphatic vessels. Minerva Chir. 1986;41:469–81. In Italian
29. Ipsen T, Pless J, Frederiksen PB. Experience with microlymphaticovenous anastomoses for congenital and acquired lymphedema. Scand J Plast Reconstr Surg Hand Surg. 1988;22:209–15.
30. Olszewski WL. The treatment of lymphedema of the extremities with microsurgical lymphovenous anastomoses. Int Angiol. 1988;7:312–21.
31. Gloviczki P, Fisher J, Hollier LH, et al. Microsurgical lymphovenous anastomosis for treatment of lymphedema: a critical review. J Vasc Surg. 1988;7: 647–52.
32. Huang GK. Results of microsurgical lymphovenous anastomoses in lymphedema – report of 110 cases. Langenbecks Arch Chir. 1989;374:194–9.
33. Campisi C, Boccardo F, Tacchella M. Reconstructive microsurgery of lymph vessels: the personal method of lymphatic-venous-lymphatic (LVL) interpositioned grafted shunt. Microsurgery. 1995;16:161–6.
34. Yamamoto Y, Sugihara T. Microsurgical lymphaticovenous implantation for the treatment of chronic lymphedema. Plast Reconstr Surg. 1998;101:157–61.
35. Wongtrungkapun R. Microsurgical lymphonodovenous implantation for chronic lymphedema. J Med Assoc Thail. 2004;87:877–82.
36. Boccardo F, Casabona F, De Cian F, et al. Lymphedema microsurgical preventive healing approach: a new technique for primary prevention of arm lymphedema after mastectomy. Ann Surg Oncol. 2009;16:703–8.
37. Olszewski WL. The lymphovenous microsurgical shunts for treatment of lymphedema of lower limbs: indications in 2011. Int Angiol. 2011;30:499–503.
38. Olszewski WL. Lymphovenous microsurgical shunts in treatment of lymphedema of lower limbs: a 45-year experience of one surgeon/one center. Eur J Vasc Endovasc Surg. 2013;45:282–90.
39. Koshima I, Inagawa K, Urushibara K, et al. Supermicrosurgical lymphaticovenular anastomosis for the treatment of lymphedema in the upper extremities. J Reconstr Microsurg. 2000;16:437–42.
40. Koshima I, Nanba Y, Tsutsui T, et al. Minimal invasive lymphaticovenular anastomosis under local anesthesia for leg lymphedema: is it effective for stage III and IV? Ann Plast Surg. 2004;53:261–6.
41. Chang DW. Lymphaticovenular bypass for lymphedema management in breast cancer patients: a prospective study. Plast Reconstr Surg. 2010;126:752–8.
42. Maegawa J, Hosono M, Tomoeda H, et al. Net effect of lymphaticovenous anastomosis on volume reduction of peripheral lymphoedema after complex decongestive physiotherapy. Eur J Vasc Endovasc Surg. 2012;43:602–8.
43. Yamamoto T, Yamamoto N, Numahata T, et al. Navigation lymphatic supermicrosurgery for the treatment of cancer-related peripheral lymphedema. J Vasc Endovascular Surg. 2014;48:139–43.
44. Olszewski WL, Zaleska M. A novel method of edema fluid drainage in obstructive lymphedema of limbs by implantation of hydrophobic silicone tubes. J Vasc Surg Venous Lymphatic. 2015;3(4):401–8.
45. Olszewski WL, Zaleska M. Treatment of postmastectomy lymphedema by bypassing the armpit with implanted silicone tubings. Int Angiol. 2017;36(1):50–8.
46. Olszewski WL, Zaleska M, Stelmach E, Swoboda-Kopec E, Jain P, Agrawal K, Gogia S, Gogia A, Andziak P, Durlik M. Cryptic bacteria of lower limb deep tissues as a possible cause of inflammatory and necrotic changes in ischemia, venous stasis and varices, and lymphedema. Surg Infect. 2015;16(3):313–22.
47. Nava VM, Lawrence WT. Liposuction on a lymphedematous arm. Ann Plast Surg. 1988;21:366–8.
48. Sando WC, Nahai F. Suction lipectomy in the management of limb lymphedema. Clin Plast Surg. 1989;16(2):369–73.

49. Brorson H, Svensson H. Complete reduction of lymphoedema of the arm by liposuction after breast cancer. Scand J Plast Reconstr Surg Hand Surg. 1997;31:137–43.
50. Brorson H, Freccero C, Ohlin K, et al. Liposuction of postmastectomy arm lymphedema completely removes excess volume: a 15-year study. Lymphology. 2010;43(Suppl):108–10.
51. Baumeister RG, Siuda S, Bohmert H, et al. Reconstruction of interrupted lymphatic pathways: autologous lymph-vessel transplantation for treatment of lymphedemas. Scand J Plast Reconstr Surg. 1986;20:141–6.
52. Becker C, Assouad J, Riquet M, et al. Postmastectomy lymphedema: long-term results following microsurgical lymph node transplantation. Ann Surg. 2006;243:313–5.
53. Li S, Cao W, Cheng K, et al. Microvascular transfer of a "lymphatic- bearing" flap in the treatment of obstructive lymphedema. Plast Reconstr Surg. 2008;121(3):150e–2e.
54. Lin CH, Ali R, Chen SC, et al. Vascularized groin lymph node transfer using the wrist as a recipient site for management of postmastectomy upper extremity lymphedema. Plast Reconstr Surg. 2009;123: 1265–75.
55. Becker C, Vasile JV, Levine JL, et al. Microlymphatic surgery for the treatment of iatrogenic lymphedema. Clin Plast Surg. 2012;39:385–98.
56. Cheng MH, Huang JJ, Nguyen DH, et al. A novel approach to the treatment of lower extremity lymphedema by transferring a vascularized submental lymph node flap to the ankle. Gynecol Oncol. 2012;126:93–8.

One-Stop Vein Clinic: The Ideal Option

21

R. Bootun, T. R. A. Lane, and A. H. Davies

21.1 Introduction

Varicose veins affect approximately one third of the population of the UK [1]. Worsening and progression of varicose veins can lead to complications such as leg ulcerations and can be costly to the health service [2]. They have an adverse effect on the quality of life of patients, which, in turn, is improved by their treatment [3]. Increasing use of endovenous methods has changed the management landscape of this ailment. Indeed, since being introduced more than a decade ago, these minimally invasive techniques are proving to be more cost-effective than more traditional means, especially when performed in an outpatient or 'office-based' setting [4, 5].

Estimates show that over 35,000 varicose vein procedures are carried out in the UK per year [1]. New National Institute for Health and Care Excellence (NICE) guidelines for the management of varicose veins were issued in July 2013, offering evidence-based guidance for more clinical and cost-effective management options, including a new set of referral criteria for treatment [1, 6]. An increase in the number of referrals has already been noted since [7], and the Department of Health anticipates that the number of procedures performed per year will increase to 50,000. Managing such a projected increase in varicose vein interventions whilst simultaneously complying with the NHS operational standards of more than 90% of patients receiving consultant-led treatment within 18 weeks from referral to treatment (RTT) could prove to be a challenge [8, 9].

At present, patients referred to the vascular unit for consideration of management of their varicose veins have to attend the outpatient clinic at least twice prior to be listed for their procedure. Patients usually have an initial appointment where the severity of the venous insufficiency is assessed clinically and, subsequently, have a venous duplex scan to evaluate the extent and cause of any venous incompetence. If any treatable lesion is found, they are then added to the waiting list to come for the eventual venous procedure. This means they have to attend at least two outpatient appointments as well as another appointment for their venous scans, before actually coming for their varicose vein procedure. Waiting for varicose vein interventions can be detrimental to the clinical and radiological severity of the condition [10]. This also has a negative impact on the quality of life of patients waiting for elective varicose vein treatment [10, 11].

An answer to the increasing number of patients and ensuing attendances is needed, and potential solutions are explored below.

R. Bootun · T. R. A. Lane · A. H. Davies (✉)
Section of Vascular Surgery, Charing Cross Hospital, Imperial College London, London, UK
e-mail: a.h.davies@imperial.ac.uk

A. K. Khanna, R. Jindal (eds.), *Venous Disorders*, https://doi.org/10.1007/978-981-13-1108-6_21

21.2 Clinic and Referral Models

Waiting times, as occurs when the demand for a particular treatment is greater than the ability of the health service to supply it, happen for a variety of reasons [12]. This discrepancy may be due either to a deficiency of capacity or inefficiencies in the service despite adequate capacity [12]. These shortcomings in healthcare provision could, in turn, be attributed to complicated booking systems, superfluous organisational steps and uneconomical usage of resources.

A number of likely solutions have been proposed including pooling of patients awaiting similar interventions onto a single list, simplifying clinical pathways or establishing 'one-stop shops' (which offer different services on a single day) [12].

In its report looking at ways to help National Health Service (NHS) providers improve their productivity when offering elective care, Monitor, an executive nondepartmental entity of the Department of Health of England (part of NHS Improvement since 1st April 2016), highlighted nine good practices when reviewing the provision of elective care in the field of ophthalmology and orthopaedics (Fig. 21.1) [13] . Five of those practices were deemed to be sufficient to enable most of the productivity gains in the NHS to be met (Table 21.1).

Patients can usually be stratified into the following categories [13]:

- Few medical problems requiring simple elective surgical procedures
- Multiple medical problems requiring simple elective procedures
- With or without multiple medical problems requiring complex elective procedures

Monitor suggests that hospitals should risk stratifying patients into high or low risk and offer different pathways accordingly [13]. Hence, teams would then be able to assess patients attending hospital outpatient clinics and provide services requiring less complex and resource-intensive practices. This may include altering the process of preassessment, anaesthesia and post-operative support. This, in turn, would allow a reduction of resources needed.

Usually, patients have to attend a number of times before a final decision for treatment is made: the initial outpatient clinic, diagnostic tests and eventual discussion for treatment [13]. Combining outpatient clinics with diagnostic services at a single outpatient visit would allow a reduction of these appointments and is often referred to in the UK and internationally as a 'one-stop' assessment. This 'one-stop' approach enables an efficient service but does require more intensive and judicious use of resources. Indeed, such 'one-stop' assessment clinics require robust relationships between diagnostic and outpatient services, availability of same-day simple diagnostic tests (e.g. ultrasound and X-rays) as well as access to a consultant, even if only for advice.

First specialist input	Outpatient care	Inpatient pre-operative care	Surgery	Inpatient post-operative care	Follow-up post-discharge
1. Stratification of patients by risk and alignment of resources to risk	2. Streamlined diagnostics, outpatients and pre-assessment	3. Day of surgery admission	4. Specialisation and extended roles within team 5. Optimised scheduling 6. Surgical teams supported to use theatres efficiently	7. Standardisation of ward care and enhanced recovery 8. Proactive management of infections and readmissions	9. Nurse/allied health professional (AHP)-led follow-up for routine patients and level of follow-up aligned to patients risk profile

Fig. 21.1 Nine practice areas where operational improvements can be made in the National Health Service [13]

Table 21.1 Five of nine practices identified by Monitor which would allow most of productivity gains in the NHS [13]

1. Risk stratification of patients and use of low-complexity pathways for patients at low-risk
2. Extension of clinical roles of lower grade staffs so they can take over tasks usually performed by consultants
3. Increase of theatre efficiency by rigorous measurement, communication and management of theatre procedures
4. Reduction of patient length of stay by improving recovery practices
5. Virtual follow-up arranged for uncomplicated patients

21.3 Refining the One-Stop Practice

The 'one-stop' assessment clinics offer a number of benefits, but an improvement of this practice could be made by the addition of treatment to the assessment, i.e. outpatient clinic, diagnosis and treatment on a single day. This different type of 'one-stop' shop ('one-stop' treatment clinic, to differentiate it from a 'one-stop' assessment clinic) is an attractive option in the health service.

This concept presents the advantages of decreasing the number of hospital visits required, reducing the waiting times to eventual treatment and allows savings to be made as a result of the previous two.

As an example, Monitor described the experience of the Newcastle upon Tyne Hospitals NHS Foundation Trust (UK) in treating patients with wet age-related macular degeneration (AMD) [13]. This one-stop treatment clinic has been able to achieve an outpatient to injection rate of 55%. The management pathway is illustrated in Fig. 21.2.

21.4 One-Stop Clinics in Other Specialties

The notion of carrying out a one-stop treatment clinic where patients are seen and treated on the same day is not new. Indeed, these already function in oncology, where a definitive diagnosis can be reached sooner. This concept has previously been reported in other surgical specialties and is as detailed below.

21.4.1 Ophthalmology: Cataract Surgery

Ophthalmology was one of the earliest specialties to embrace this concept of one-stop clinic initially for the treatment of cataracts. A one-stop cataract service was set up and operated between 1997 and 1999 at the Bristol Eye Hospital [14]. Over that period, 190 patients referred for consideration of cataract surgery were selected from their referral letter and invited to attend the service, with the letter explaining that they might be operated on the same day. Assessments were conducted in the morning, with procedures performed in the afternoon.

Approximately 82% of patients (156 patients) invited to the 'one-stop' clinic underwent same-day surgery [14]. Satisfaction with the service was high (94%), though not statistically significant compared to patients attending a more conventional pathway. All patients also felt they were given enough time to decide about whether they should go ahead with the procedure or not. This indicates the question as to whether patients needed a 'cooling off' period before deciding about their procedure did not arise. Moreover, neither the General Medical Council (GMC, UK) nor the Medical Protection Society (MPS, UK) raised any concerns regarding this issue either.

Since not all patients attending the clinic were operated on, theatres were often used inefficiently (as low as 50% of the time). To improve on these figures, patients attending the conventional clinics were added to the theatre list and asked to attend as there was a chance they could be operated that day.

The authors suggested that this type of service could lead to a reduction of total hospital visits, freeing up resources that could be used elsewhere [14]. In addition, it eliminated waiting lists since patients were seen and operated on the same day. This type of service provision

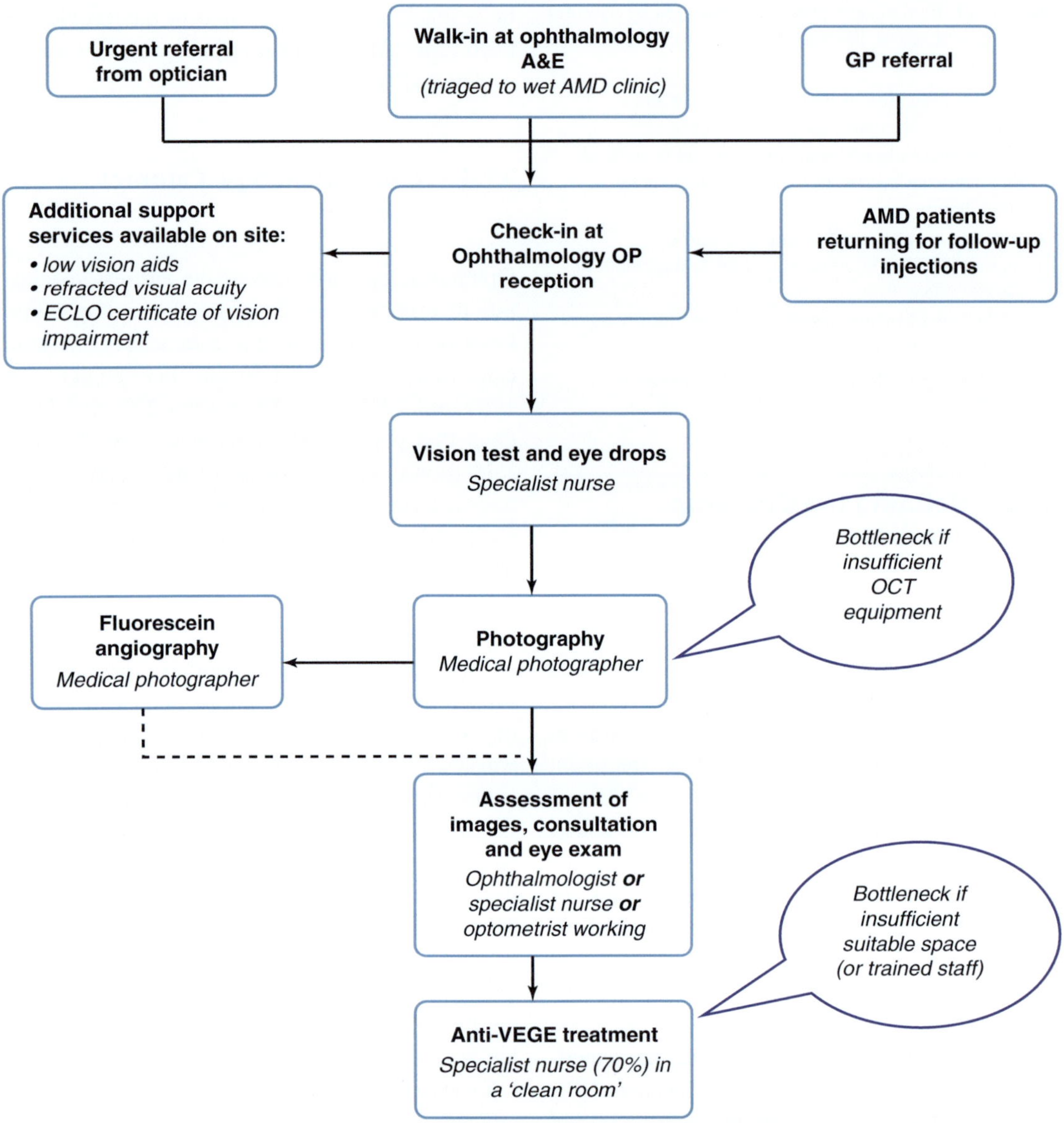

Fig. 21.2 Modified diagram showing a one-stop clinic for the diagnosis, assessment and treatment of wet AMD at the Newcastle upon Tyne Hospitals NHS Foundation Trust (*AMD* age-related macular degeneration, *ECLO* eye clinic liaison office, *OTC* optical coherence tomography, *VEGF* vascular endothelial growth factor)

also seemed to be popular with patients. They do point out though that inefficient use of theatres could mean that all the benefits of this one-stop treatment clinic would be negated and may not actually be superior to a one-stop diagnosis clinic.

To this day, the Bristol Eye Hospital continues to provide a one-stop service for the management of ophthalmic conditions.

21.4.2 Orthopaedics: Carpal Tunnel Syndrome

Reid et al. [15] looked into improving the waiting times for patients with carpal tunnel syndrome (CTS). This followed the publication of the NHS plan (in 2000) and the NHS Improvement Plan (2005) which encouraged a different approach to deliver care. They conducted a study to assess whether a one-stop CTS clinic for diagnosis and treatment of the condition on the same day would reduce the waiting time for patients whilst maintaining clinical outcome and patient satisfaction [15].

Patients were selected from their GP referral letter and were invited to the clinic. On the day, patients were seen and examined. Based on the history and examination findings, patients either went on to have carpal tunnel decompression or further investigations. All procedures were carried out under local anaesthesia, and patients were discharged home on the same day.

In total, 49 patients, with mean age of 52 years, were included. Ninety-four percent of patients underwent surgery. The mean waiting time from referral to the one-stop clinic was 9 weeks. None of the patients required a day-case bed or overnight admission. Post-procedure, patients had better functional scores, and satisfaction was high. Once again, no patients felt that they needed more time to consider having their surgery.

The authors concluded that the one-stop carpal tunnel clinic appears to be more efficient and cost-effective way of treating this common condition [15].

21.4.3 General Surgery: Inguinal Hernia

Open Repair

Patients referred by their GPs to a London hospital (UK) for the management of unilateral inguinal hernias were considered for a one-stop hernia repair clinic [16]. Based on their referral letter, patients with no clear contraindication to day surgery were sent information material about the proposed treatment plan and a health questionnaire that their GP needed to fill. Based on the responses obtained, patients deemed suitable for day-case surgery were invited to attend a special clinic for both assessment by the operating surgeon and possible definitive surgery. The procedure undertaken was an open, tension-free Lichtenstein mesh repair and carried out under general or local anaesthesia.

One-hundred and ten patients were included in the study. Out of them, 98 were deemed suitable for day-case procedure and invited to the clinic. All patients were males with a mean age of 49.5 years and ASA grade I or II.

Overall, 92 patients (94% of total) of those invited underwent day-case procedure, mostly under general anaesthesia (90 patients). One patient required admission because of urinary retention, but all the others were discharged on the same day [16].

The authors concluded that patients with primary unilateral inguinal hernia could be treated efficiently in a one-stop clinic with low levels of cancellations and complications.

Laparoscopic Repair

A similar approach was taken at a Dutch hospital where the safety and feasibility of setting up a one-stop total extraperitoneal (TEP) inguinal hernia repair was undertaken [17].

GPs were informed about the alternative one-stop treatment available, with the inclusion and exclusion criteria provided. Once selected, patients made contact with the hospital. Further information about the condition and its management were given on three separate occasions: by their GPs, by receipt of a leaflet about the procedure and by the general surgeons on the day of their procedures. Having been adequately counselled, patients, then, underwent the TEP repair and were discharged on the same day. Patients were contacted again 2 weeks later and were offered an outpatient appointment if indicated.

Fifty-two patients were recruited in 12 months, and 50 of them received a TEP repair [17]. Three patients were required overnight stay. At 2 weeks, 11 patients (22%) had symptoms of pain or swelling and 8 of them were followed up in clinic. Satisfaction was high with 98% of patients rating the one-stop set-up as 'good' or 'excellent'.

Further analysis and comparison with patients treated on the conventional pathway showed that 35% of them, and approximately half of all the referred patients, would also have been suitable for the one-stop pathway.

This study demonstrated that the one-stop concept appears safe, reduces the waiting time for intervention, is less costly and well accepted [17]. The authors do highlight potential issues such as patients with incorrect diagnoses presenting for treatment, those unfit for day-case procedures, patients not attending their appointment, inefficient use of theatre time and unsatisfied patients [17].

21.5 Application of the One-Stop Pathway to Phlebology: The One-Stop Vein Clinic

Similar concepts to the ones mentioned above can be applied to varicose veins. Many vascular centres already operate a one-stop diagnostic pathway, whereby patients are seen and receive a vascular scan, including a varicose vein scan, on a single day in the outpatient clinic [18, 19]. Treatment is then provided on another day.

A possible enhancement to this model would, therefore, involve the addition of a definitive therapeutic intervention to this one-stop set-up (Fig. 21.3). This has been largely aided by the introduction of endovenous ablation more than a decade ago. These techniques have revolutionised the management of varicose veins disease, enabling procedures to be carried out under local anaesthetic and as day cases. Interventions carried out in such a manner in an outpatient or 'office-based' setting have also been deemed to be cost-effective [5].

Organising such a one-stop treatment pathway is dependent on several factors as previously detailed [13].

21.5.1 Risk Stratification of Patients

Similar to Monitor's risk stratification, three categories can be recognised when stratifying patients with varicose veins:

1. Patients with no or simple medical conditions requiring simple treatment

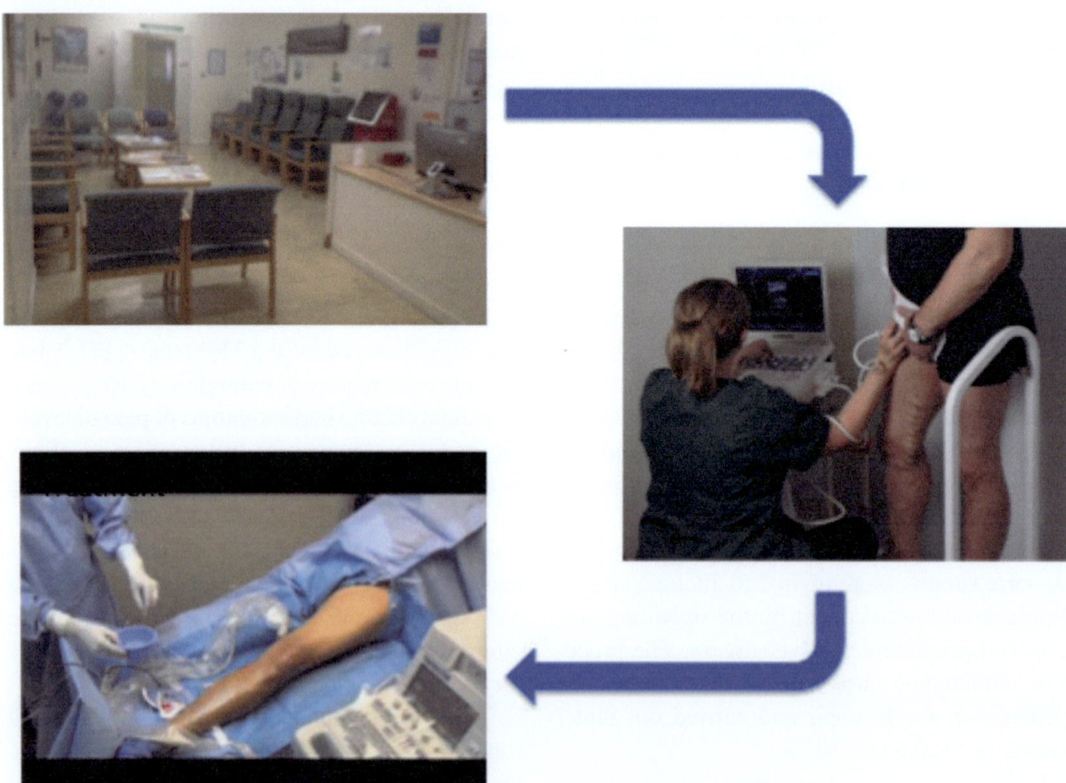

Fig. 21.3 The stages in a one-stop vein clinic offering same day diagnosis and treatment

2. Patients with complex medical conditions requiring simple treatment
3. Patients with no, simple or complex medical conditions requiring complex treatment

Varicose vein treatment is dependent on first determining whether they are of primary, secondary (e.g. following deep vein thrombosis) or recurrent origin. Secondary and recurrent varicose veins often have a complicated pattern and are notoriously more difficult to treat. On the other hand, primary varicose veins are considered generally relatively less complex and easier to manage. Hence, the latter often only require simple interventions which are increasingly being carried out as day cases using local anaesthesia. Utilisation of local anaesthetic provides the advantage of allowing patients with complex medical problems to be treated.

21.5.2 Streamlining Outpatients, Diagnostics and Treatment

Another step is to ensure that there is enough capacity for patients to be seen in the outpatient clinic, receive a varicose vein scan and be treated. Good communication links between all these departments is also essential to allow a smooth and timely transfer of patients from one department to another and avoiding delays.

Patients found to be eligible candidates for single-day treatment on their scans could receive further counselling regarding the proposed intervention and will be consented for the procedure.

21.5.3 Improving Theatre Efficiency

A 'one-stop' pathway is very reliant upon ensuring there are enough spare theatre slots to accommodate patients as well as quick patient turn around. Patients could be added to an elective list or to lists dedicated to those attending the 'one-stop' clinic.

Elective lists do allow for the latter patients to have their intended procedures and avoids the loss of theatre space as elective patients are already being operated on. However, depending on the number of patients attending the 'one-stop' clinic, there is a possibility that theatres might overrun or even that patients may get cancelled. A quick turnaround, which might help avoid this problem, could be facilitated by having staff familiar with the procedure scrub for the varicose vein interventions.

Dedicated lists also pose a different type of problem with possible under usage of theatres, especially, if none or only a few of the 'one-stop' patients are suitable for same-day treatment.

21.5.4 Patient Recovery

Varicose vein interventions are increasingly being carried out under local anaesthesia, simplifying the recovery procedure. After spending an appropriate amount of complication-free time in the recovery area, patients could be discharged with instructions about what to expect over the following days and to return to activities as soon as they felt able to.

21.5.5 Follow-Up

Routine follow-up, especially after an uncomplicated varicose vein procedure, is probably unnecessary. Most complications, if they occur, tend to happen within the first 2 weeks of treatment [20–22]. Around the time of their procedures, the complication rate is 5.1%, but this increases to nearly 70% by 6 weeks [23]. Most of those complications, however, tend to be minor, and it would be difficult to justify the associated extra costs of such outpatient appointments. It has been argued that routinely following up patients after uncomplicated interventions is neither necessary nor cost-effective and that easier access to outpatient clinics might be more appropriate for those developing complications [24]. Provision of information leaflets detailing likely complications and time to improvement could potentially avoid unnecessary follow-up [24].

21.6 Benefits and Drawbacks of a One-Stop Vein Clinic

There are several potential advantages of organising a one-stop vein clinic. Along with the possibility of eliminating waiting times, it enables abolishment of unnecessary outpatient appointments. Provision of same-day assessment and treatment may lead to improved patient satisfaction and an earlier improvement in patient quality of life. Another likely advantage is potential cost savings made by avoiding the unnecessary appointments.

However, a number of possible problems are also evident. Patients invited to such a clinic may not necessarily have varicose veins as the main cause of their symptoms, or they may have more complicated varicose veins disease than expected. The lack of a 'cooling off' period to consider the options available could be an issue, even though this can be dealt with by providing patients with information material prior to their appointments. Another potential pitfall could be the inefficient use of theatre facilities which could invalidate any benefits accrued from such a one-stop clinic.

Conclusion

Strategies to improve the efficiency in the health service are always welcome. A one-stop approach to diagnosing and treating simple conditions is very attractive to all concerned, and managing varicose veins in this manner appears to be an ideal solution. Both potential advantages and drawbacks exist, and, hopefully, studies looking at the feasibility and cost implications of this concept being applied to varicose vein disease would be able to elucidate the merits of such an undertaking.

References

1. Marsden G, Perry M, Kelley K, Davies AH. Diagnosis and management of varicose veins in the legs: summary of NICE guidance. BMJ. 2013;f4279:347.
2. Gohel MS, Epstein DM, Davies AH. Cost-effectiveness of traditional and endovenous treatments for varicose veins. Br J Surg. 2010;97:1815–23.
3. Smith JJ, Garratt AM, Guest M, Greenhalgh RM, Davies AH. Evaluating and improving health-related quality of life in patients with varicose veins. J Vasc Surg. 1999;30:710–9.
4. Marsden G, Perry M, Bradbury A, et al. A cost-effectiveness analysis of surgery, endothermal ablation, ultrasound-guided foam sclerotherapy and compression stockings for symptomatic varicose veins. Eur J Vasc Endovasc Surg. 2015;50(6):794–801.
5. van den Bos R, Arends L, Kockaert M, Neumann M, Nijsten T. Endovenous therapies of lower extremity varicosities: a meta-analysis. J Vasc Surg. 2009;49:230–9.
6. National Institute of Clinical Excellence, NICE Clinical Guideline Centre. Varicose veins in the legs - the diagnosis and management of varicose veins (clinical guideline 168). London: NICE; 2013.
7. Davies HO, Popplewell M, Bate G, Kelly L, Darvall K, Bradbury AW. The impact of 2013 UK NICE guidelines on the management of varicose veins at the heart of England NHS foundation trust, Birmingham, UK. Phlebology. 2016;31(9):612–6.
8. Department of Health. The operating framework for the NHS in England 2012/13. London: Department of Health; 2011.
9. NHS England. NHS standard contract 2014/15 - particulars. Leeds: NHS England; 2013.
10. Sarin S, Shields DA, Farrah J, Scurr JH, Coleridge-Smith PD. Does venous function deteriorate in patients waiting for varicose vein surgery. J R Soc Med. 1993;86:21–3.
11. Oudhoff JP, Timmermans DR, Knol DL, Bijnen AB, van der Wal G. Waiting for elective general surgery: impact on health related quality of life and psychosocial consequences. BMC Public Health. 2007;7:164.
12. Kreindler SA. Policy strategies to reduce waits for elective care: a synthesis of international evidence. Br Med Bull. 2010;95:7–32.
13. Monitor. Helping NHS providers improve productivity in elective care. London: Monitor; 2015.
14. Hughes EH, Forrest F, Diamond JP. 'One-stop' cataract surgery: the Bristol Eye Hospital experience 1997-1999. Eye (Lond). 2001;15:306–8.
15. Reid MJ, David LA, Nicholl JE. A one-stop carpal tunnel clinic. Ann R Coll Surg Engl. 2009;91:301–4.
16. Putnis S, Merville-Tugg R, Atkinson S. 'One-stop' inguinal hernia surgery--day-case referral, diagnosis and treatment. Ann R Coll Surg Engl. 2004;86:425–7.
17. Jutte EH, Cense HA, Dur AHM, Hunfeld MAJM, Cramer B, Breederveld RS. A pilot study for one-stop endoscopic total extraperitoneal inguinal hernia repair. Surg Endosc. 2010;24:2730–4.
18. Sandison AJ, King DH, Padayachee TS, Taylor PR. A one-stop vascular clinic: a practical proposition with non-invasive assessment. Ann R Coll Surg Engl. 1997;79:447–50.
19. Makris SA, Karkos CD, Awad S, London NJ. An "all-comers" venous duplex scan policy for patients with lower limb varicose veins attending a one-stop vas-

cular clinic: is it justified? Eur J Vasc Endovasc Surg. 2006;32:718–24.
20. Shepherd AC, Gohel MS, Brown LC, Metcalfe MJ, Hamish M, Davies AH. Randomized clinical trial of VNUS ClosureFAST radiofrequency ablation versus laser for varicose veins. Br J Surg. 2010;97:810–8.
21. Rasmussen LH, Lawaetz M, Bjoern L, Vennits B, Blemings A, Eklof B. Randomized clinical trial comparing endovenous laser ablation, radiofrequency ablation, foam sclerotherapy and surgical stripping for great saphenous varicose veins. Br J Surg. 2011;98:1079–87.
22. Darvall KA, Bate GR, Adam DJ, Bradbury AW. Recovery after ultrasound-guided foam sclerotherapy compared with conventional surgery for varicose veins. Br J Surg. 2009;96:1262–7.
23. Brittenden J, Cotton SC, Elders A, et al. A randomized trial comparing treatments for varicose veins. N Engl J Med. 2014;371:1218–27.
24. Bailey J, Roland M, Roberts C. Is follow up by specialists routinely needed after elective surgery? A controlled trial. J Epidemiol Community Health. 1999;53:118–24.

MIX
Papier aus verantwortungsvollen Quellen
Paper from responsible sources
FSC® C105338

If you have any concerns about our products,
you can contact us on
ProductSafety@springernature.com

In case Publisher is established outside the EU,
the EU authorized representative is:
Springer Nature Customer Service Center GmbH
Europaplatz 3, 69115 Heidelberg, Germany

Printed by Libri Plureos GmbH
in Hamburg, Germany